A Thousand
Coloured Castles

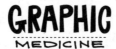

GRAPHIC MEDICINE

Books in the Graphic Medicine series are inspired by a growing awareness of the value of comics as an important resource for communicating about a range of issues broadly termed "medical." For healthcare practitioners, patients, families, and caregivers dealing with illness and disability, graphic narrative enlightens complicated or difficult experience. For scholars in literary, cultural, and comics studies, the genre articulates a complex and powerful analysis of illness, medicine, and disability and a rethinking of the boundaries of "health." The series includes original comics from artists and non-artists alike, such as self-reflective "graphic pathographies" or comics used in medical training and education, as well as monographic studies and edited collections from scholars, practitioners, and medical educators.

Other titles in the series:

MK Czerwiec, Ian Williams, Susan Merrill Squier, Michael J. Green, Kimberly R. Myers, and Scott T. Smith, *Graphic Medicine Manifesto*

Ian Williams, *The Bad Doctor: The Troubled Life and Times of Dr. Iwan James*

Peter Dunlap-Shohl, *My Degeneration: A Journey Through Parkinson's*

Aneurin Wright, *Things to Do in a Retirement Home Trailer Park: . . . When You're 29 and Unemployed*

Dana Walrath, *Aliceheimers: Alzheimer's Through the Looking Glass*

Lorenzo Servitje and Sherryl Vint, eds., *The Walking Med: Zombies and the Medical Image*

Henny Beaumont, *Hole in the Heart: Bringing Up Beth*

MK Czerwiec, *Taking Turns: Stories from HIVIAIDS Care Unit 371*

Paula Knight, *The Facts of Life*

A
THOUSAND
COLOURED
CASTLES

Gareth Brookes

The Pennsylvania State University Press
University Park, Pennsylvania

Cataloging-in-publication data is on file with
the Library of Congress.

Copyright © Gareth Brookes 2017

All rights reserved

Printed in Poland

Published by The Pennsylvania State University Press,

University Park, PA 16802-1003

First published by Myriad Editions,

www.myriadeditions.com

The Pennsylvania State University Press is a member of the
Association of American University Presses.

It is the policy of The Pennsylvania State University Press to
use acid-free paper. Publications on uncoated stock satisfy
the minimum requirements of American National Standard
for Information Sciences—Permanence of Paper for Printed
Library Material, ANSI Z39.48–1992.

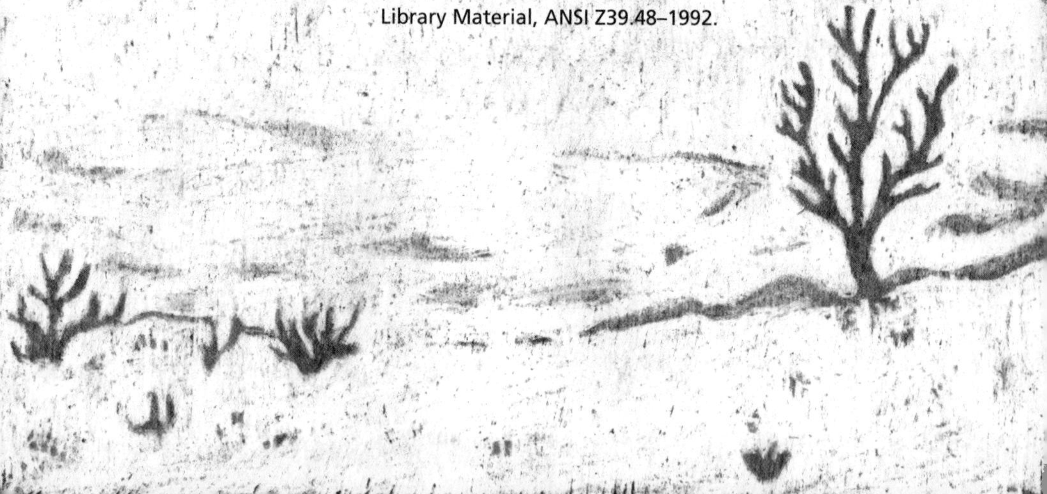

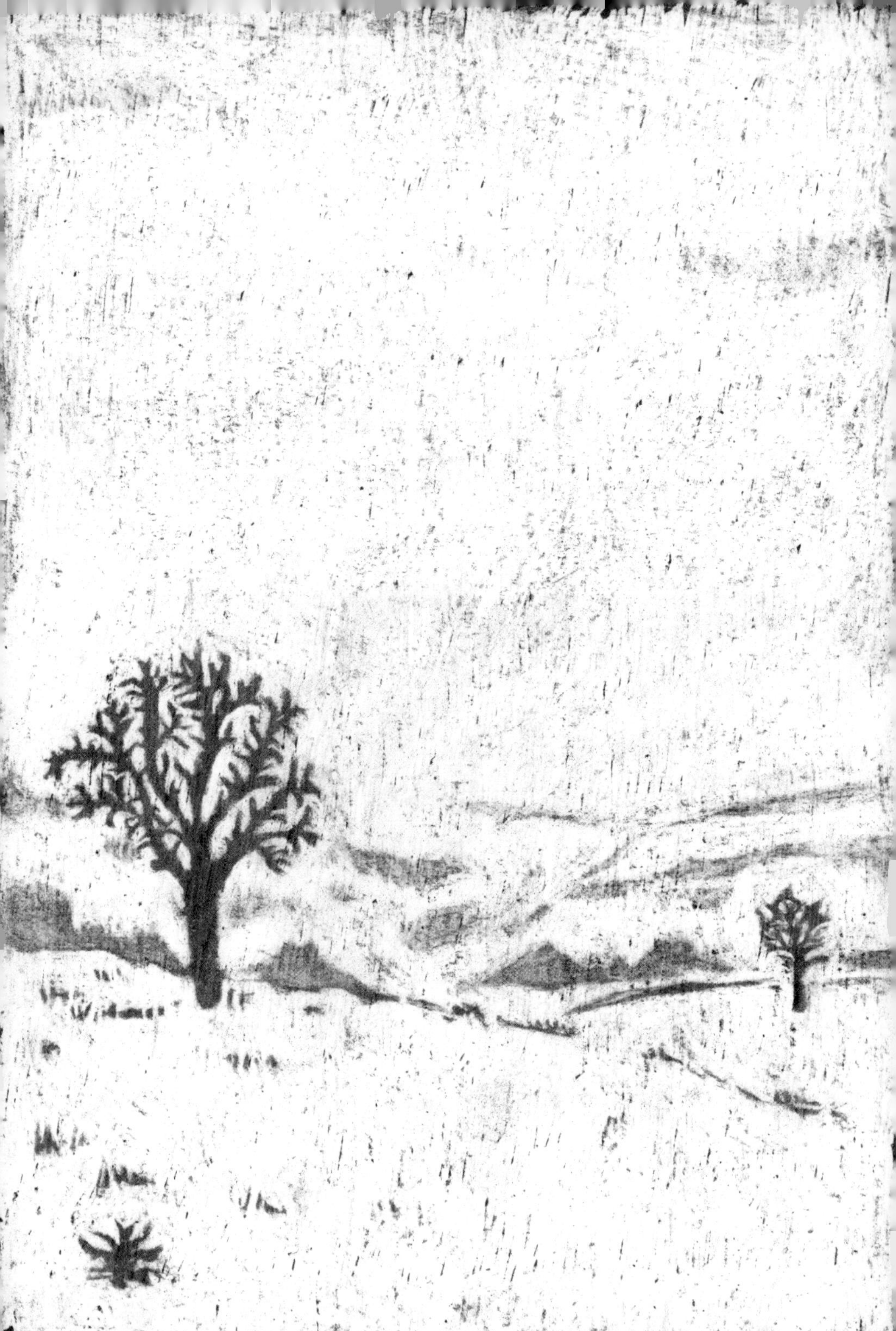

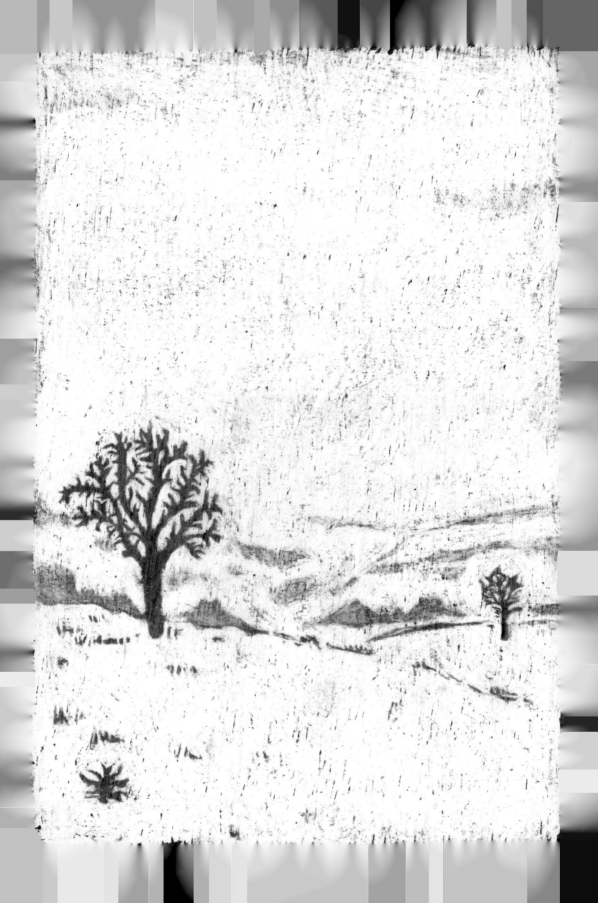

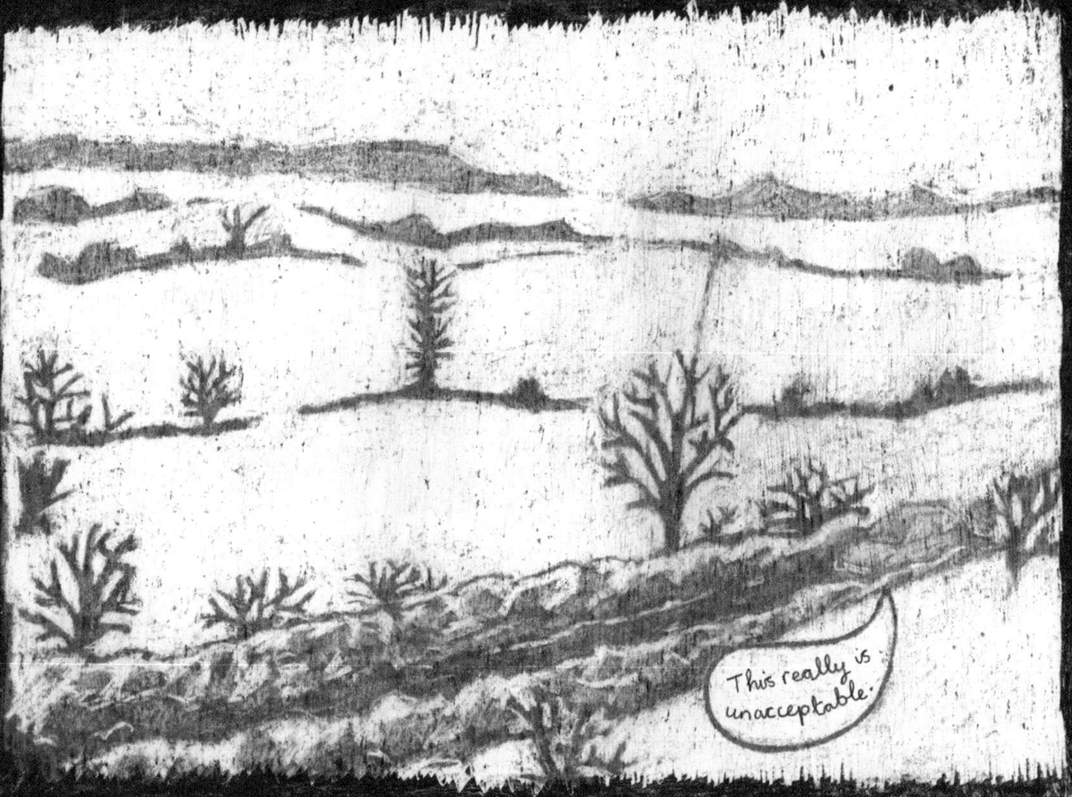
This really is unacceptable.

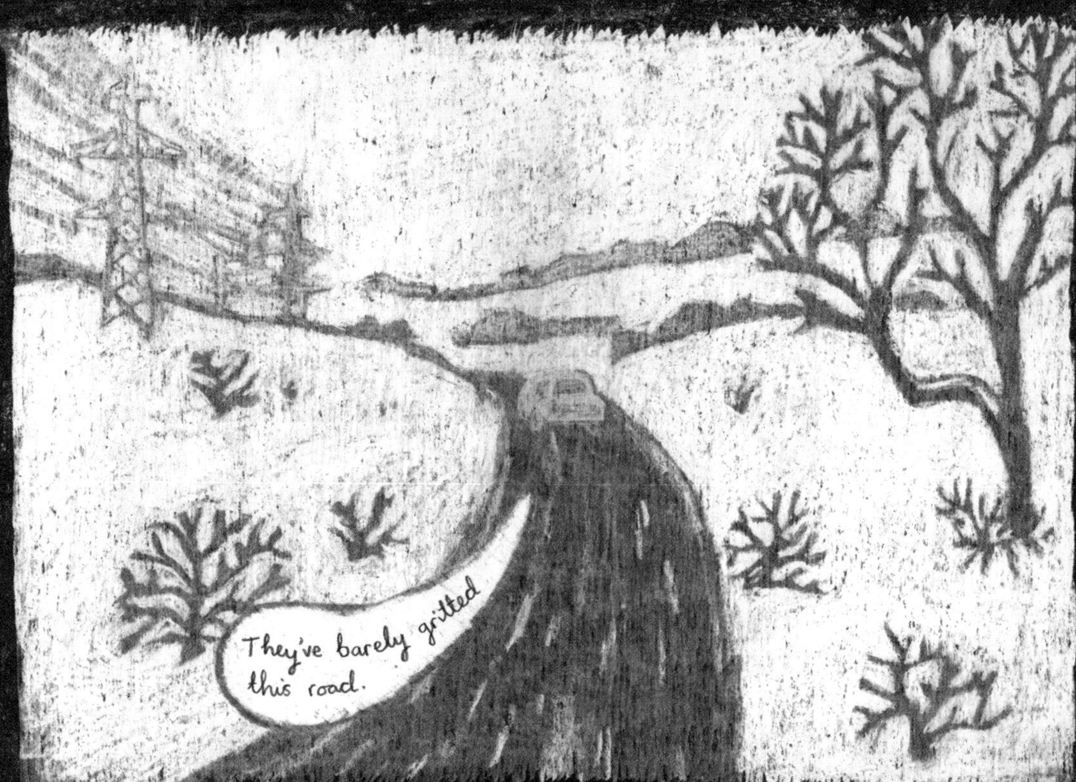
They've barely gritted this road.

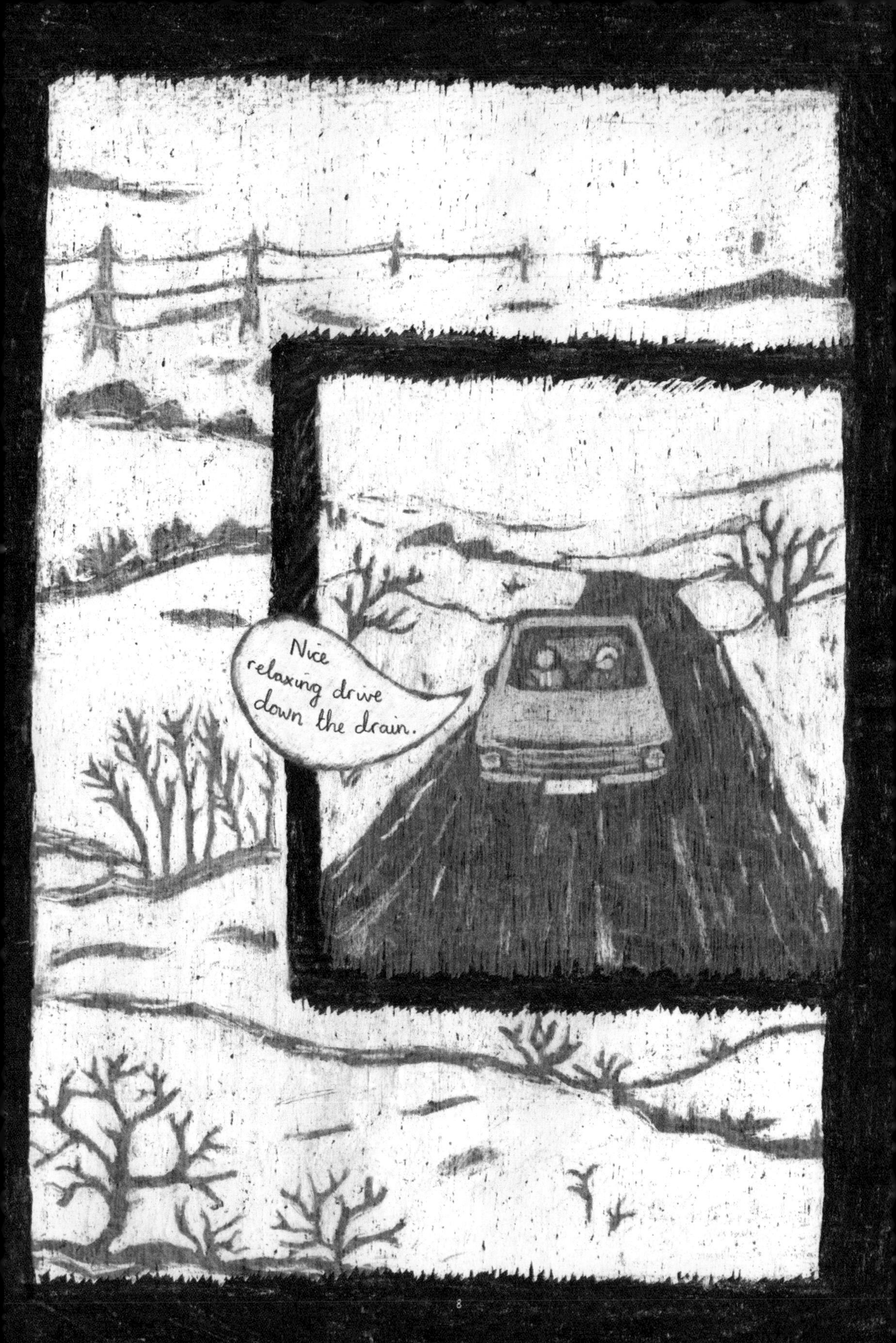
Nice relaxing drive down the drain.

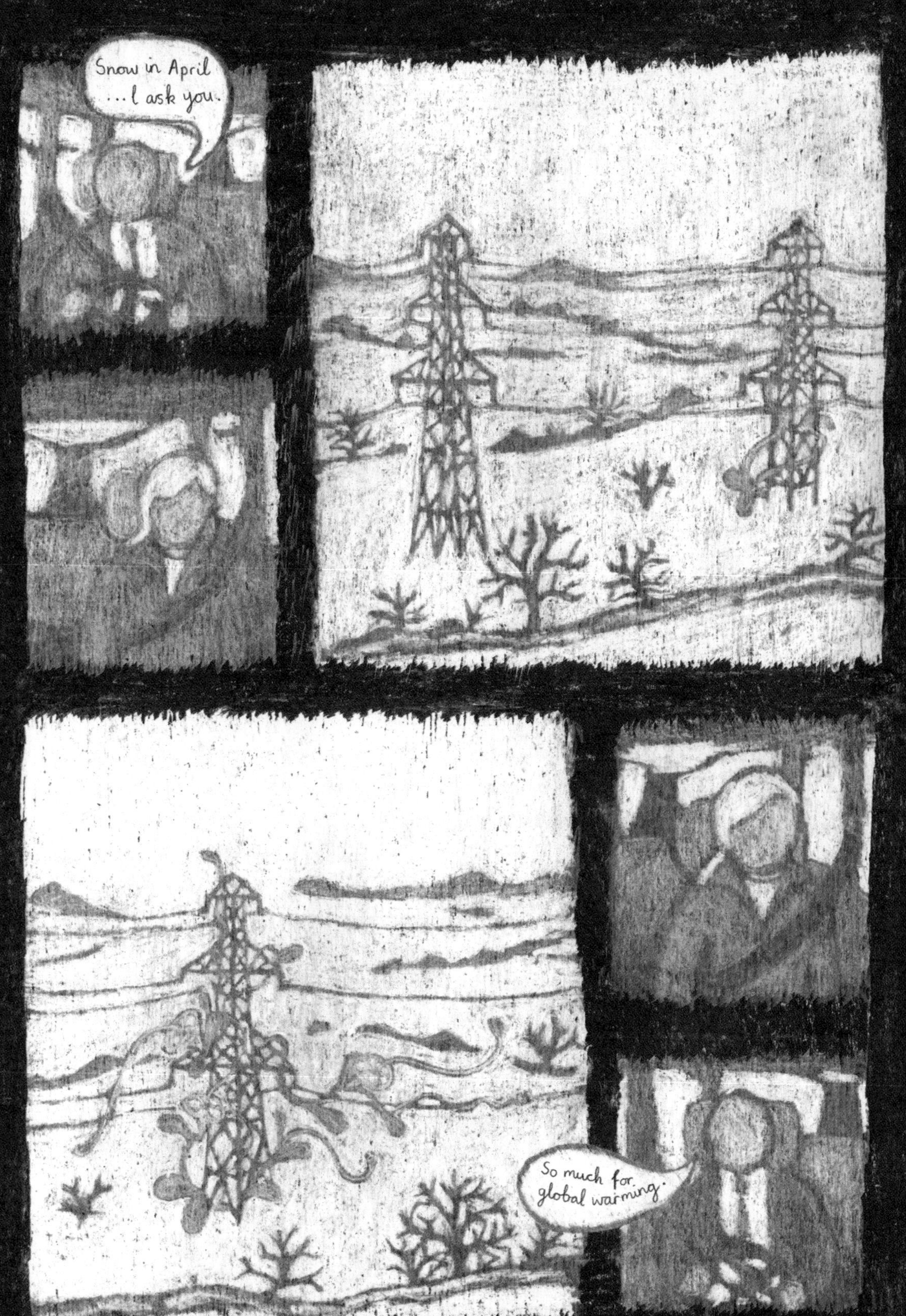
Snow in April
...I ask you.
So much for global warming.

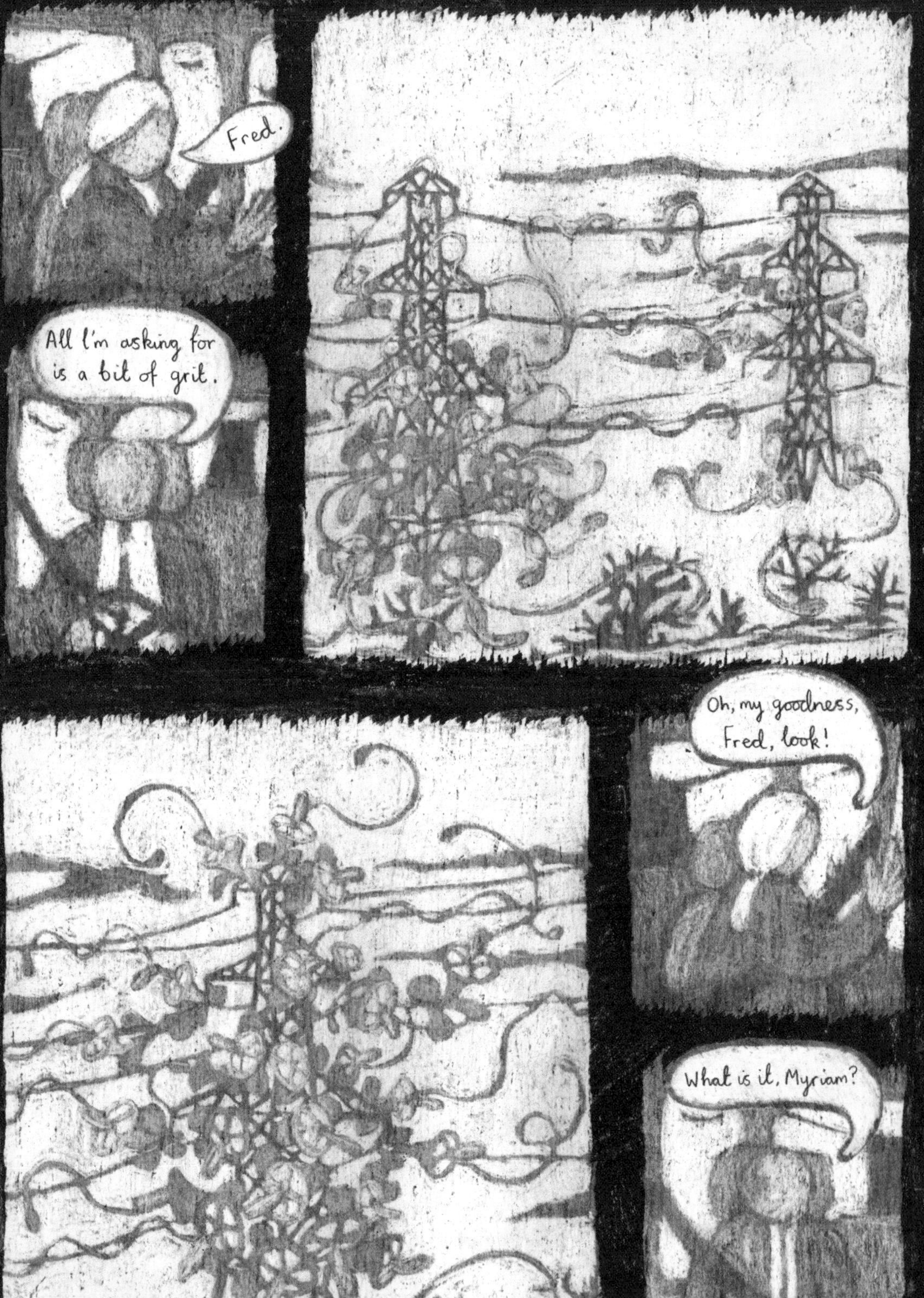
Fred.
All I'm asking for is a bit of grit.
Oh, my goodness, Fred, look!
What is it, Myriam?

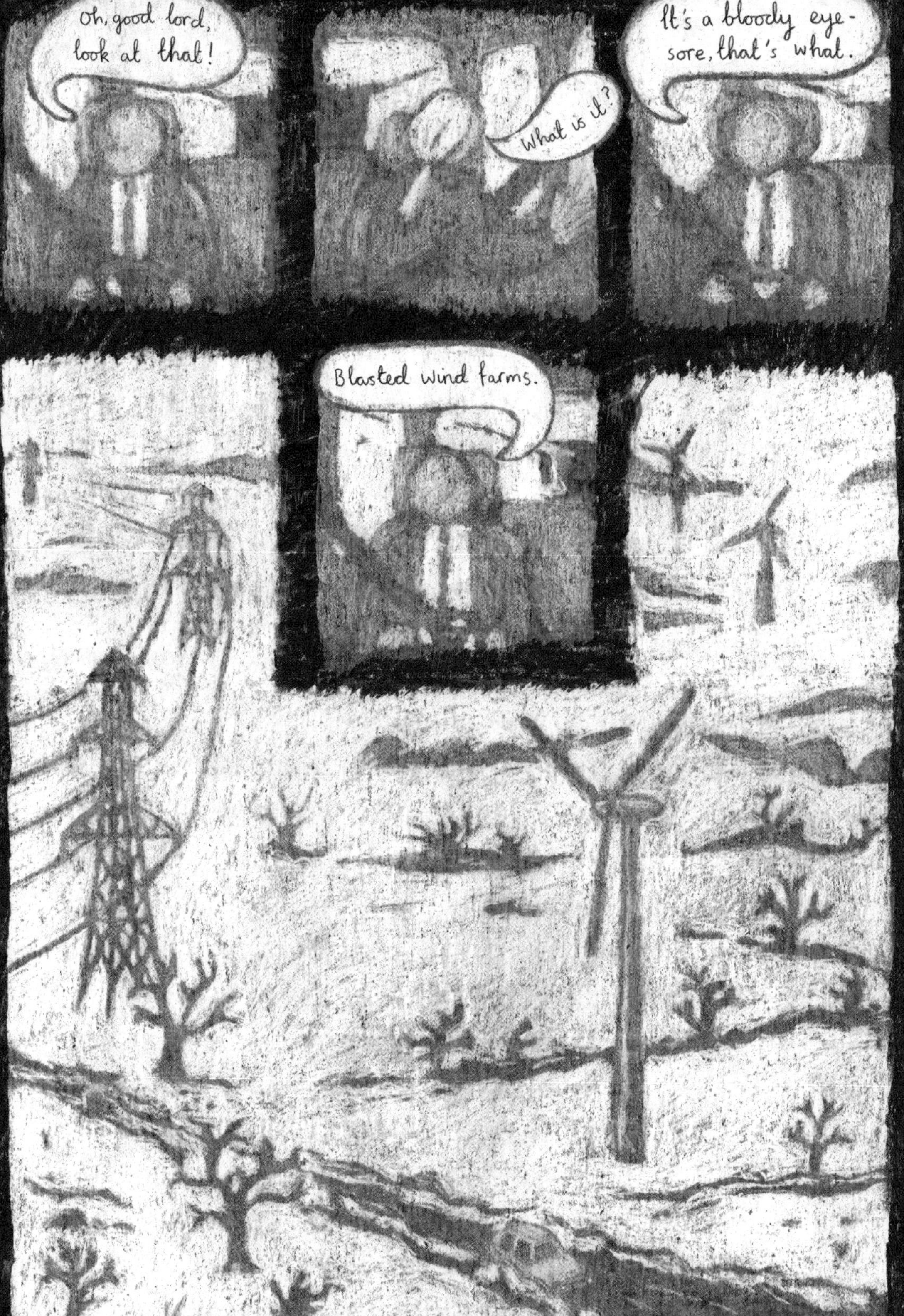
Oh, good lord, look at that!
What is it?
It's a bloody eye-sore, that's what.
Blasted wind farms.

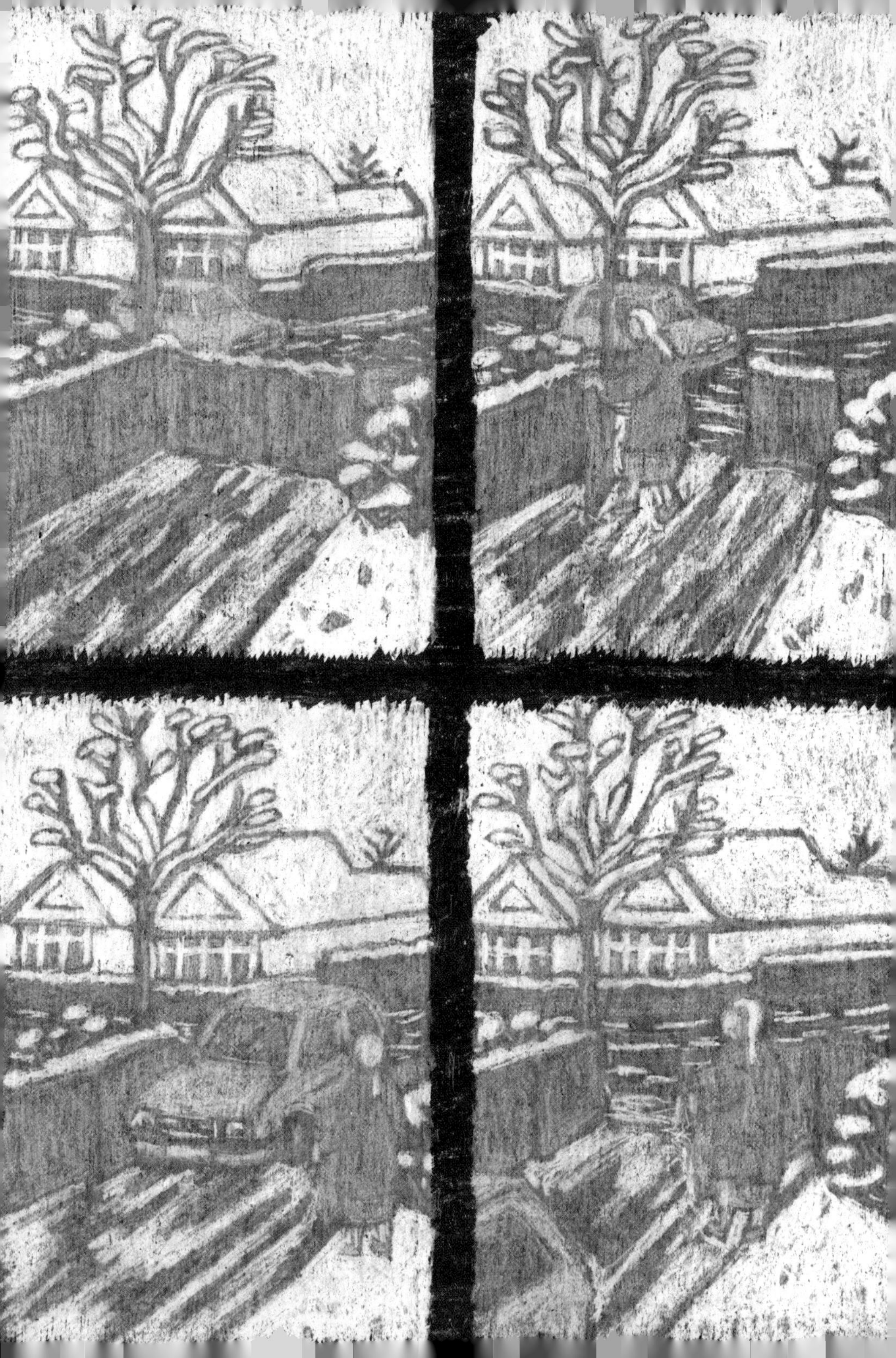

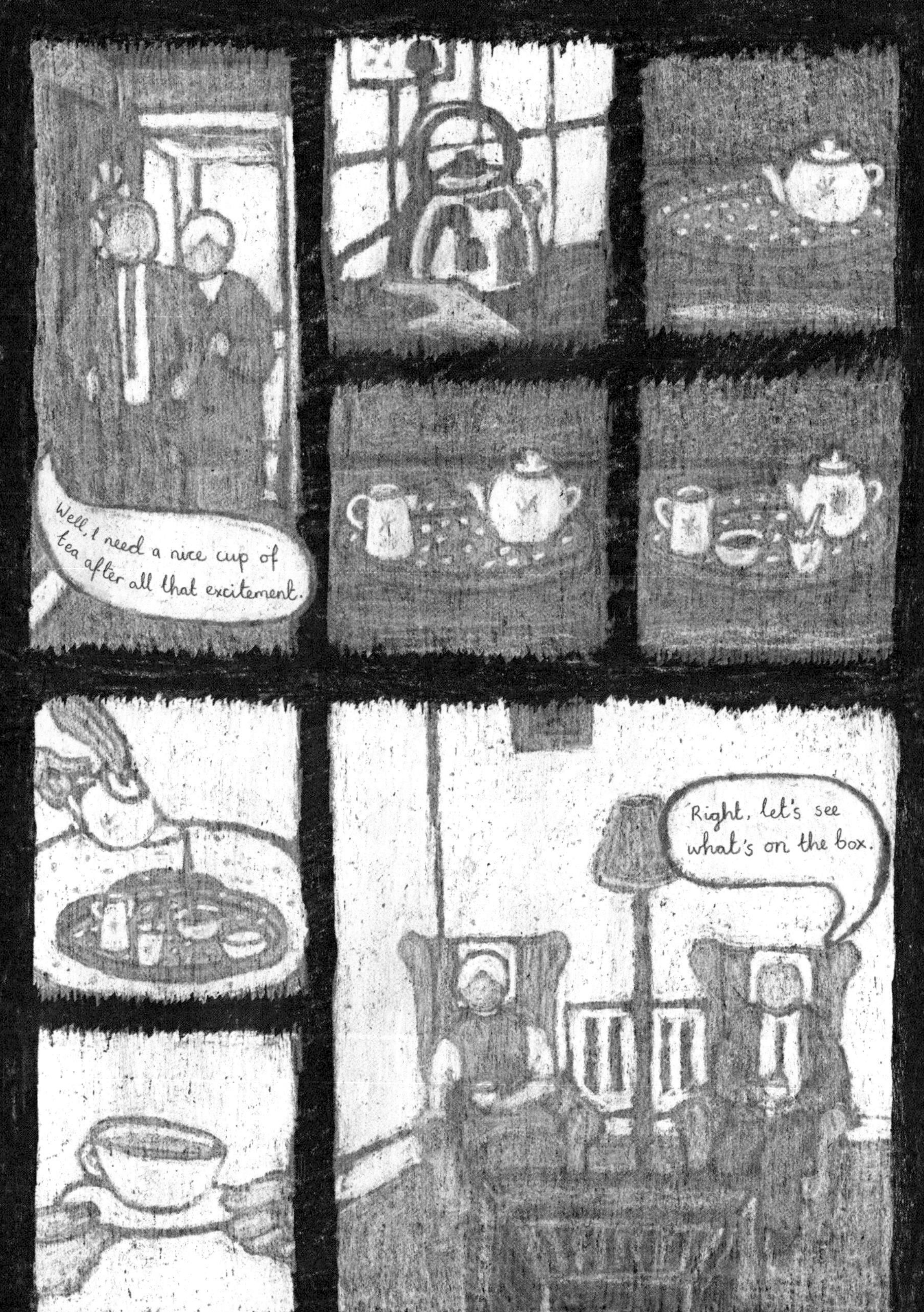
Well, I need a nice cup of tea after all that excitement.
Right, let's see what's on the box.

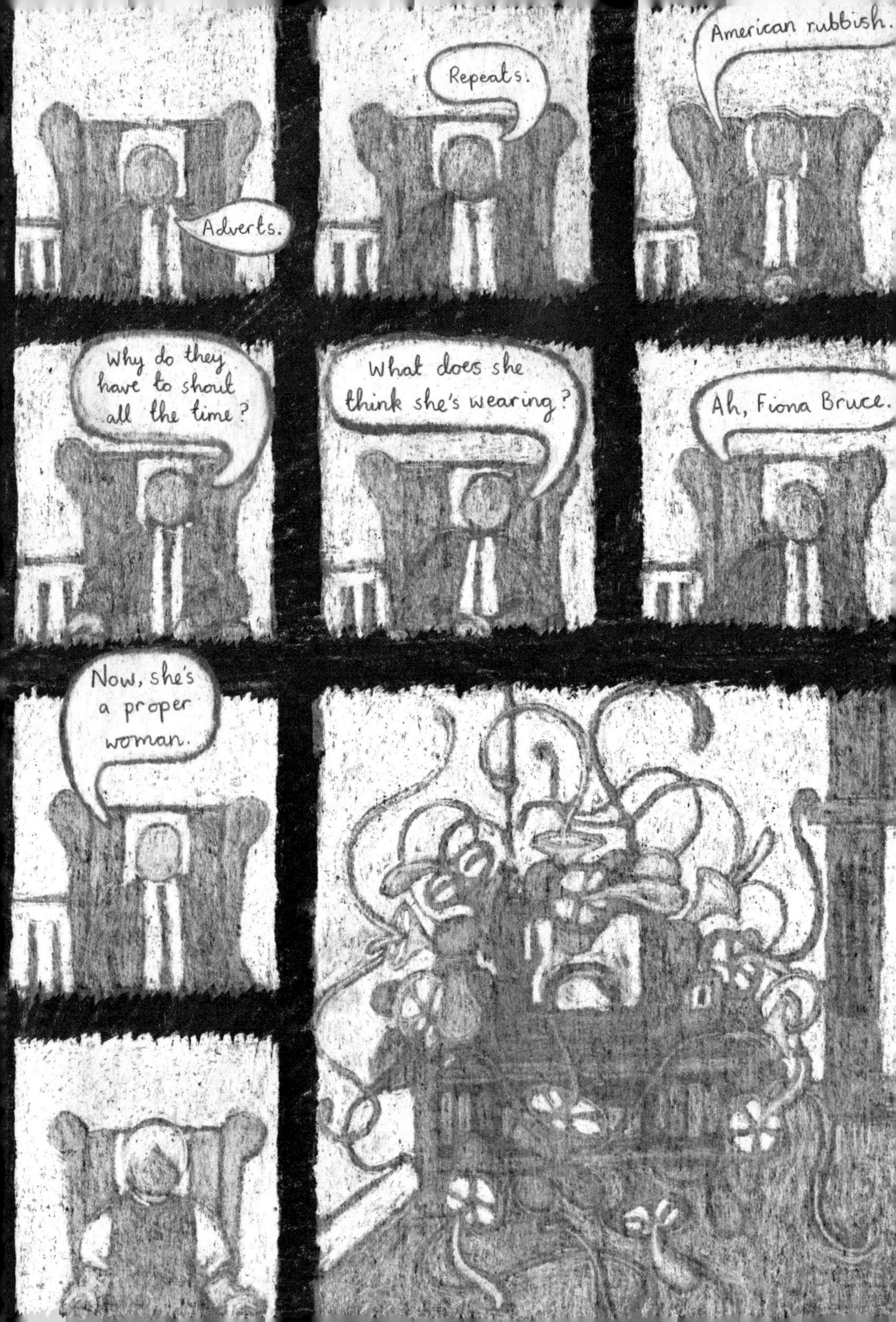
Adverts.
Repeats.
American rubbish.
Why do they have to shout all the time?
What does she think she's wearing?
Ah, Fiona Bruce.
Now, she's a proper woman.

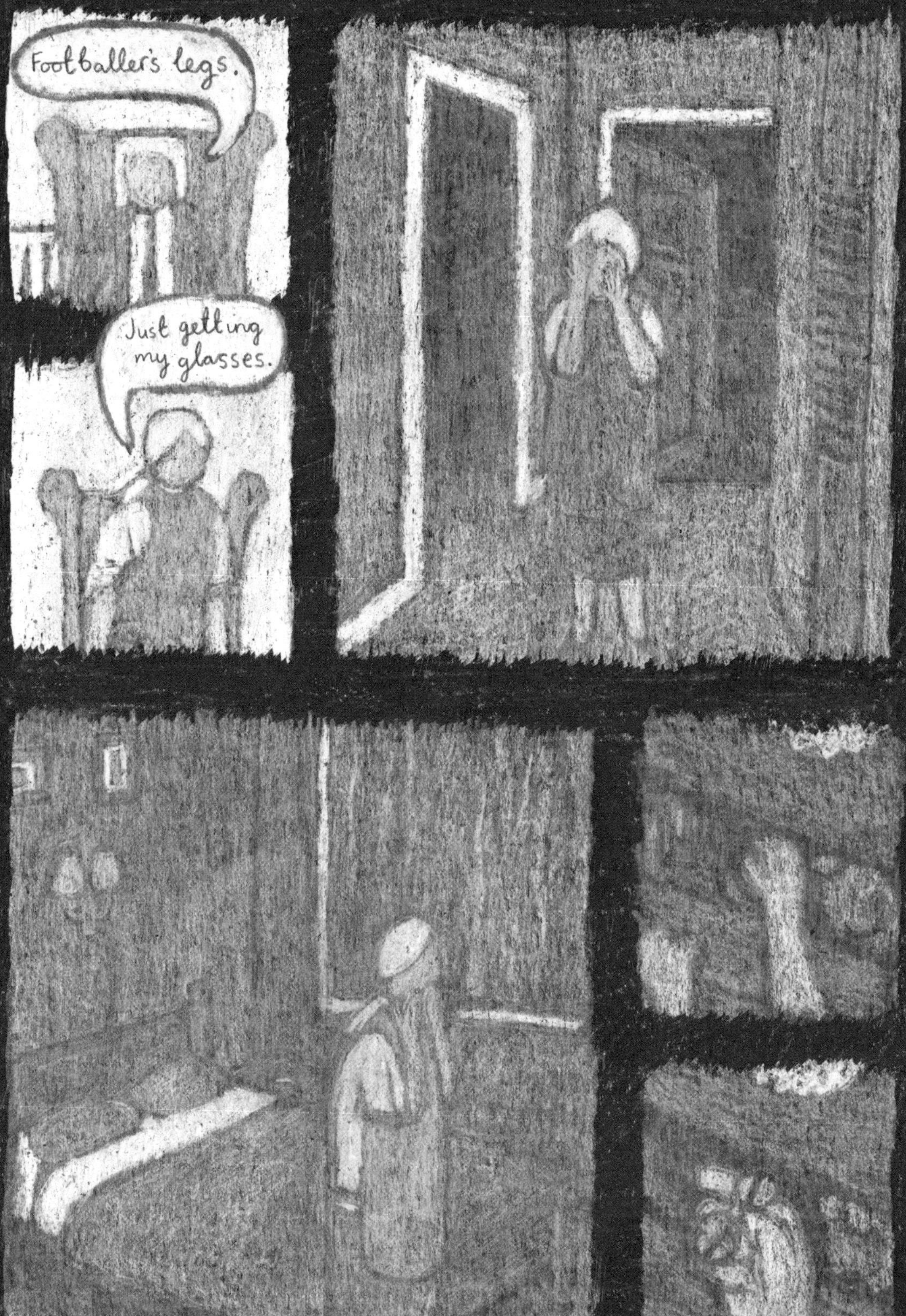
Footballer's legs.
Just getting my glasses.

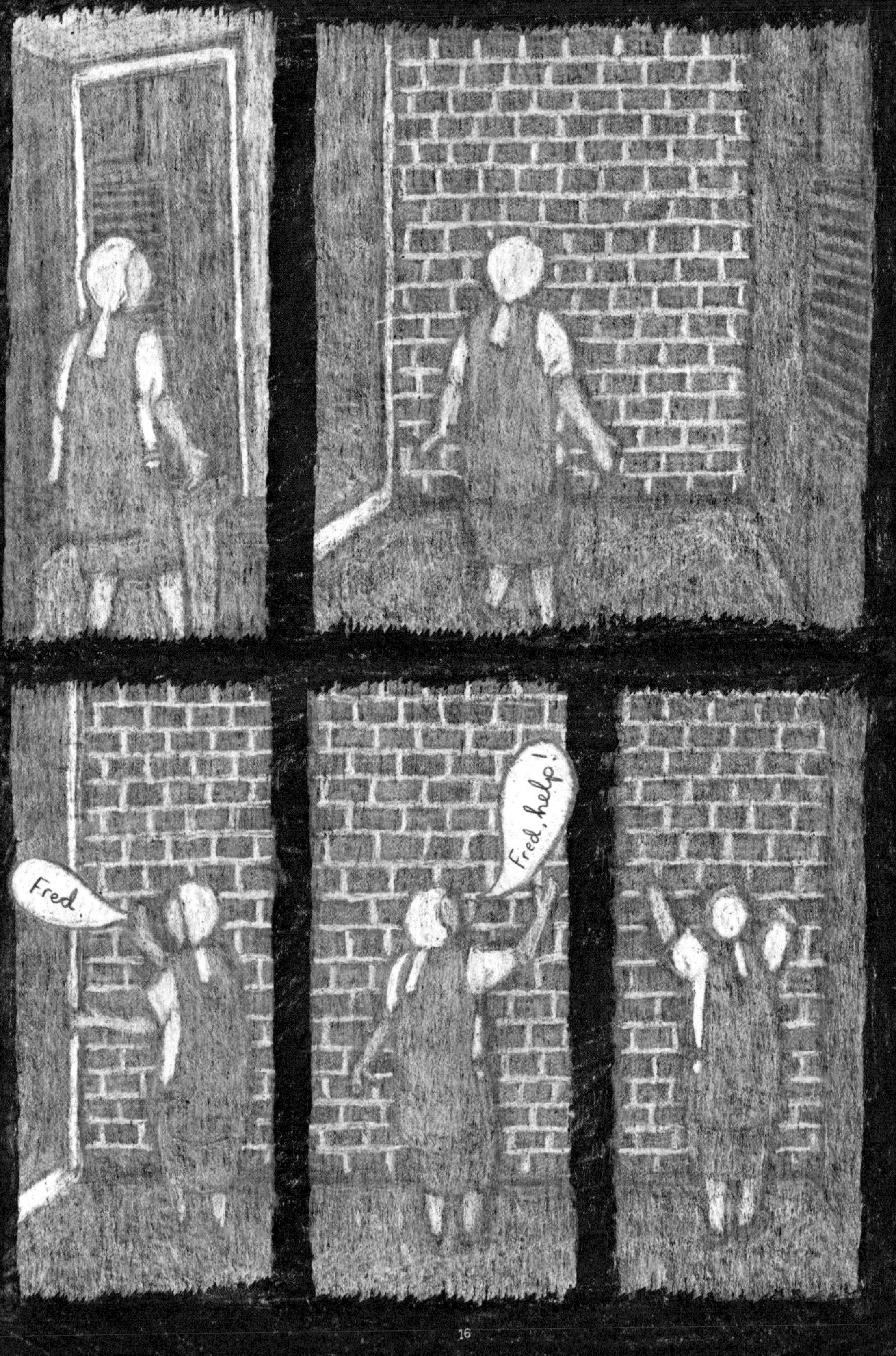
Fred.
Fred, help!

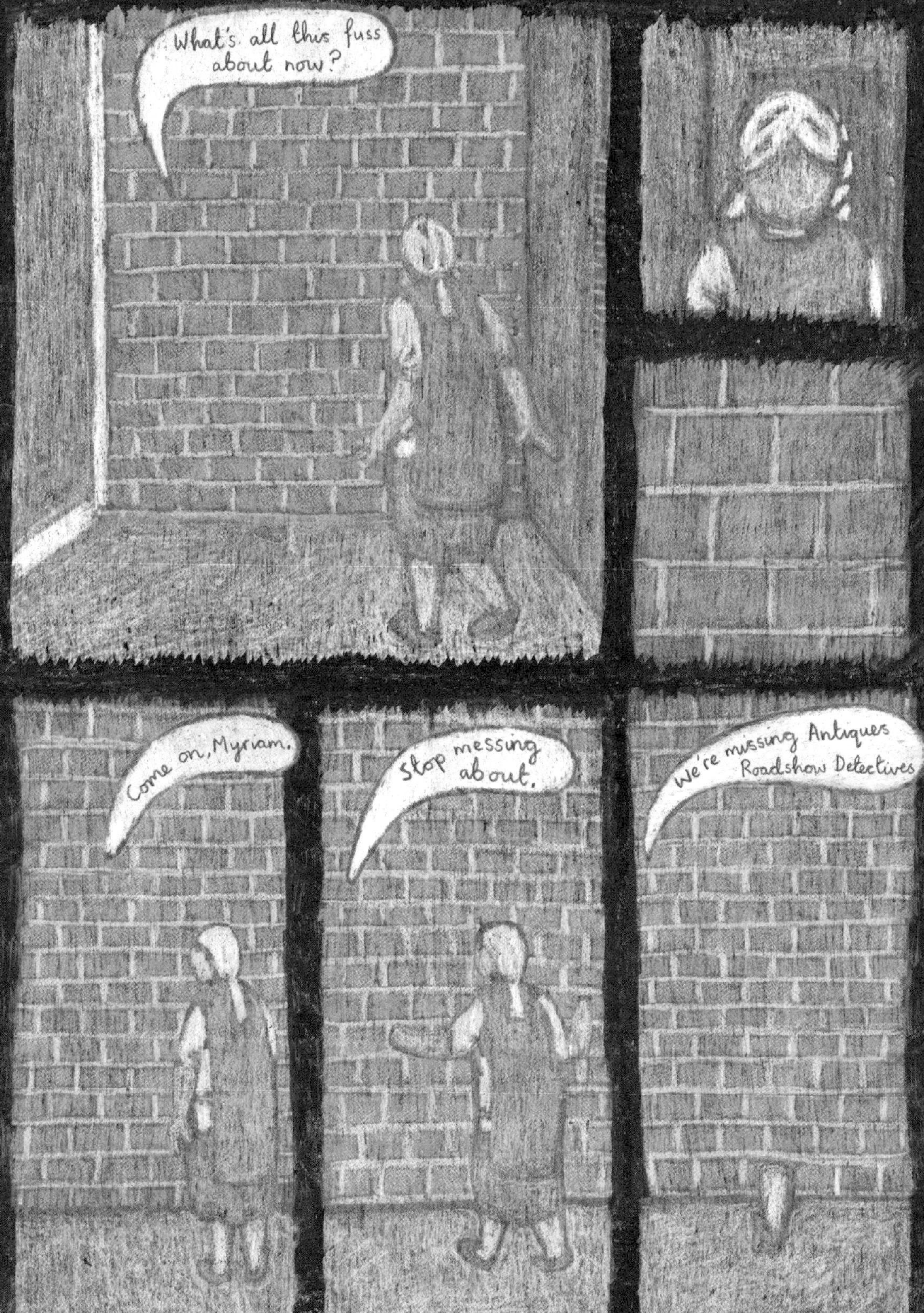
What's all this fuss about now?
Come on, Myriam.
Stop messing about.
We're missing Antiques Roadshow Detectives

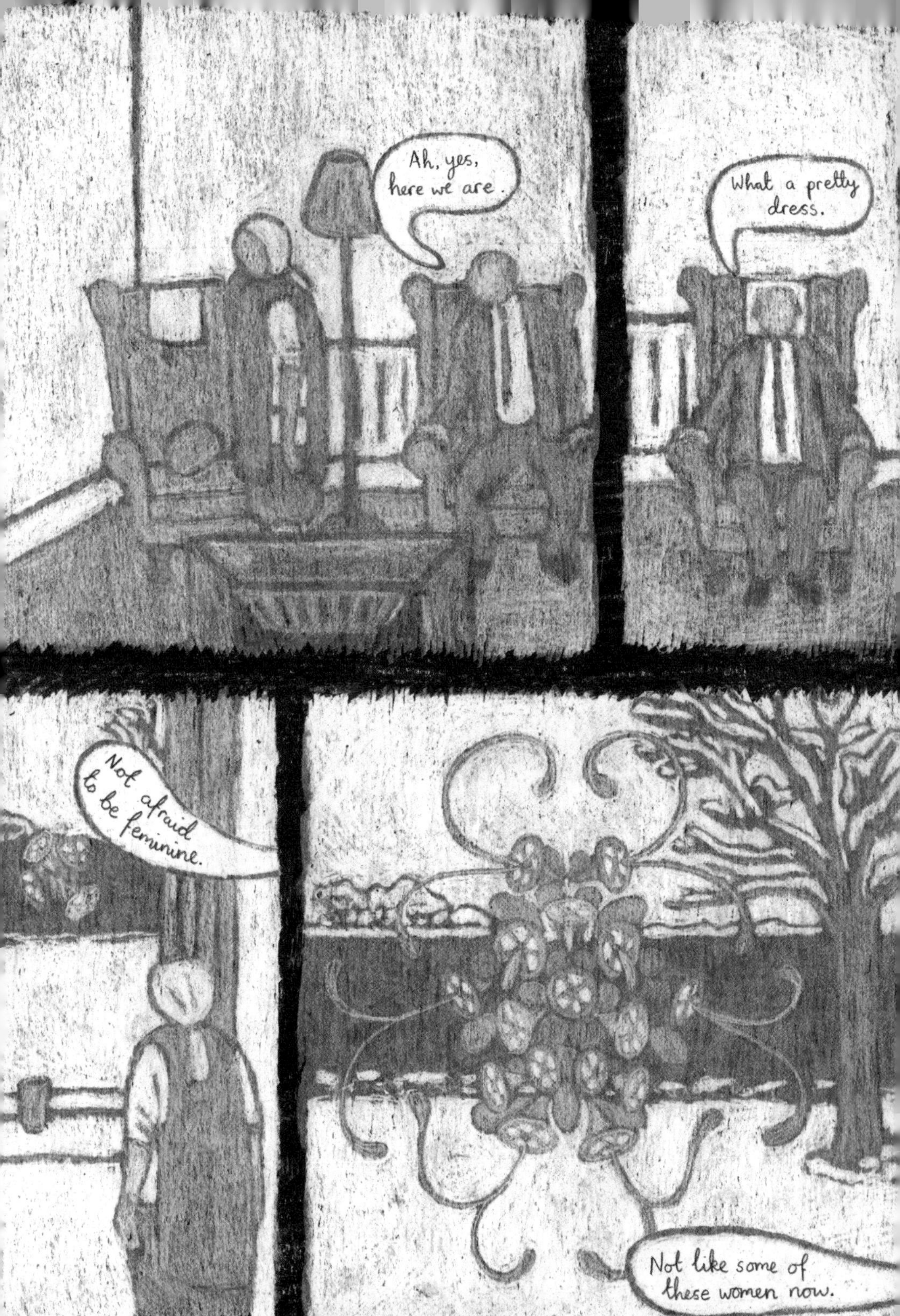
Ah, yes, here we are.
What a pretty dress.
Not afraid to be feminine.
Not like some of these women now.

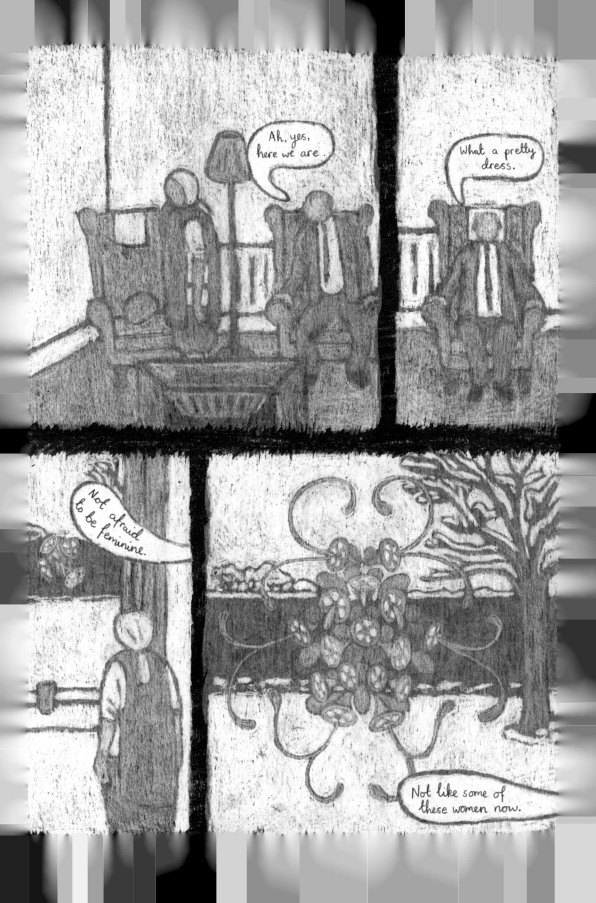

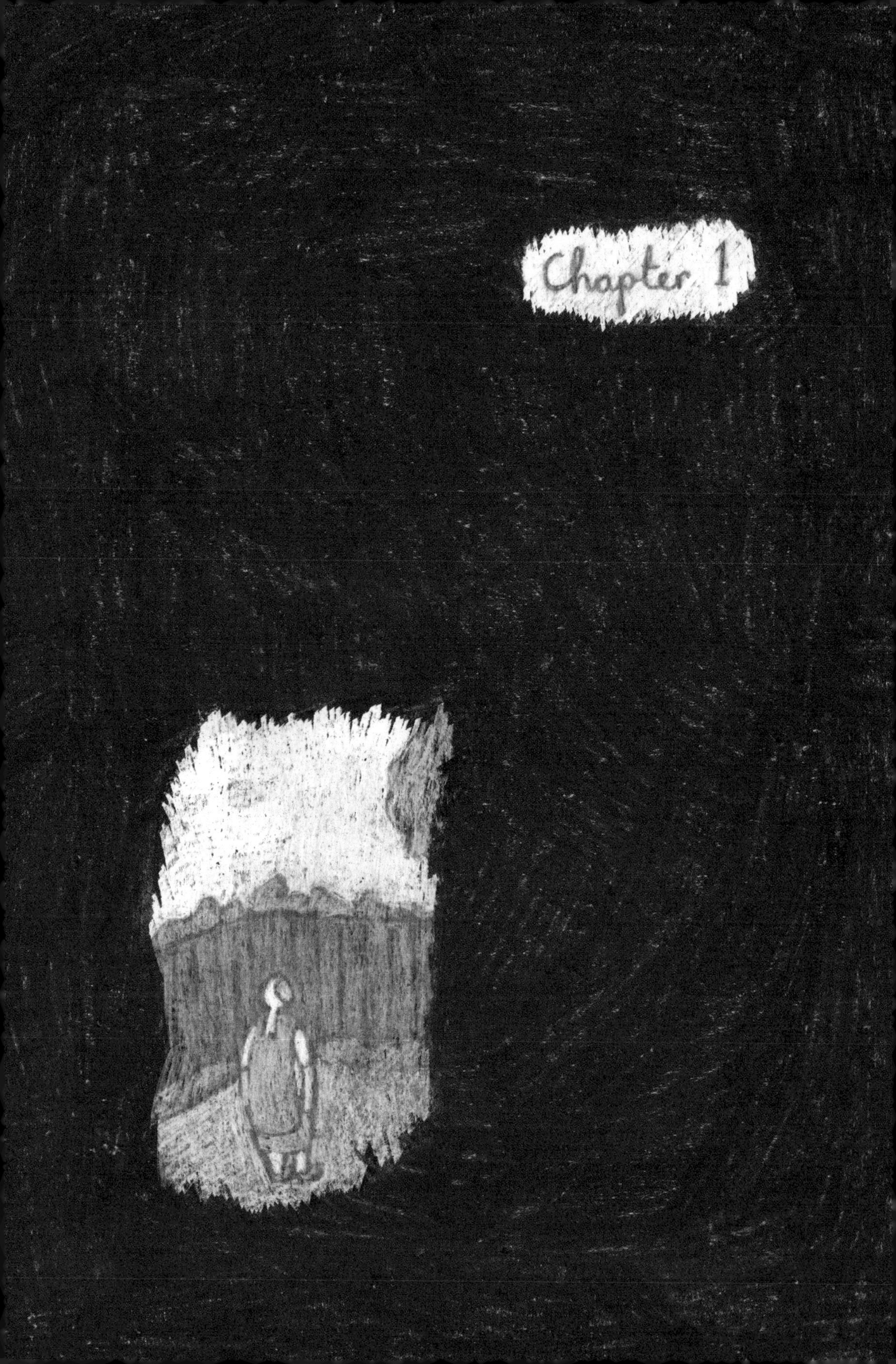
Chapter 1

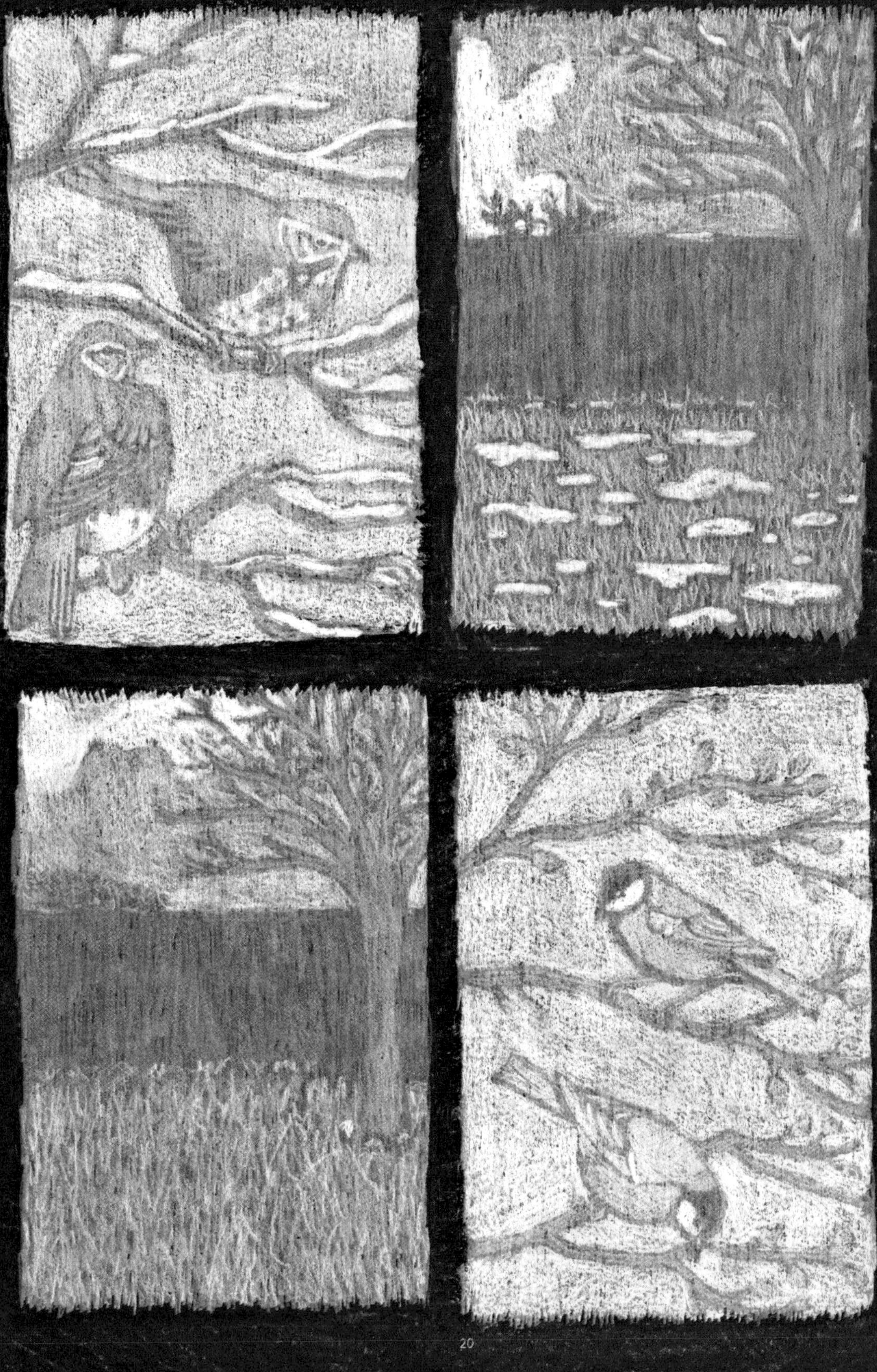

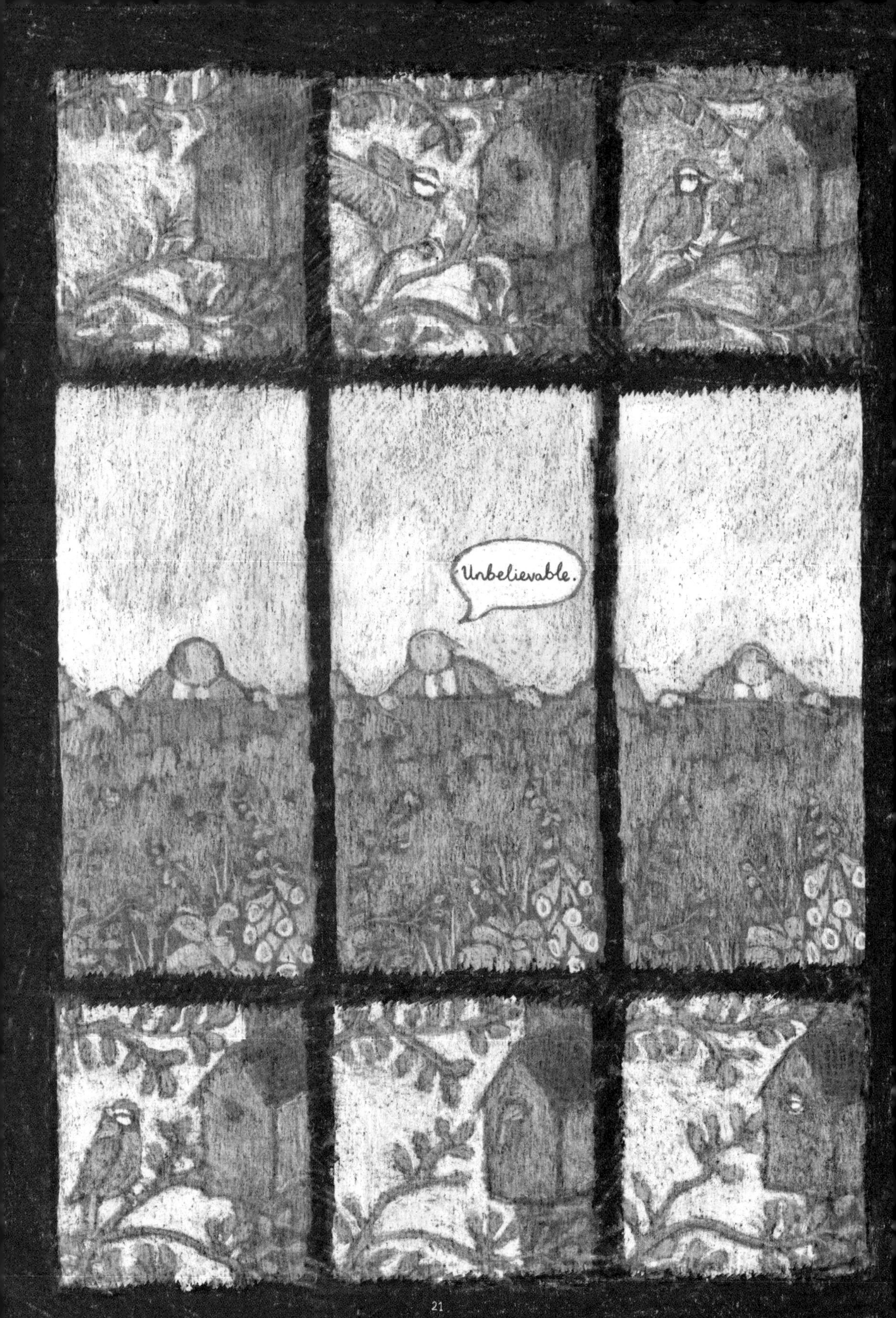
Unbelievable.

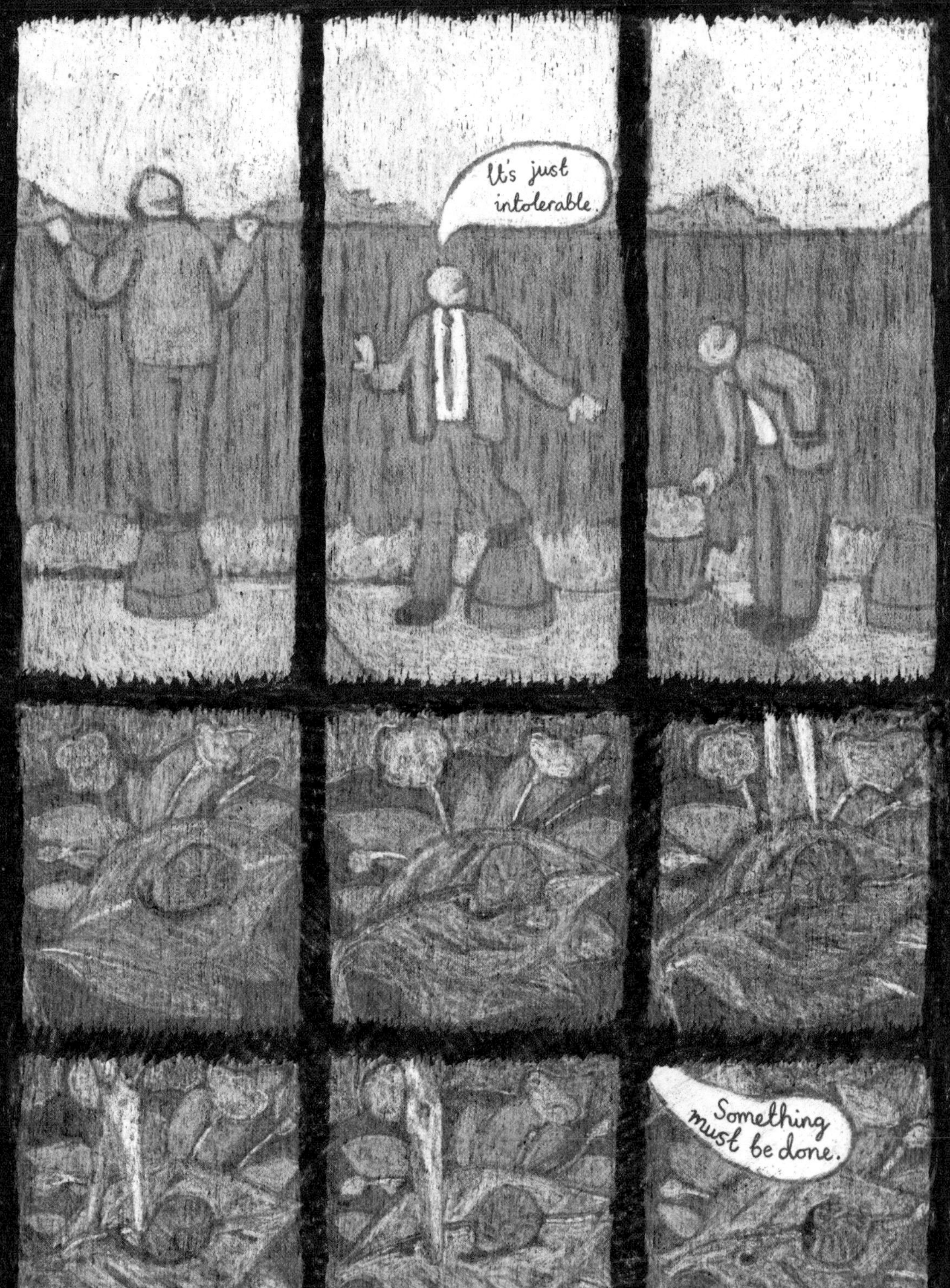
It's just intolerable.
Something must be done.

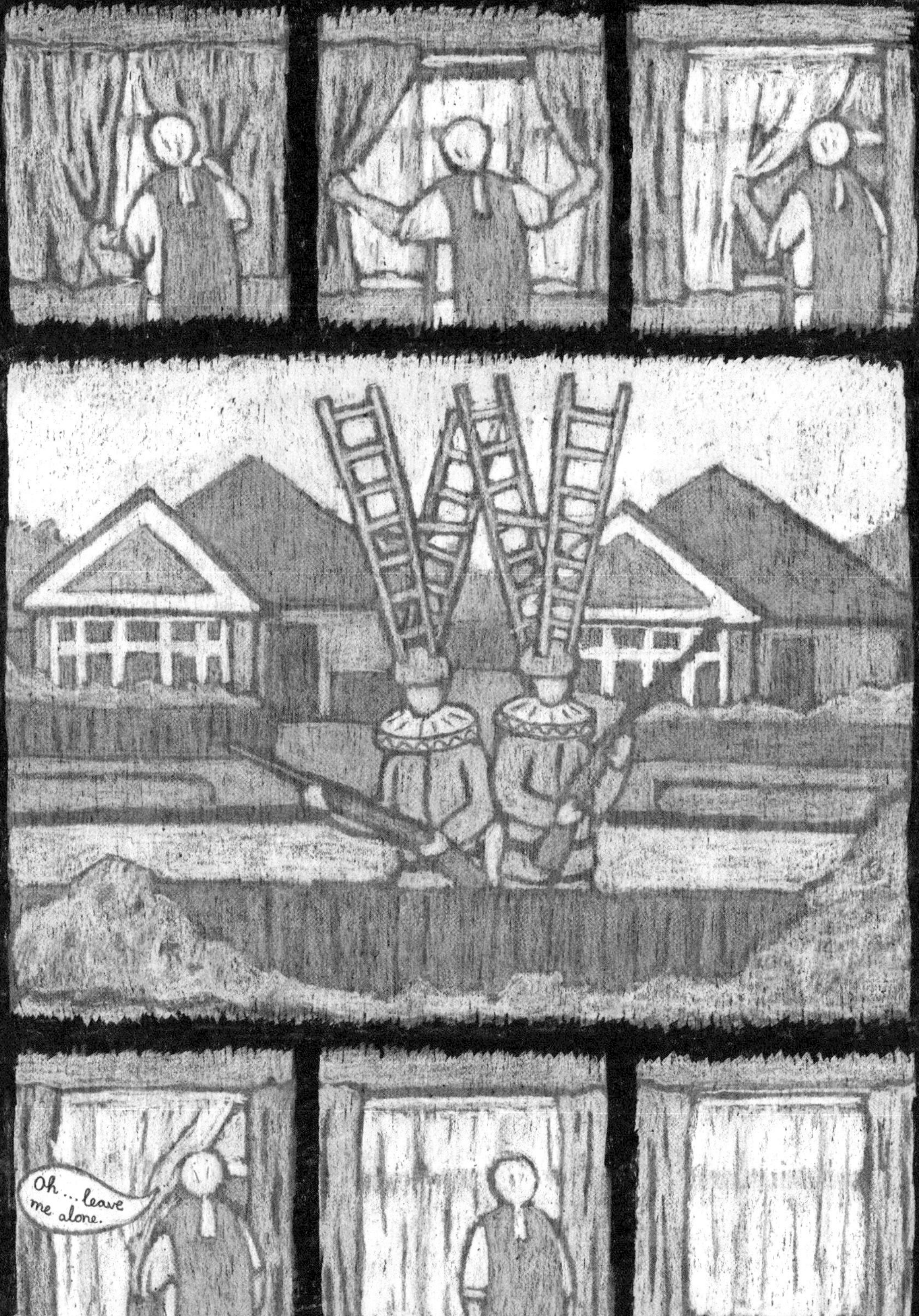
Oh ... leave me alone.

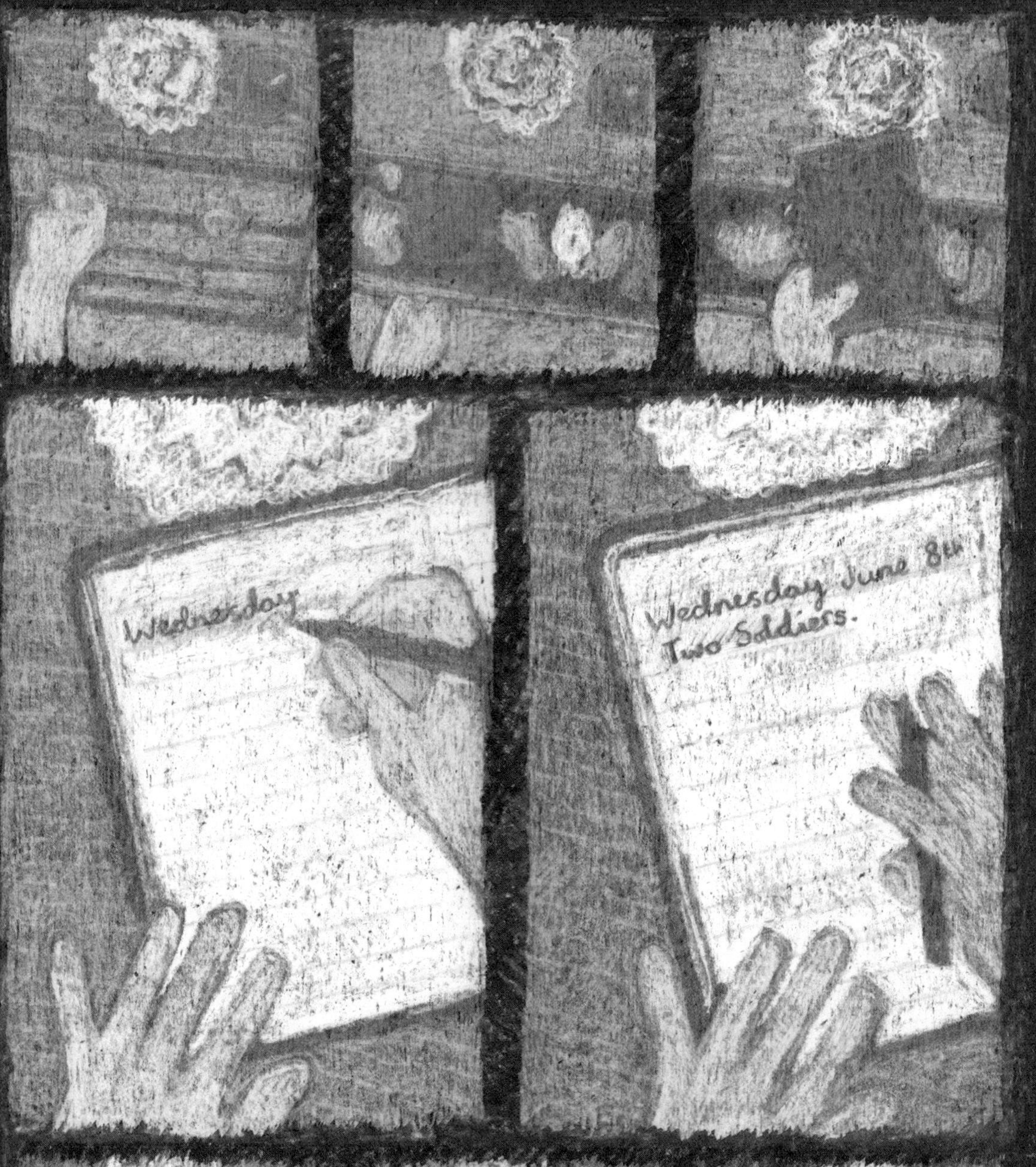
Wednesday
Wednesday June 8th
Two Soldiers.

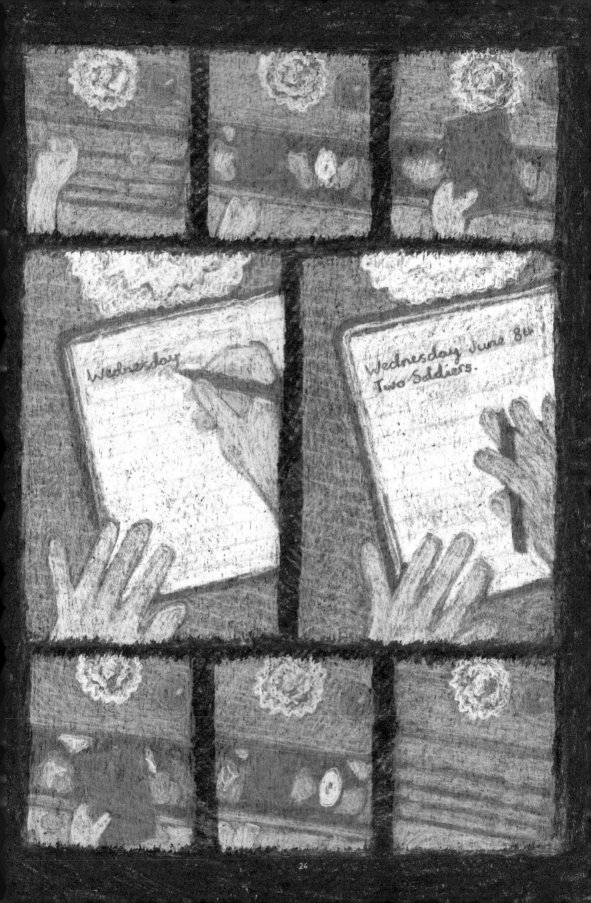

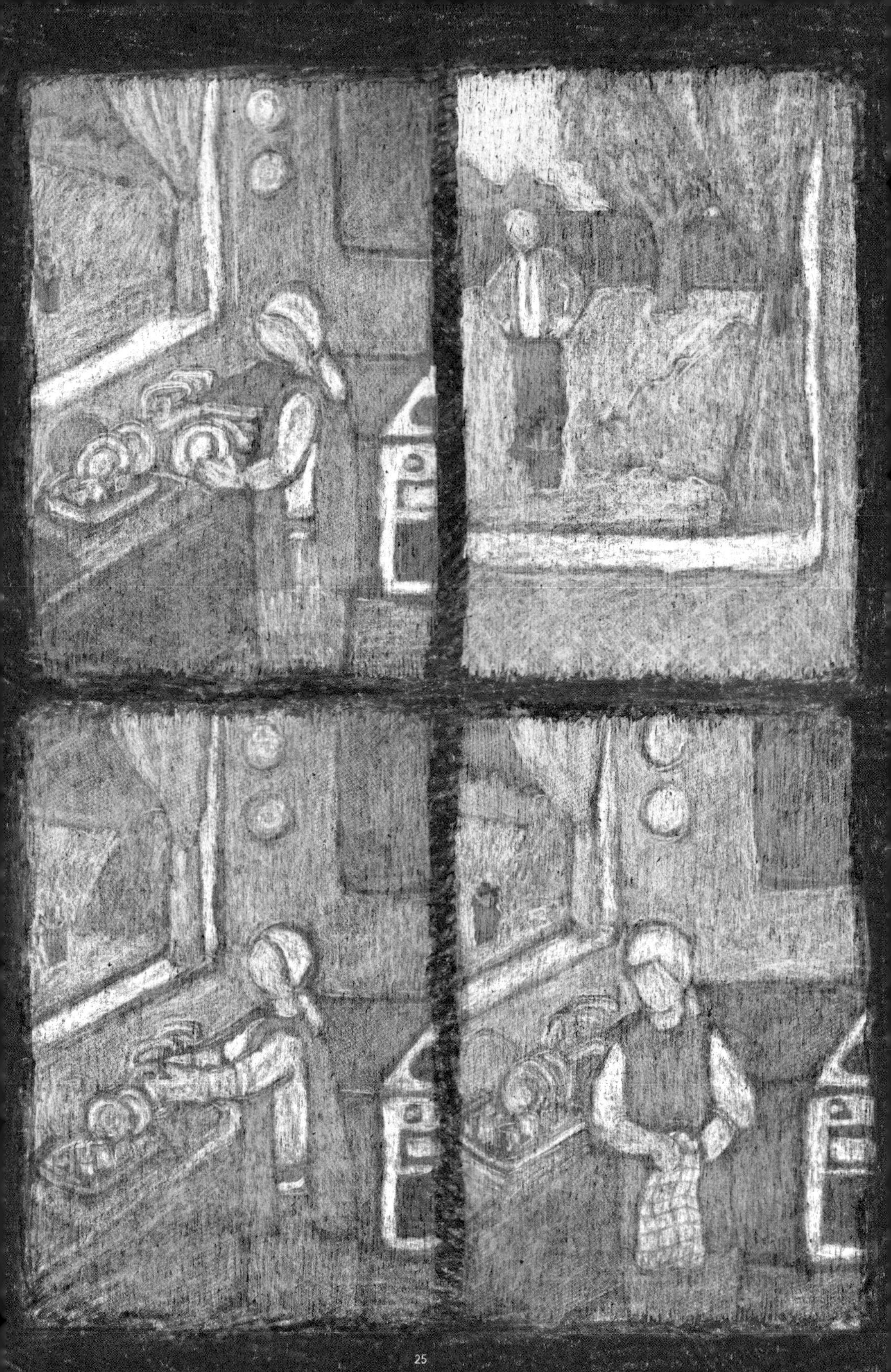

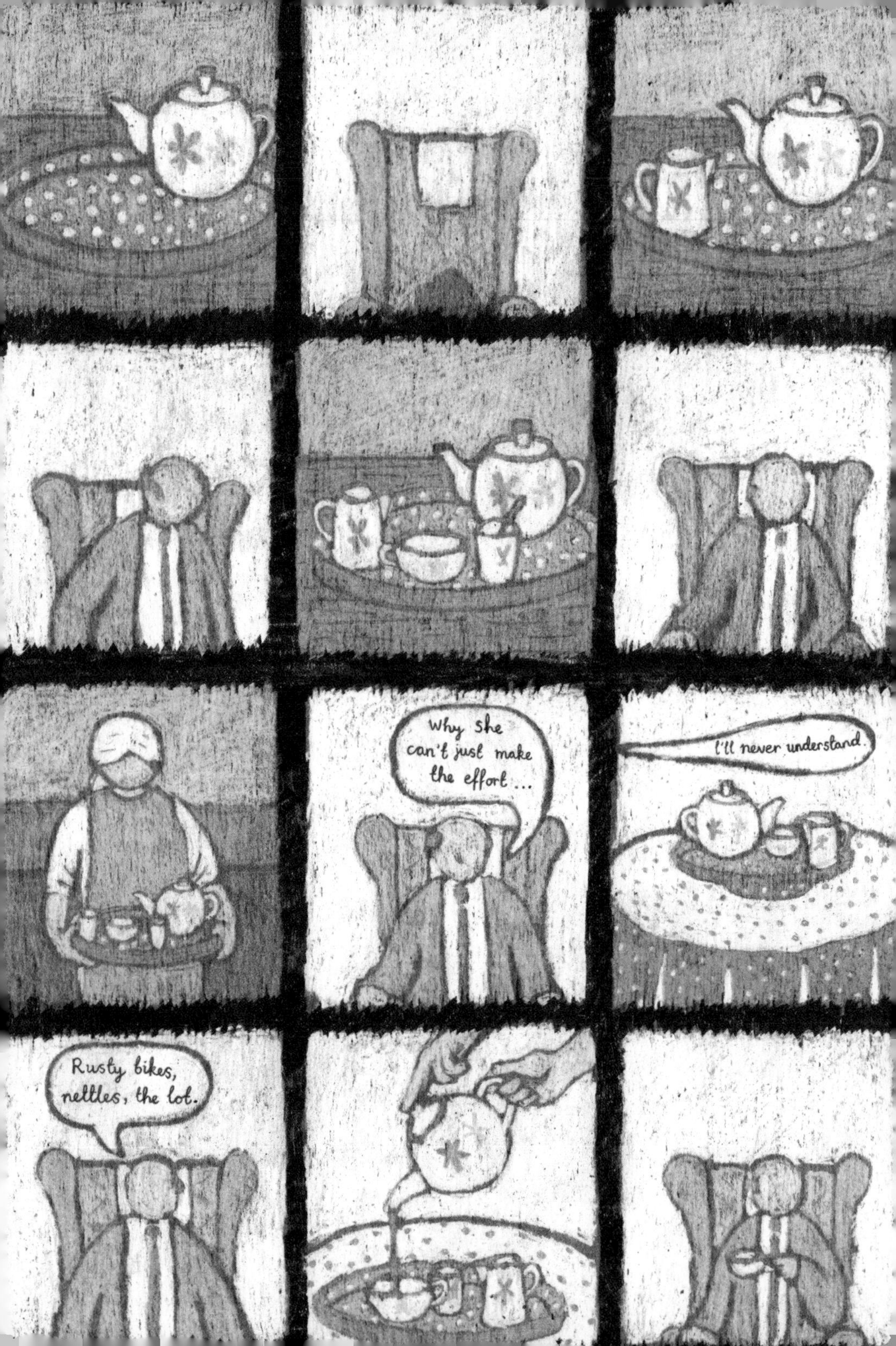
Why she can't just make the effort...
I'll never understand.
Rusty bikes, nettles, the lot.

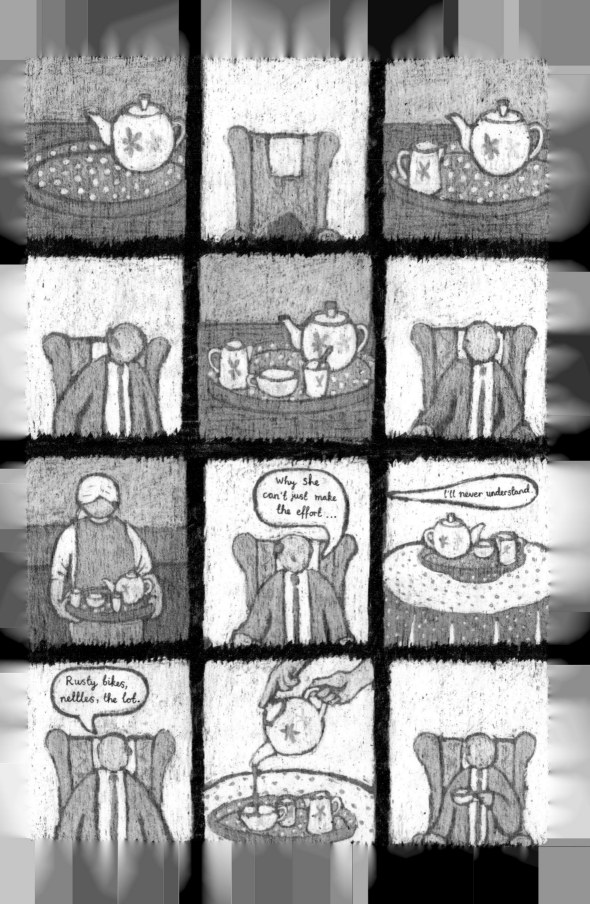

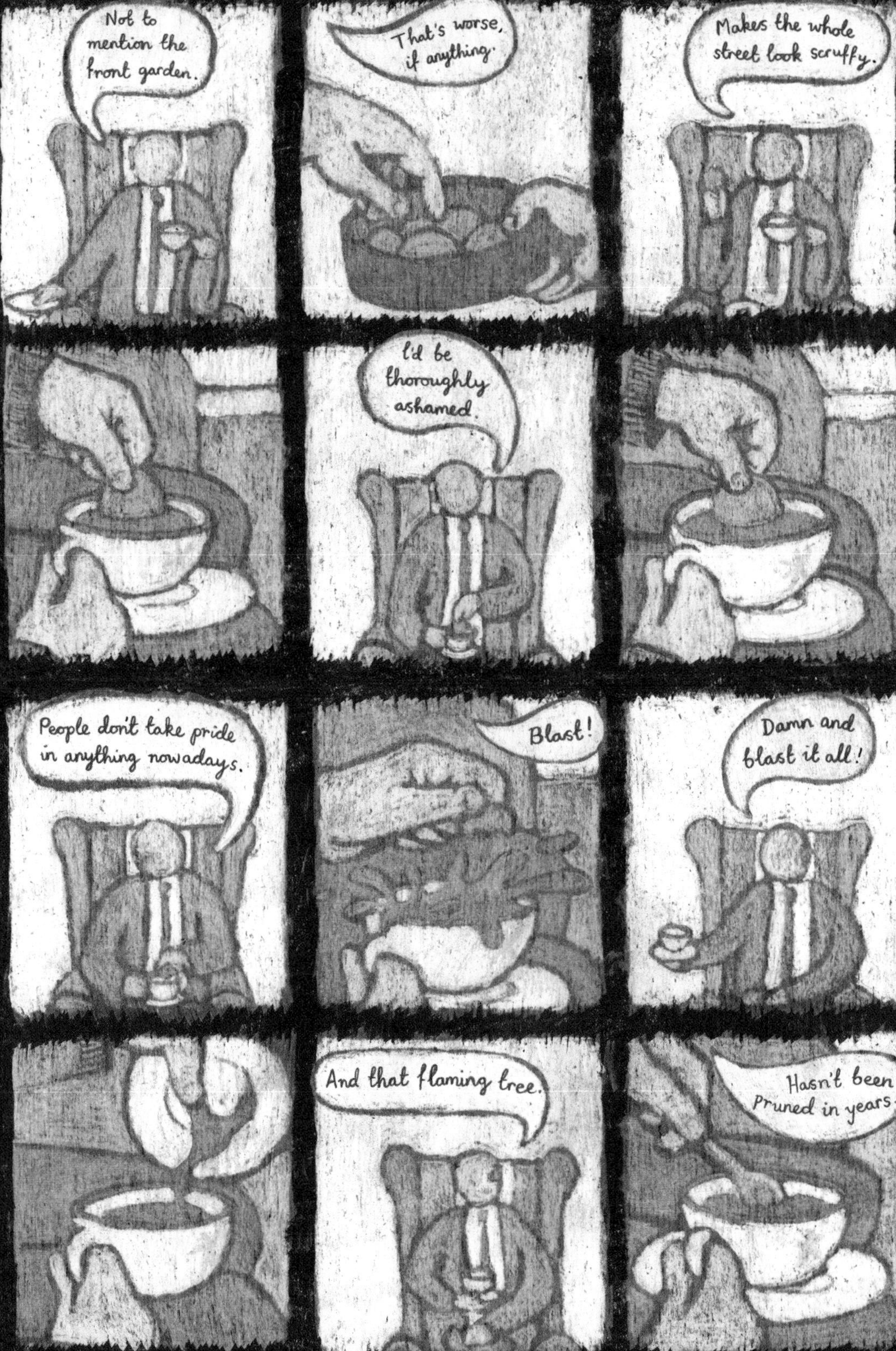
Not to mention the front garden.
That's worse, if anything.
Makes the whole street look scruffy.
I'd be thoroughly ashamed.
People don't take pride in anything nowadays.
Blast!
Damn and blast it all!
And that flaming tree.
Hasn't been pruned in years.

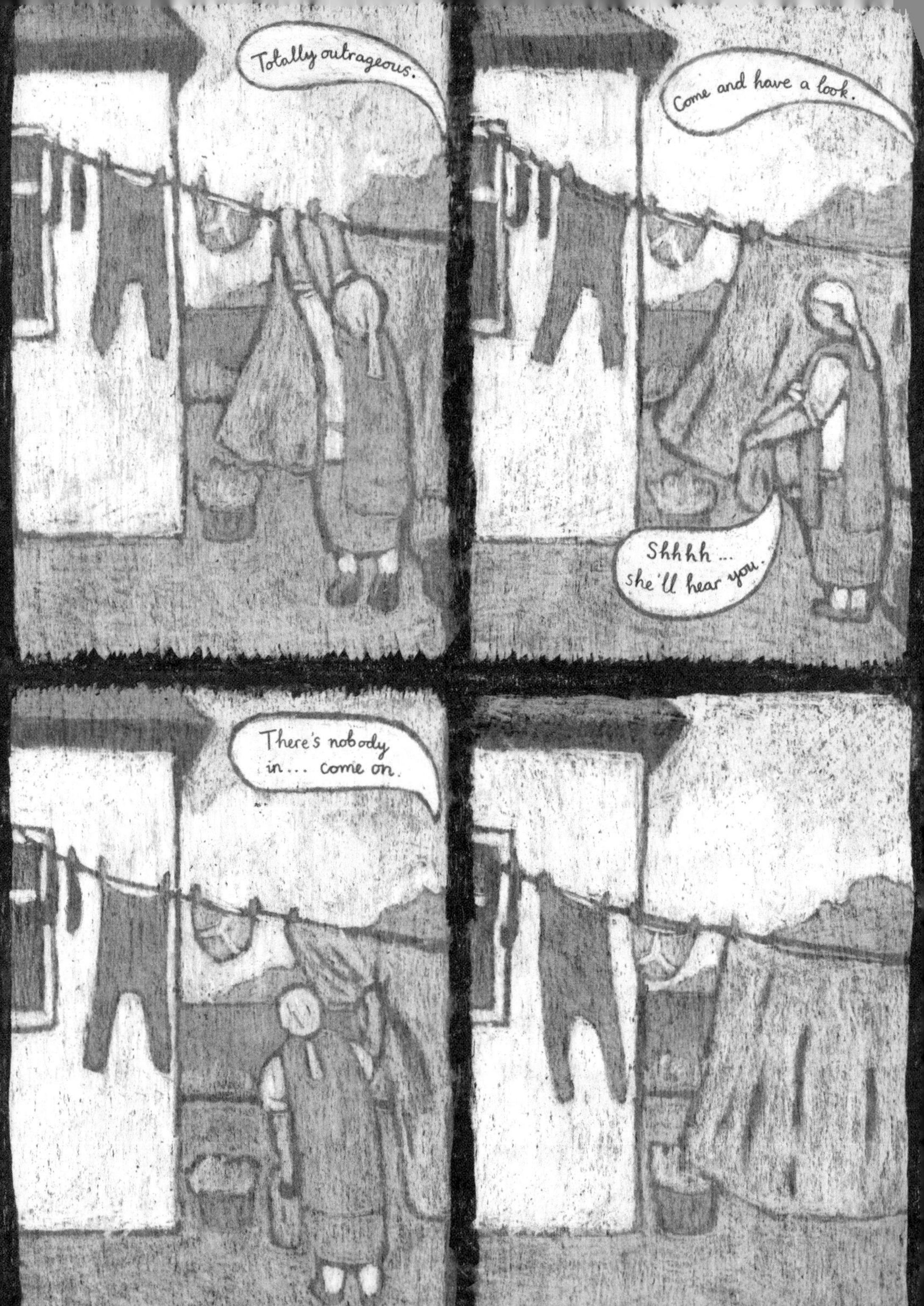
Totally outrageous.
Come and have a look.
Shhhh ... she'll hear you.
There's nobody in ... come on.

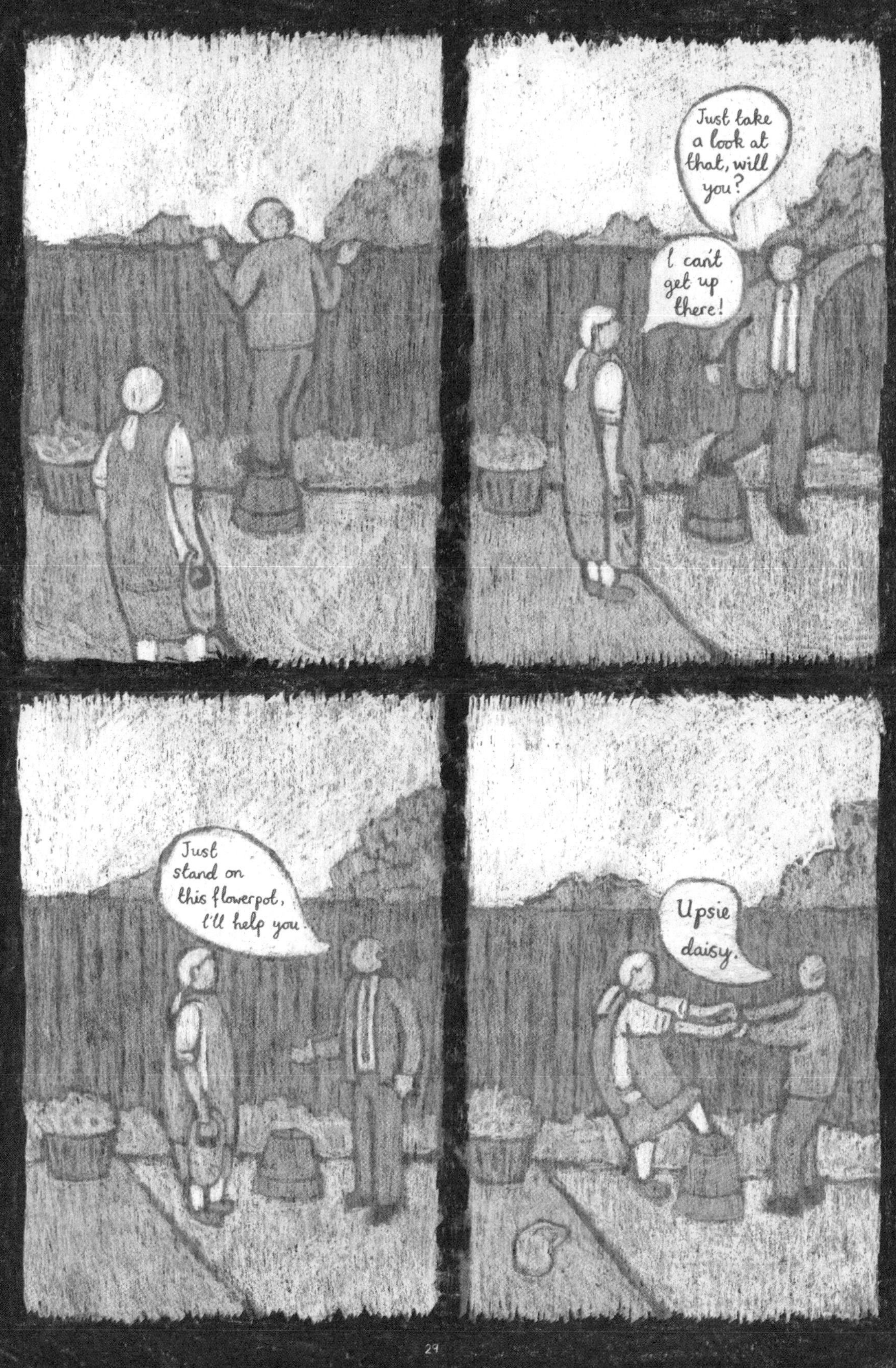
Just take a look at that, will you?
I can't get up there!
Just stand on this flowerpot, I'll help you.
Upsie daisy.

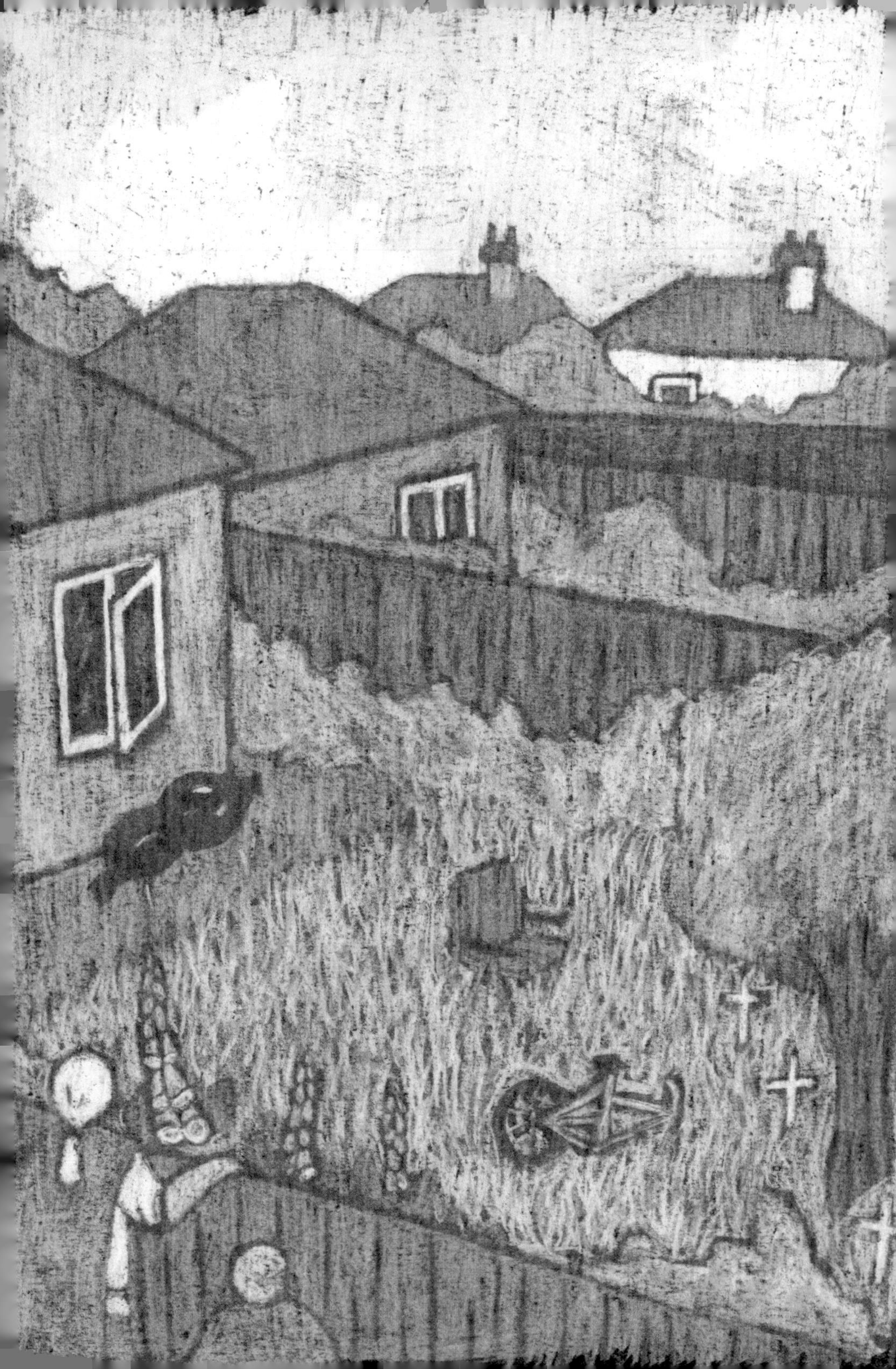

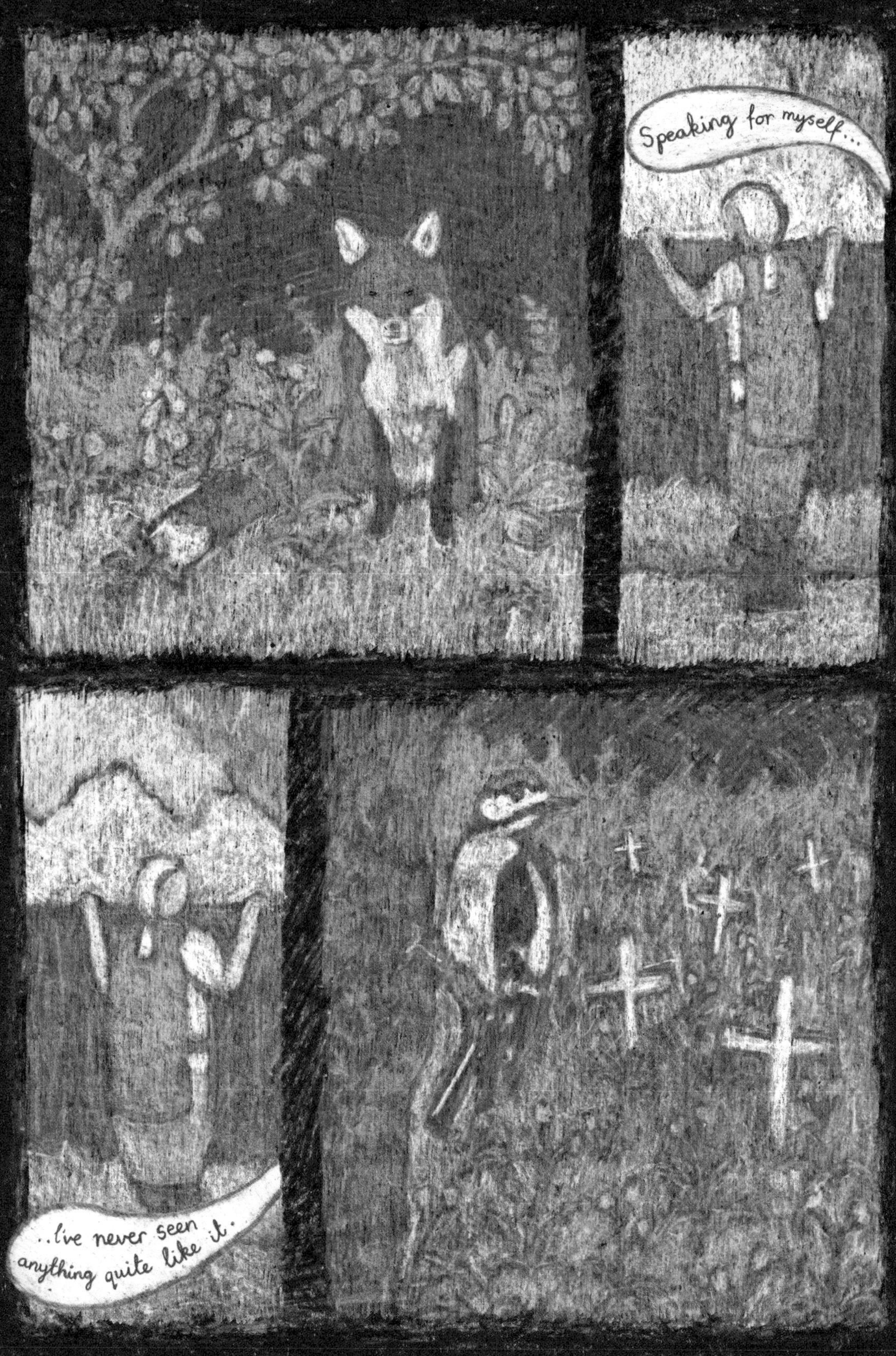
Speaking for myself...
..I've never seen anything quite like it.

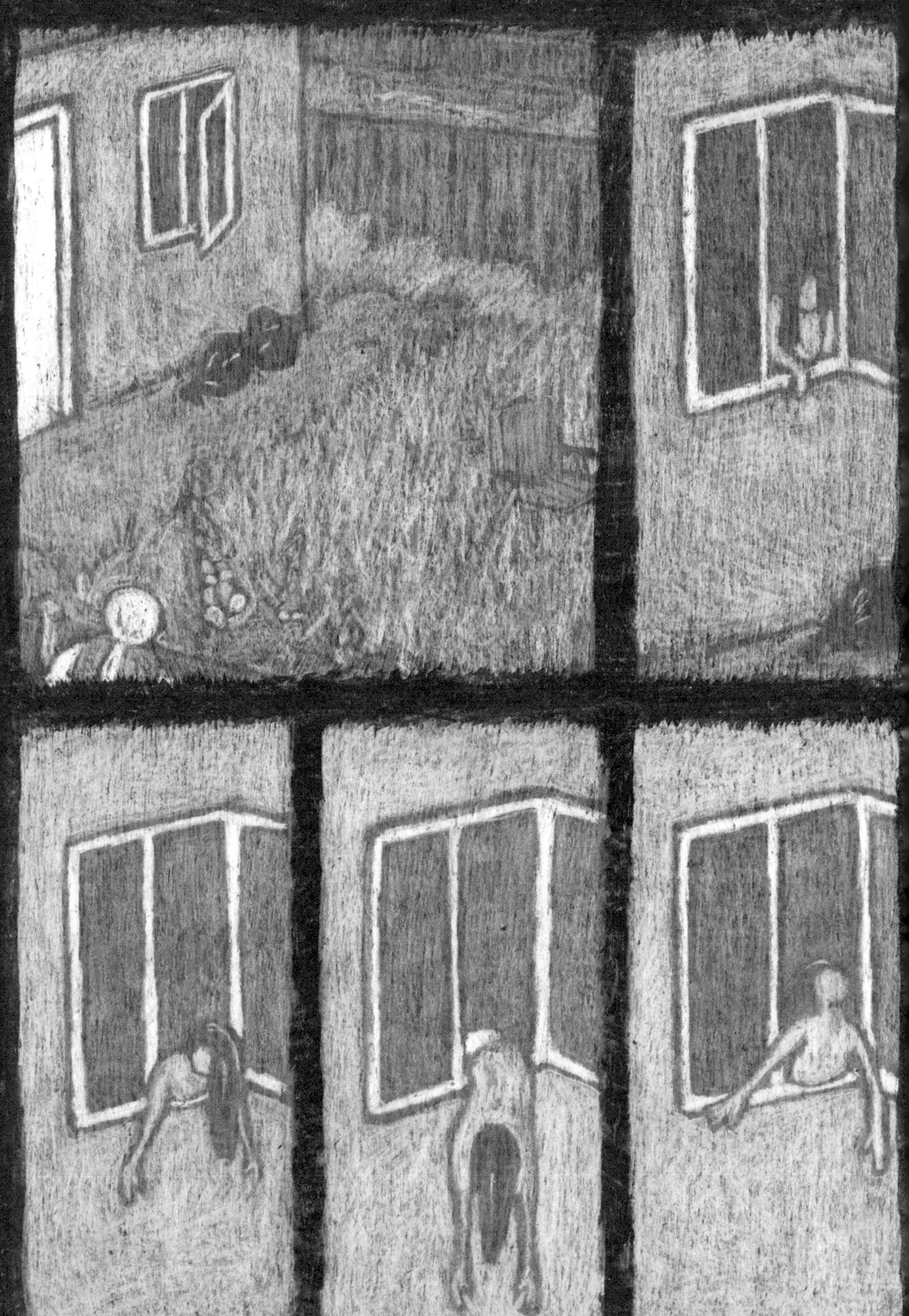

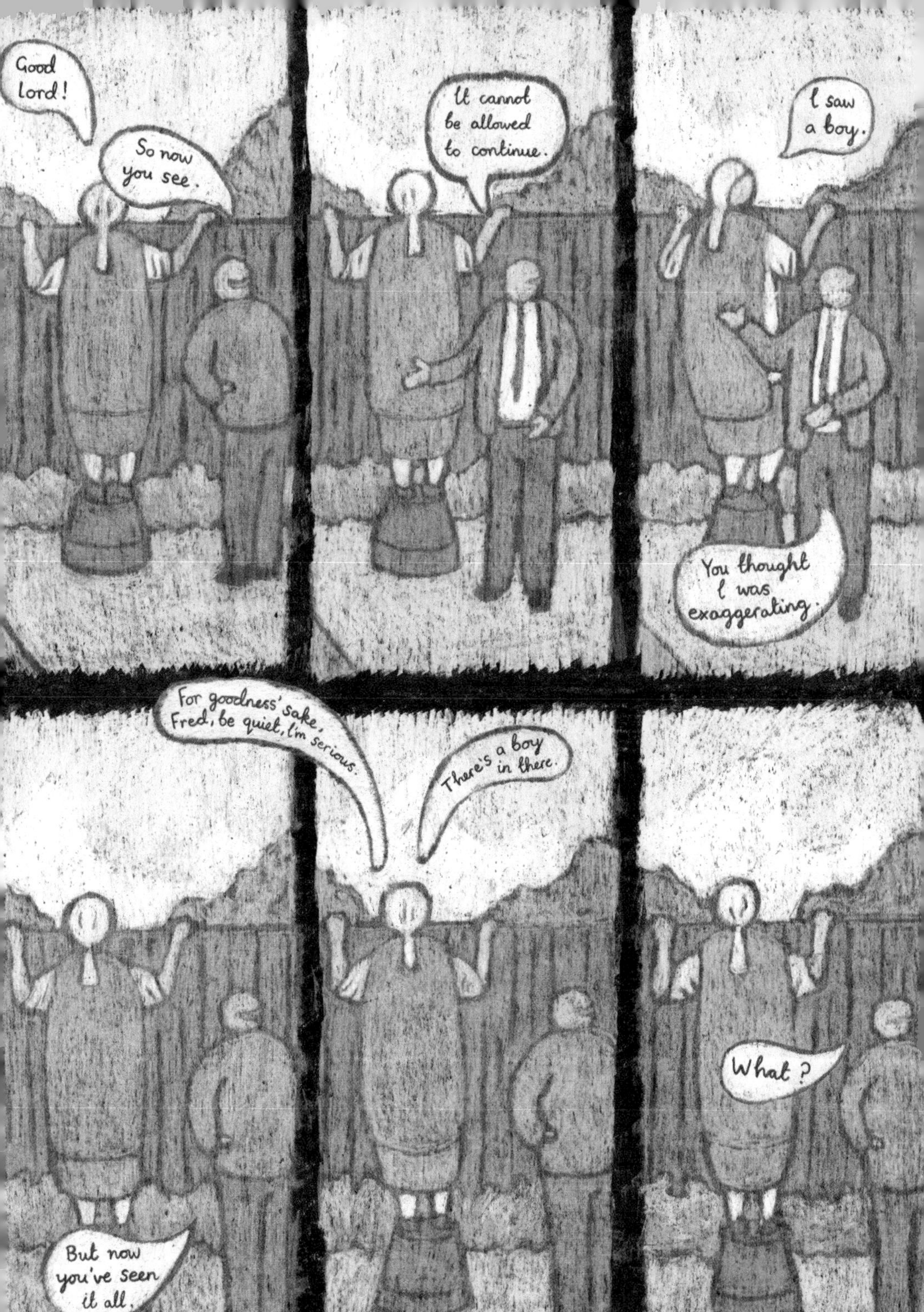
Good lord!
So now you see.
It cannot be allowed to continue.
I saw a boy.
You thought I was exaggerating.
But now you've seen it all.
For goodness' sake, Fred, be quiet, I'm serious.
There's a boy in there.
What?

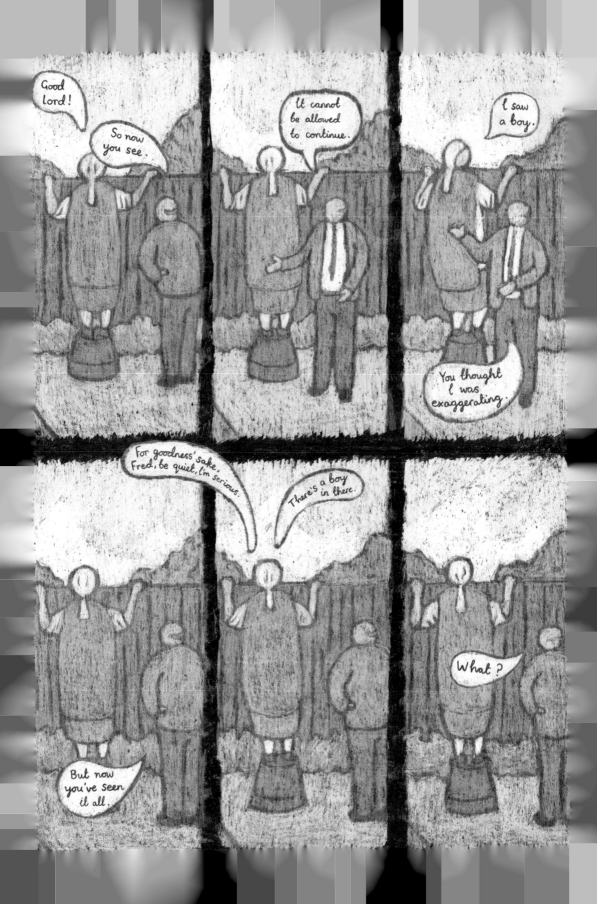

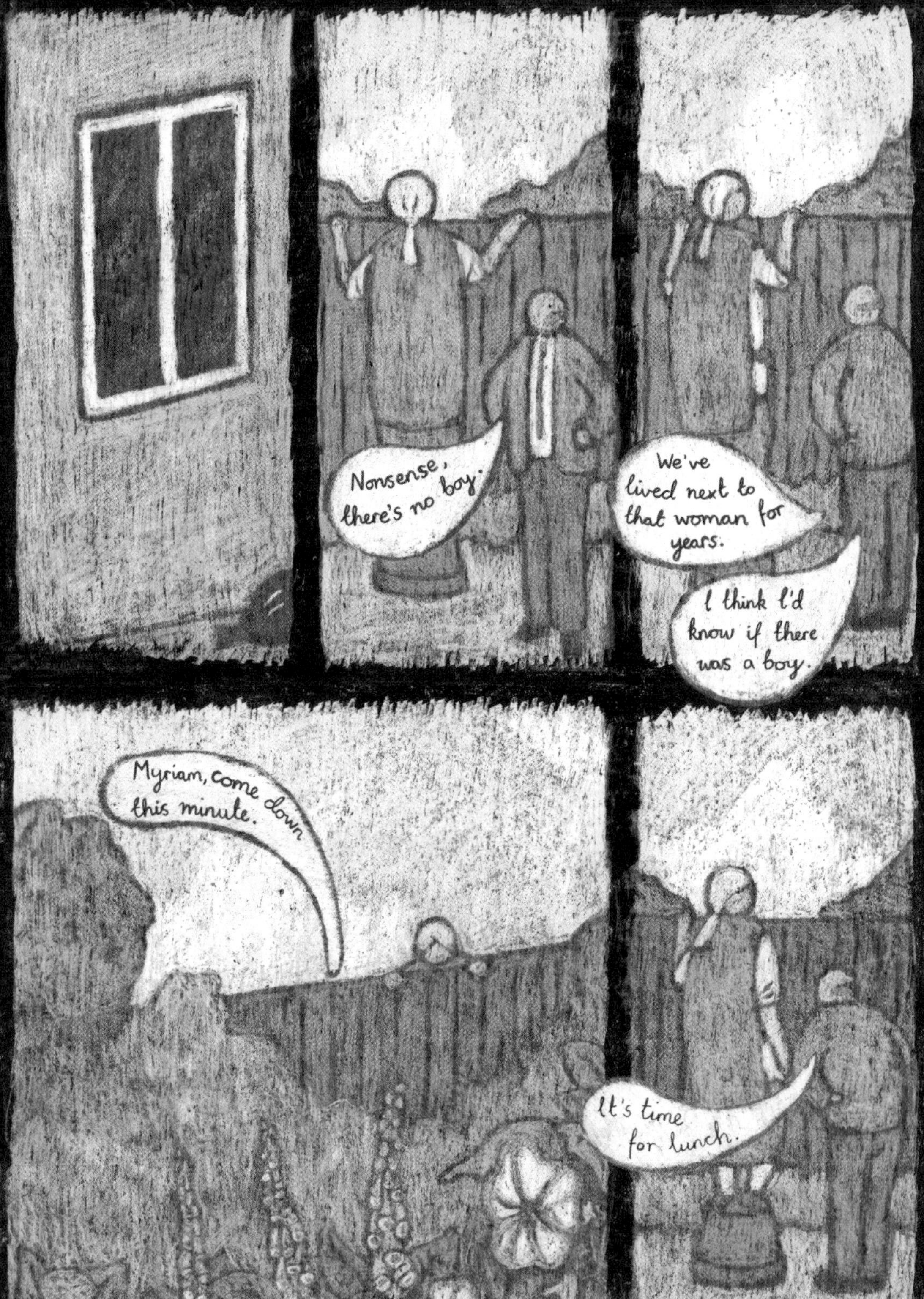
Nonsense, there's no boy.
We've lived next to that woman for years.
I think I'd know if there was a boy.
Myriam, come down this minute.
It's time for lunch.

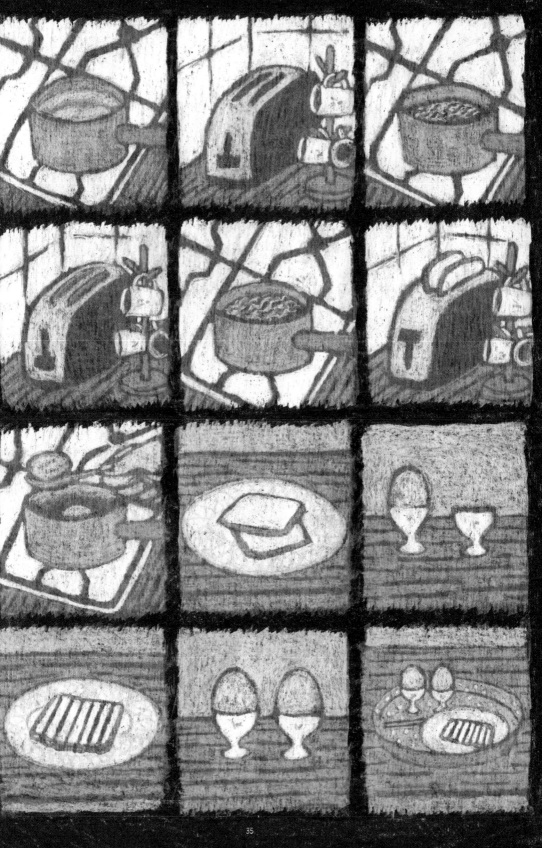

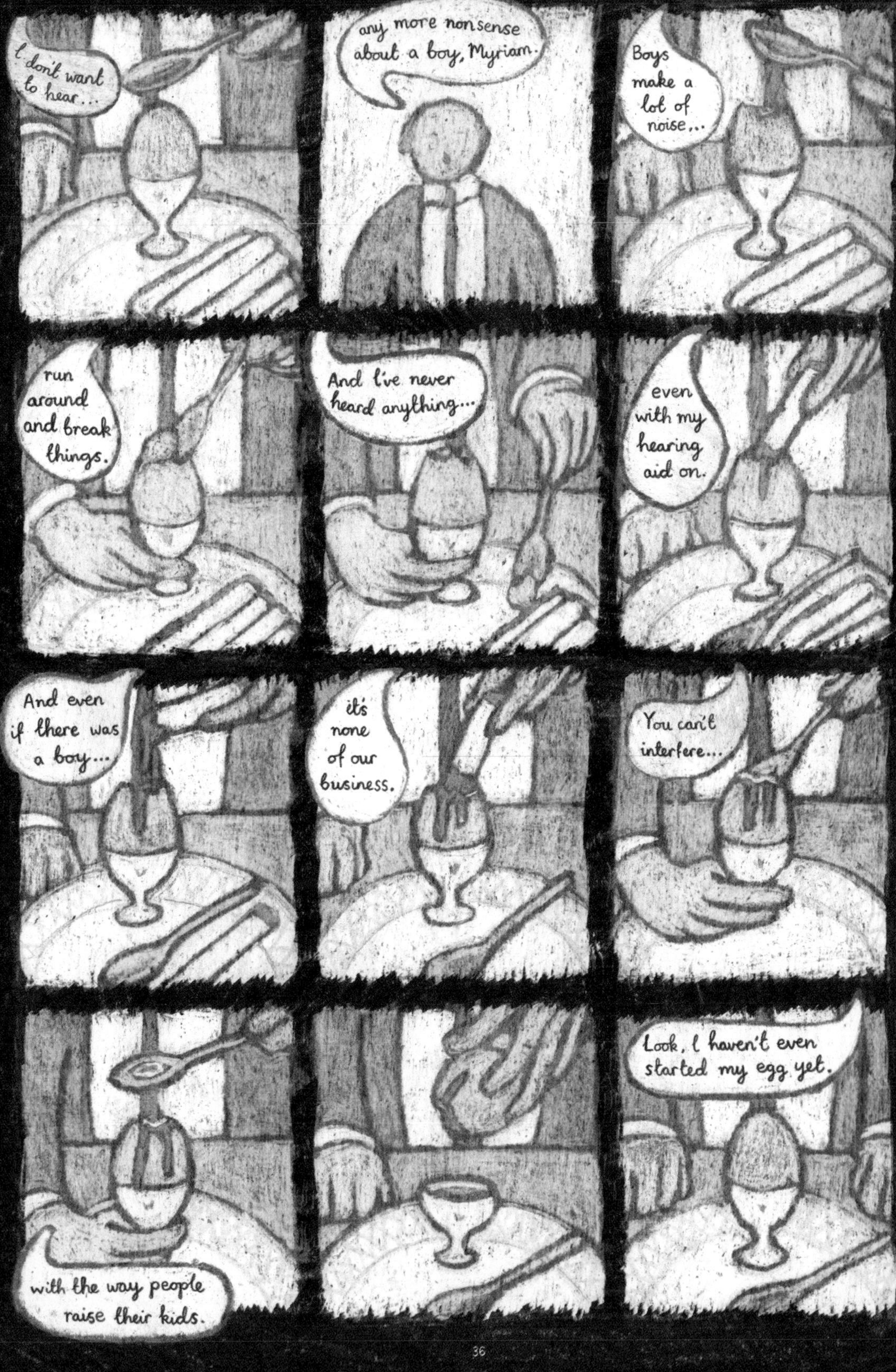
I don't want to hear...
any more nonsense about a boy, Myriam.
Boys make a lot of noise,...
run around and break things.
And I've never heard anything...
even with my hearing aid on.
And even if there was a boy...
it's none of our business.
You can't interfere...
with the way people raise their kids.
Look, I haven't even started my egg yet.

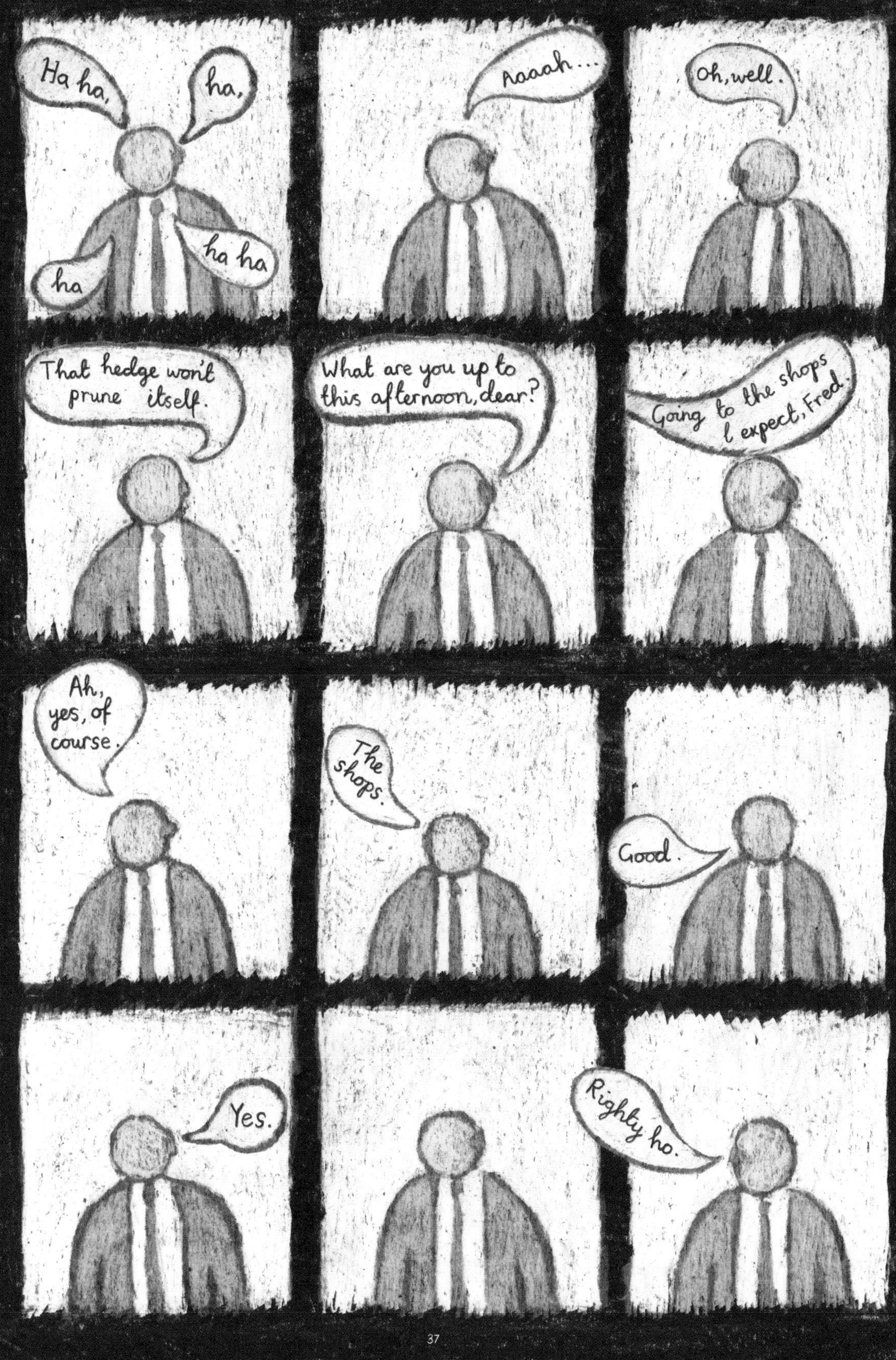
Ha ha,
ha,
ha ha
ha
Aaaah...
Oh, well.
That hedge won't prune itself.
What are you up to this afternoon, dear?
Going to the shops I expect, Fred.
Ah, yes, of course.
The shops.
Good.
Yes.
Righty ho.

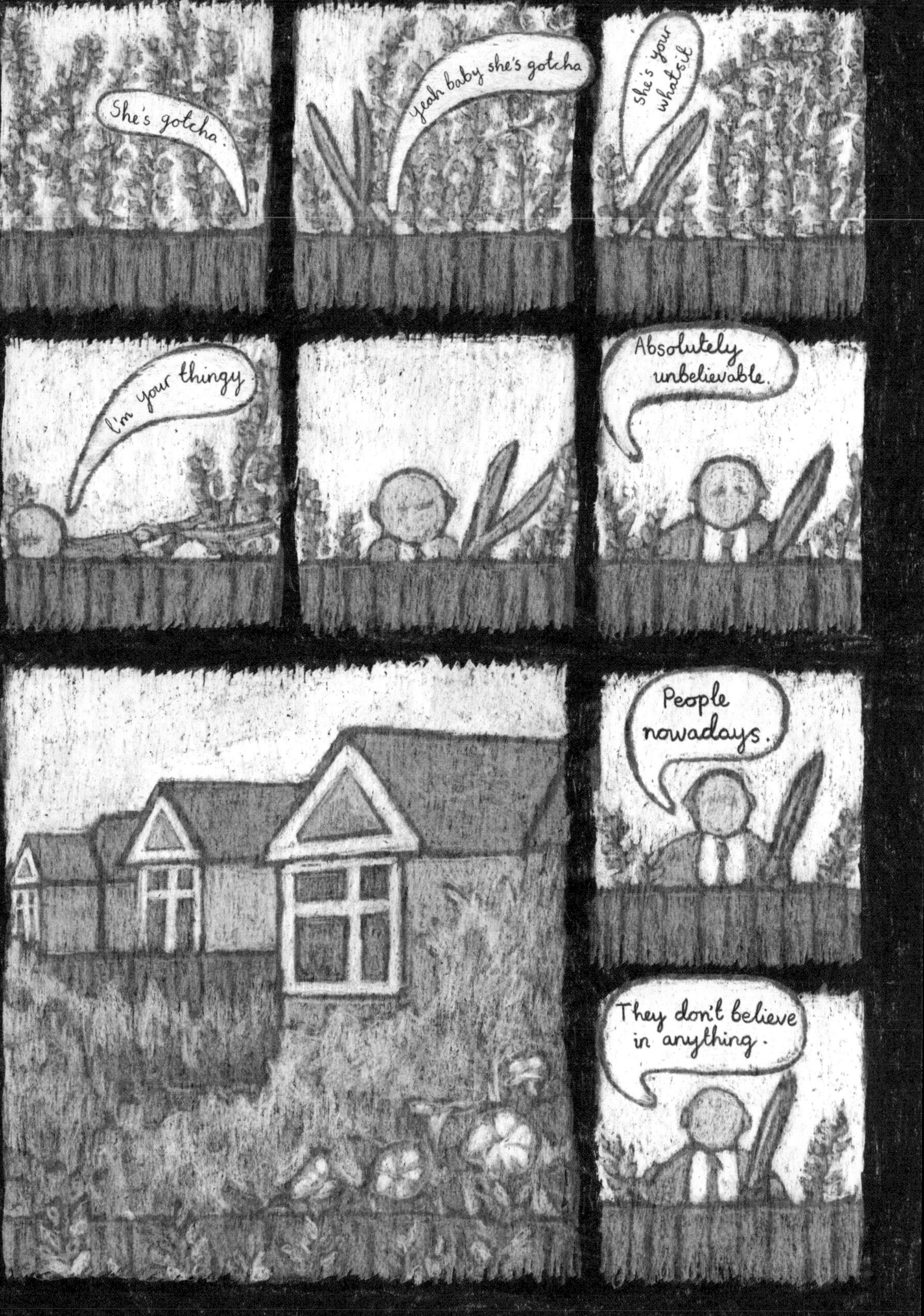
She's gotcha.
yeah baby she's gotcha
she's your whatsit
I'm your thingy
Absolutely unbelievable.
People nowadays.
They don't believe in anything.

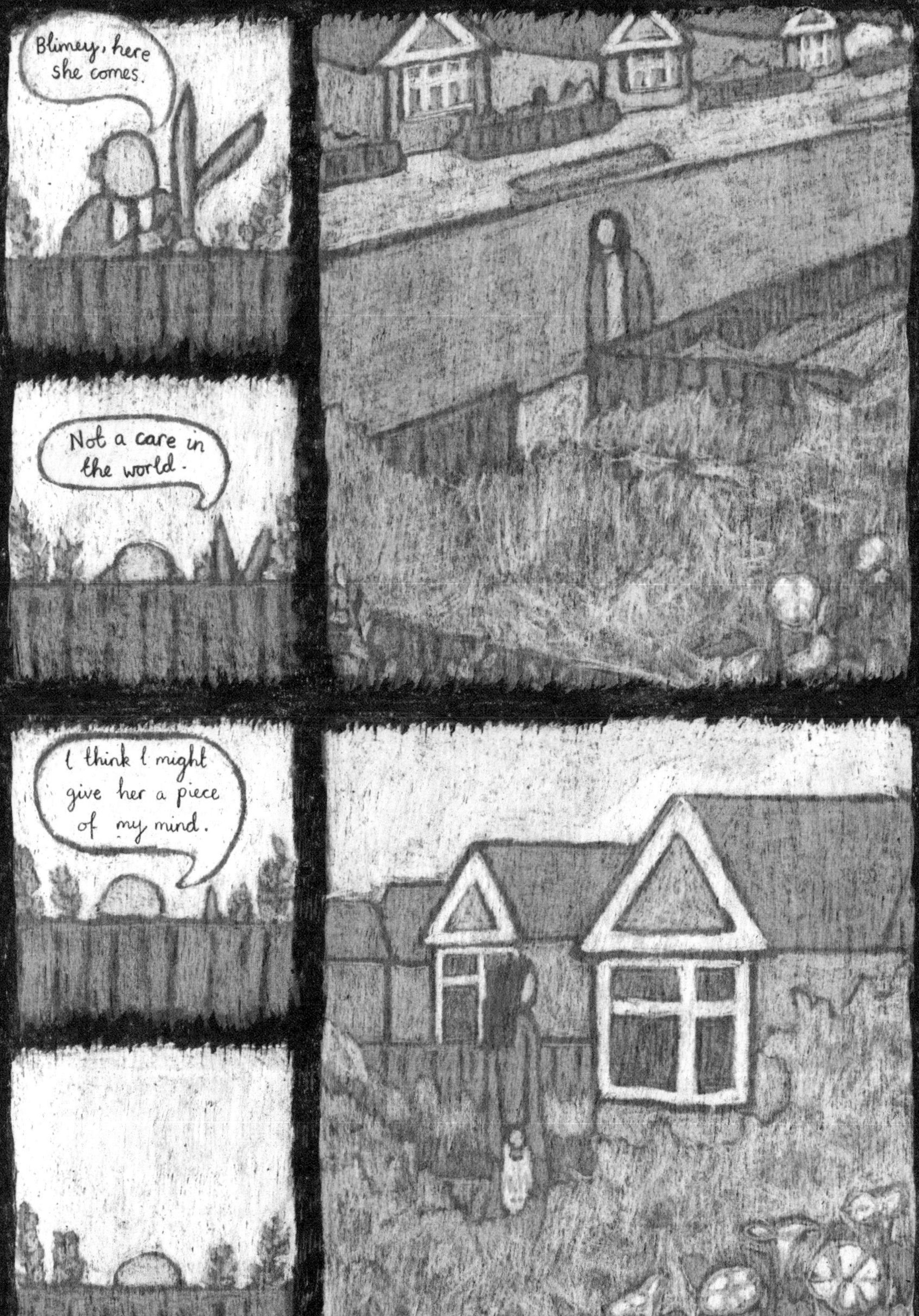

Blimey, here she comes.
Not a care in the world.
I think I might give her a piece of my mind.

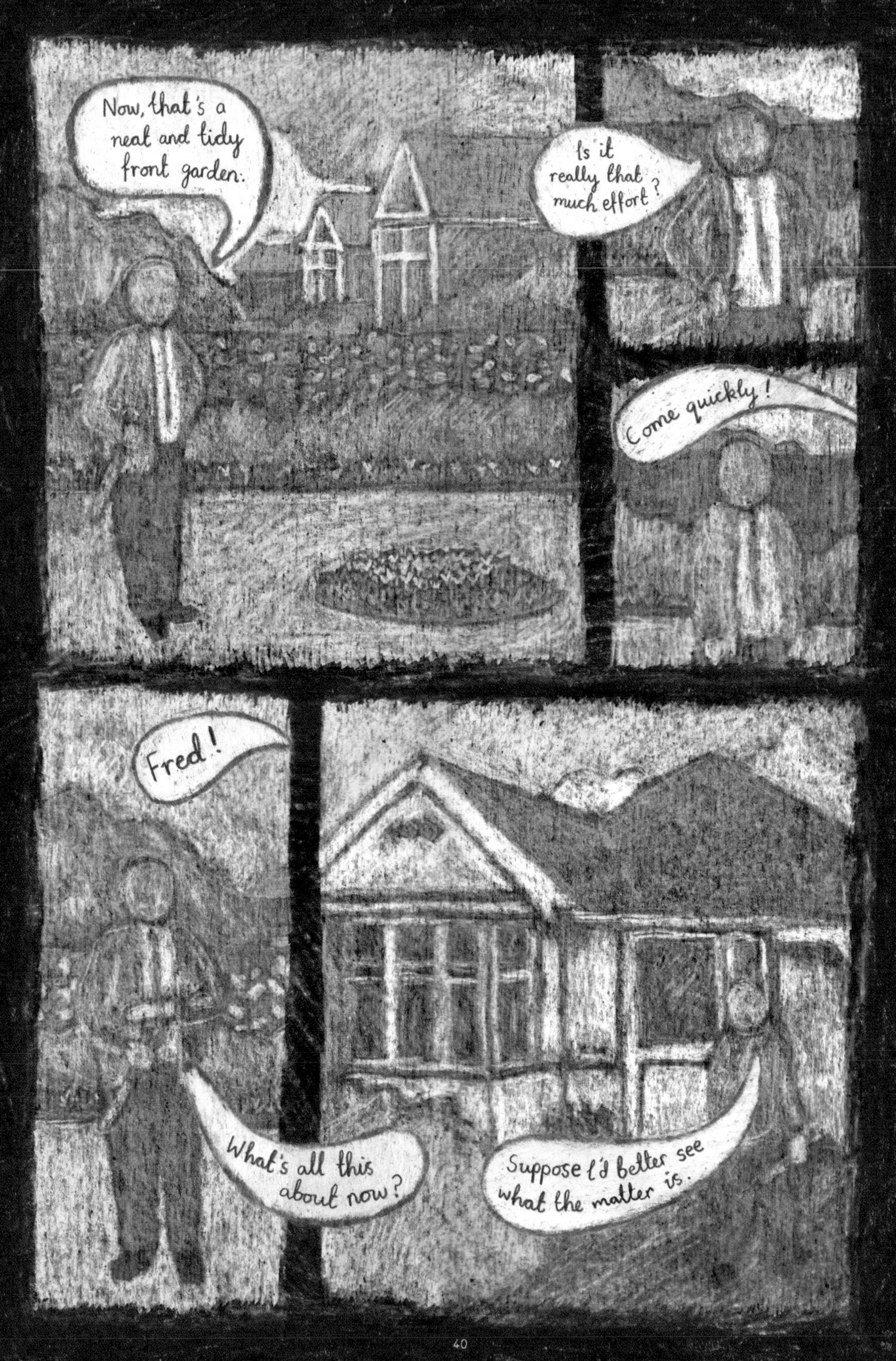
Now, that's a neat and tidy front garden.
Is it really that much effort?
Come quickly!
Fred!
What's all this about now?
Suppose I'd better see what the matter is.

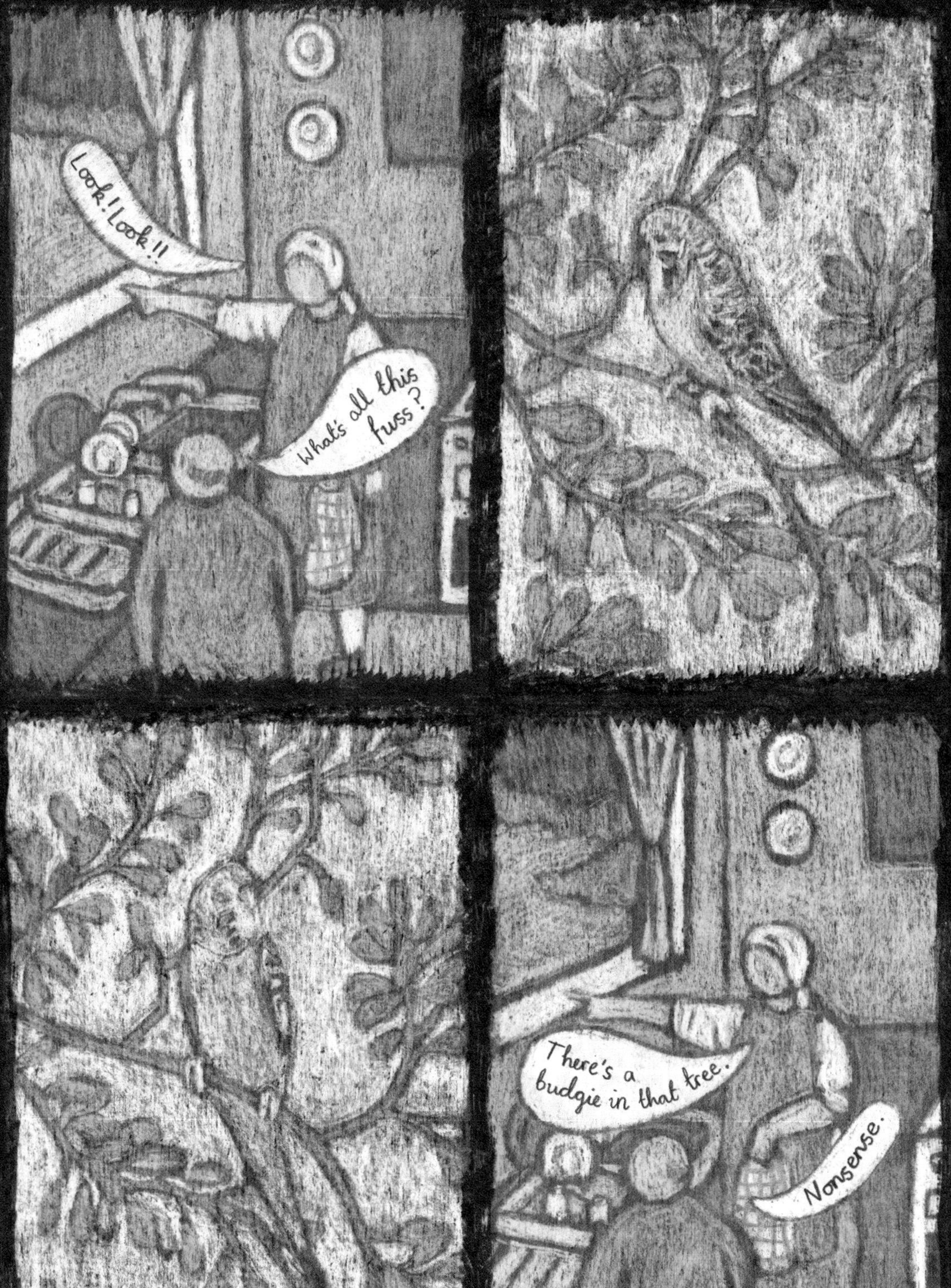
Look! Look!!
What's all this fuss?
There's a budgie in that tree.
Nonsense.

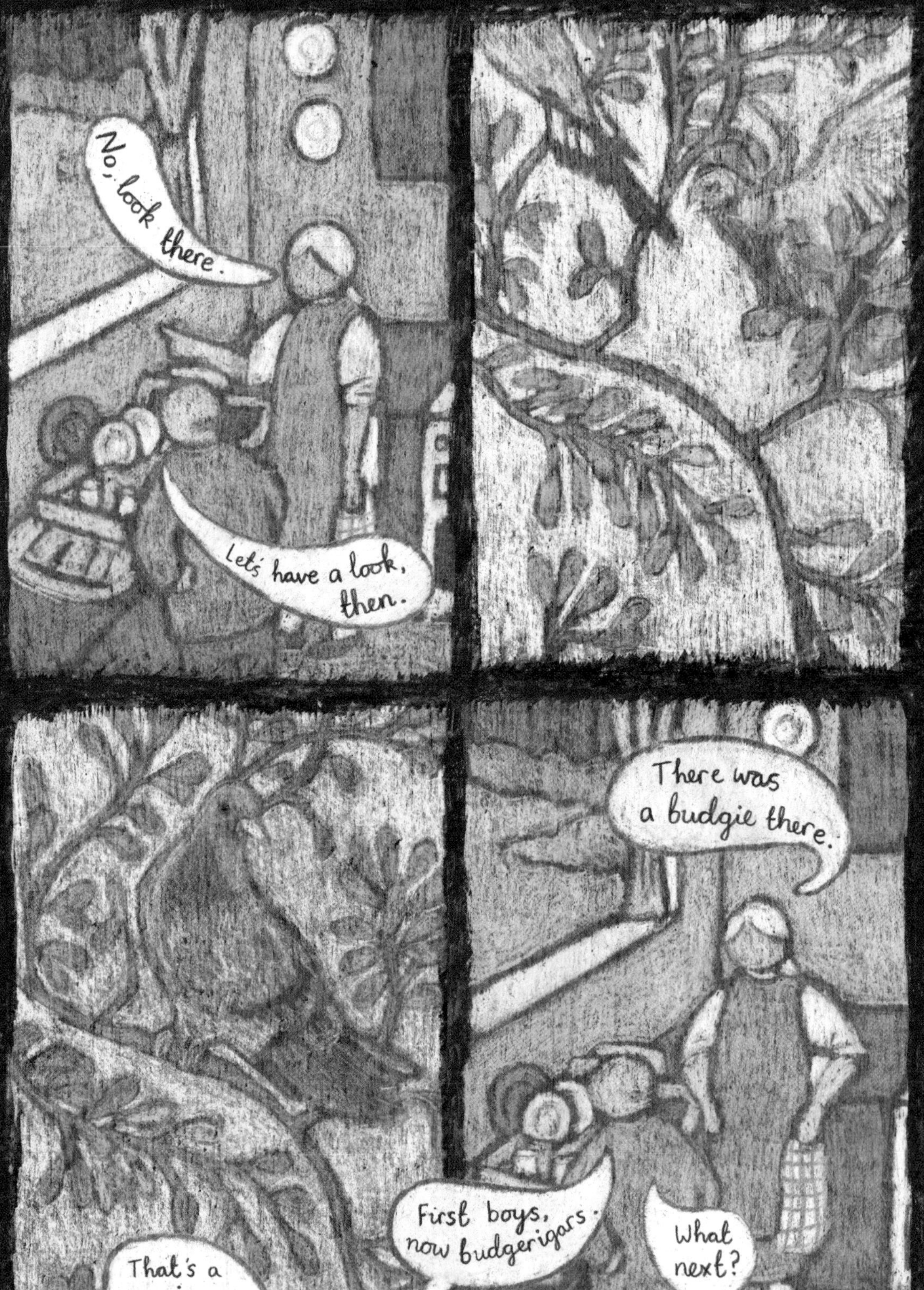
No, look there.
Let's have a look, then.
There was a budgie there.
That's a pigeon.
First boys, now budgerigars.
What next?

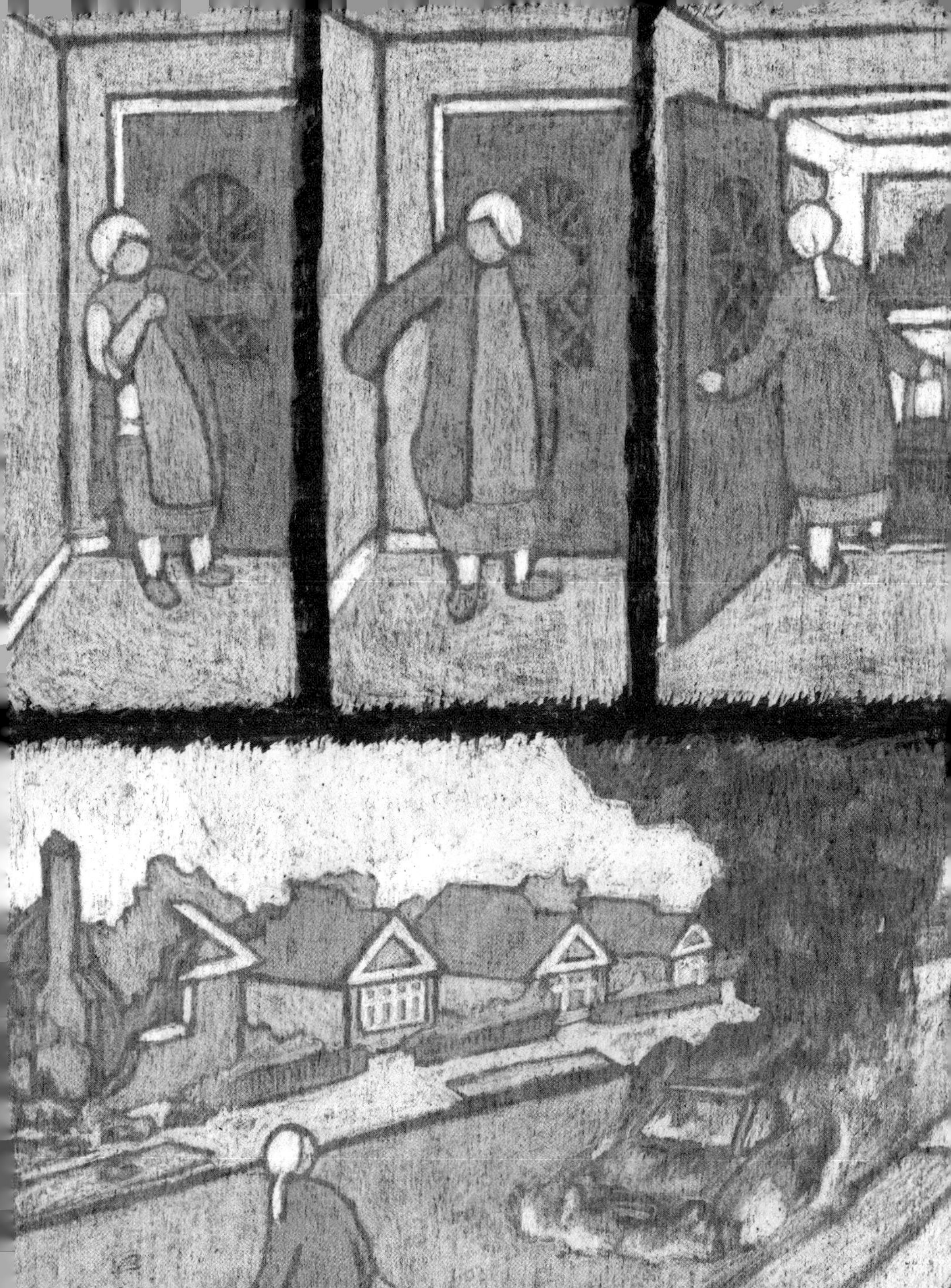

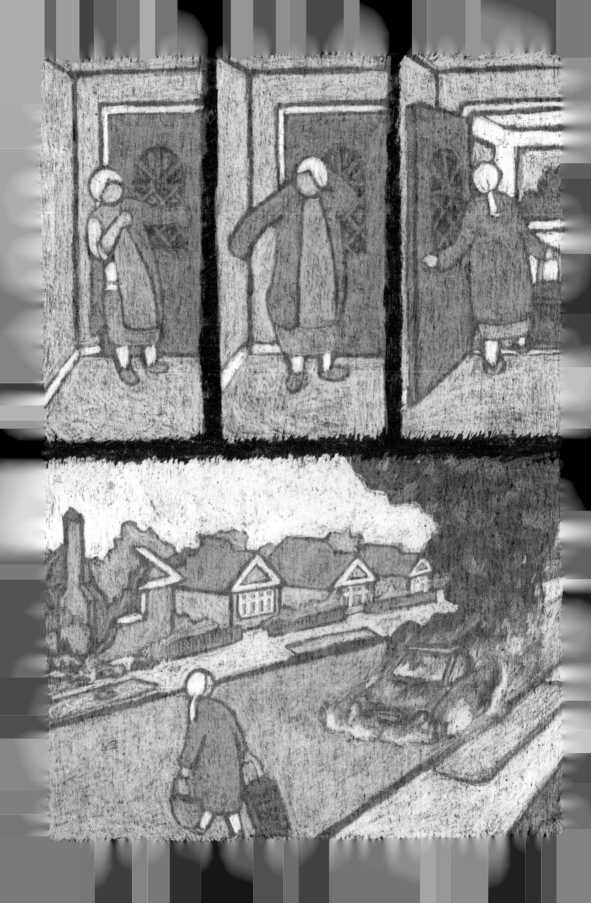

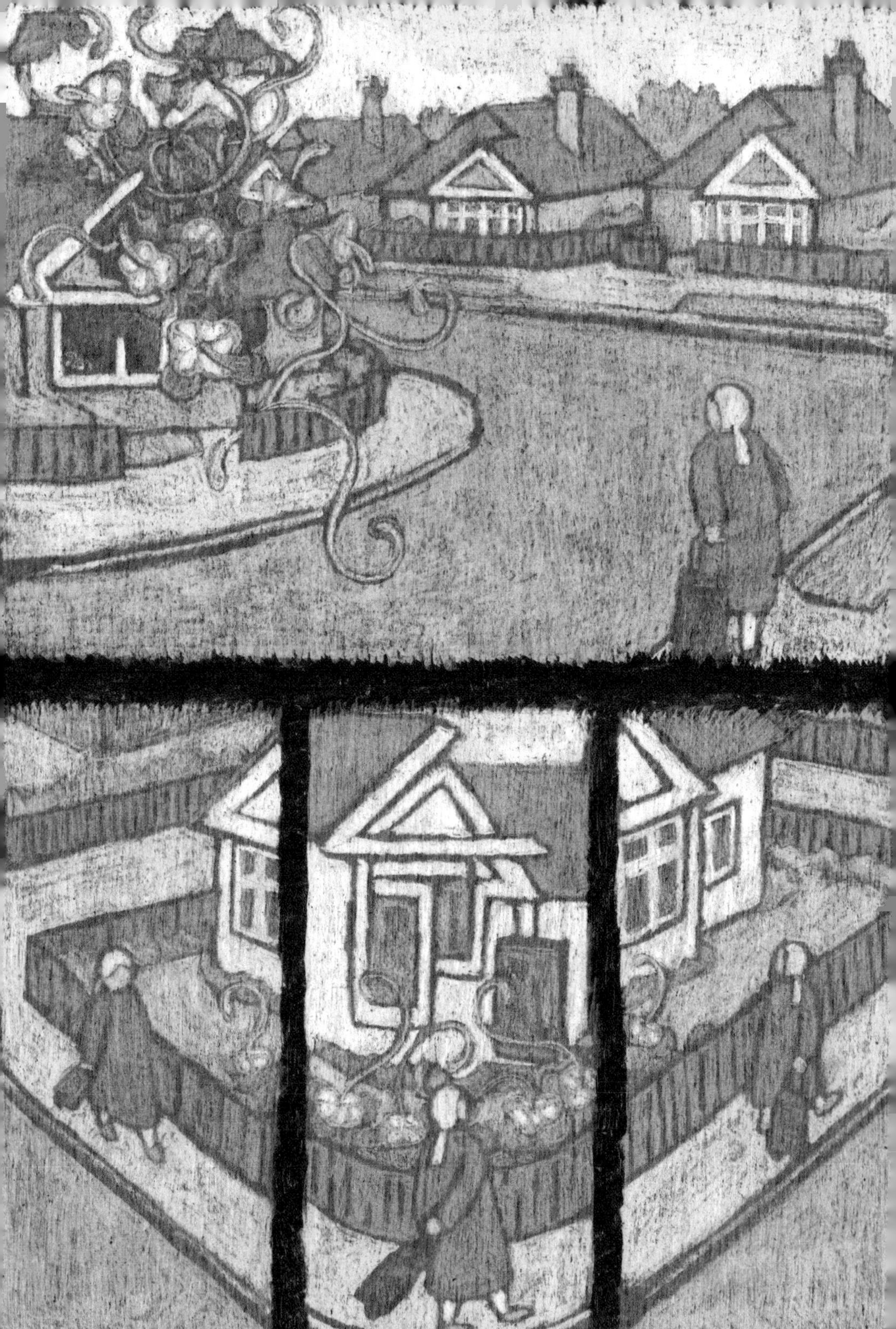

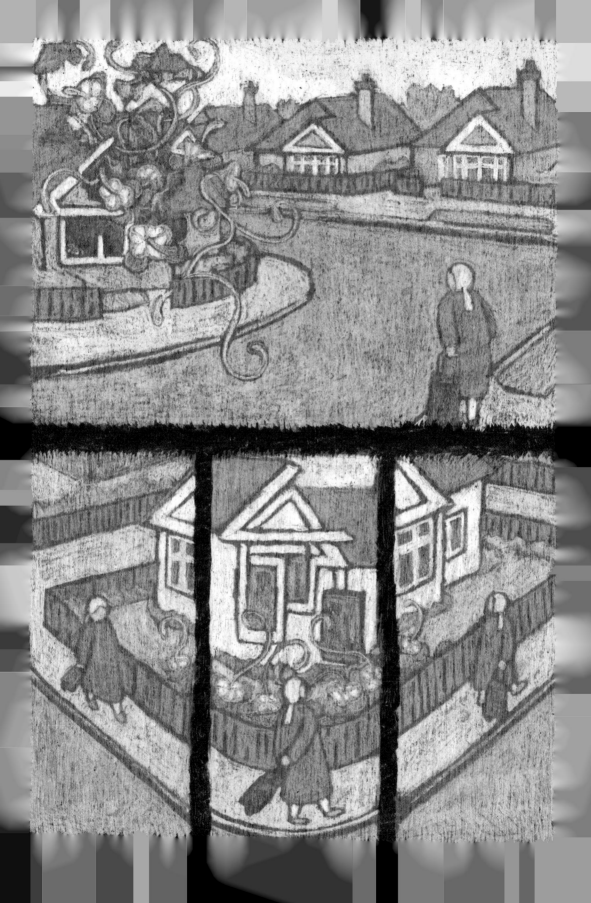

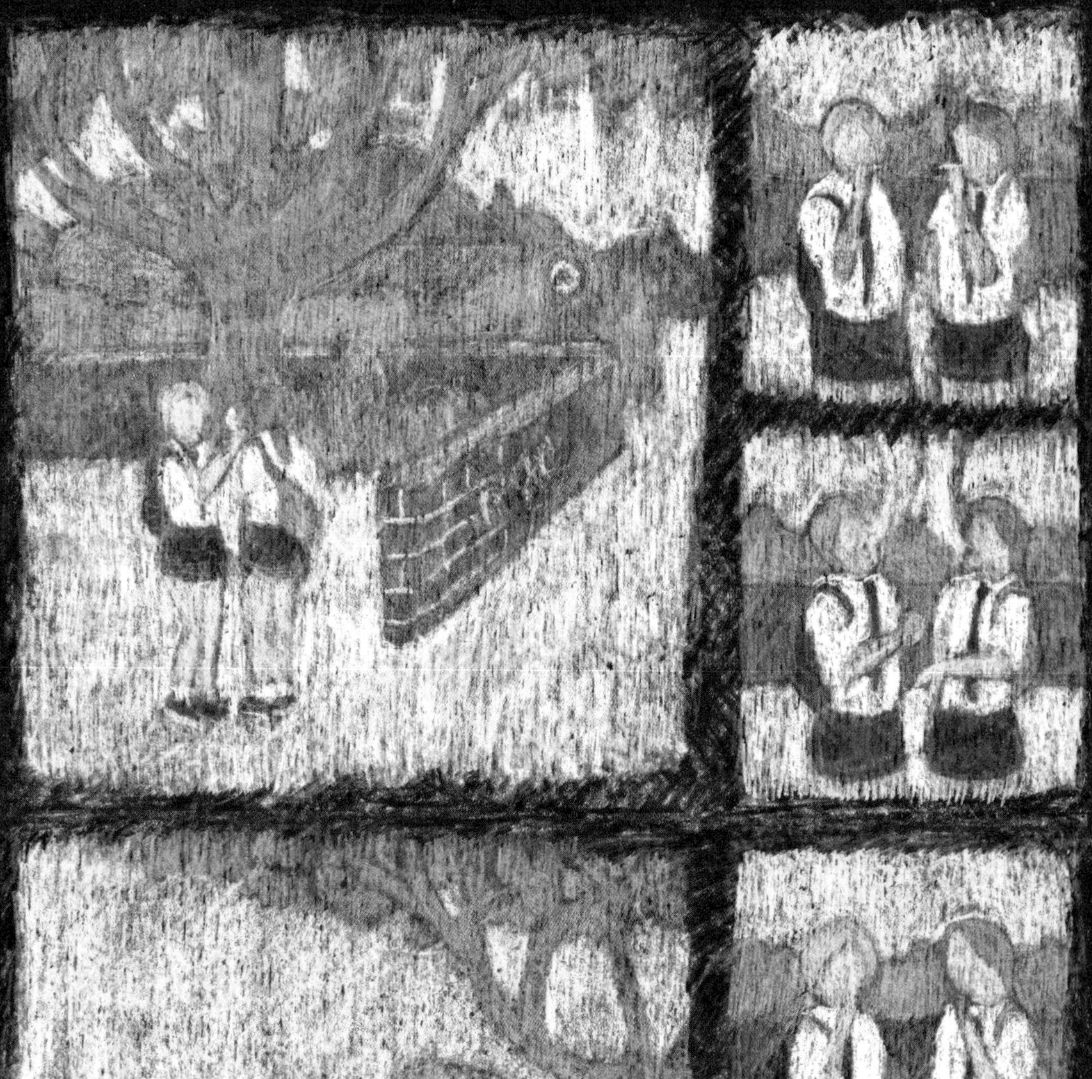
KIRSTY
IS A SLAG

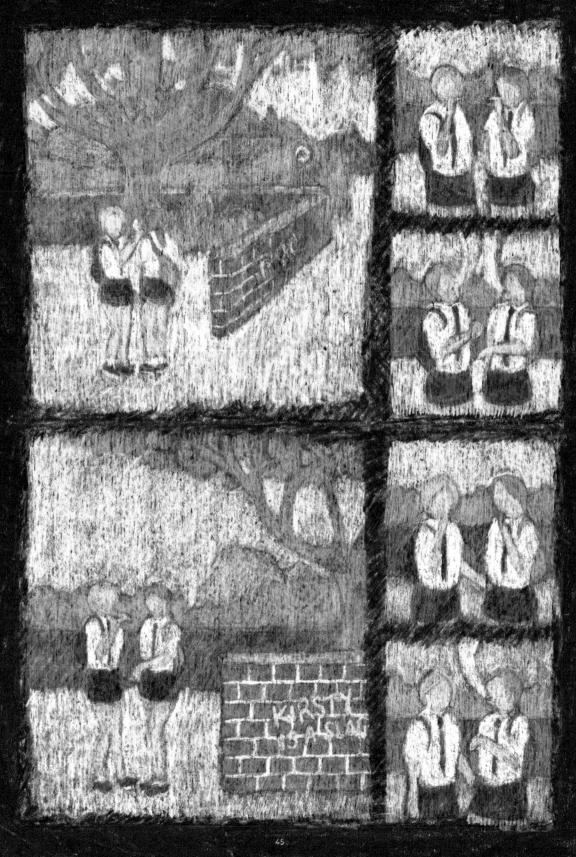

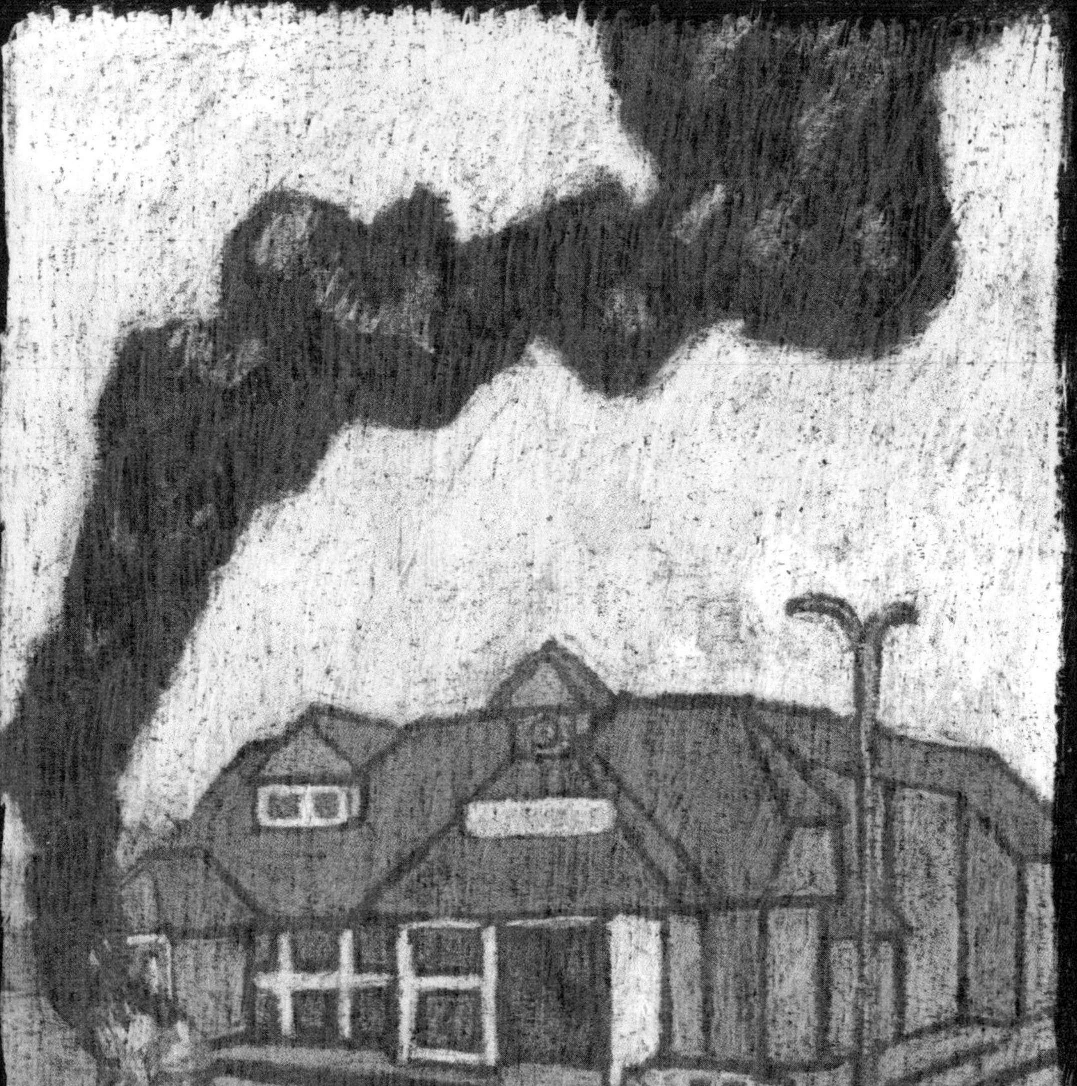

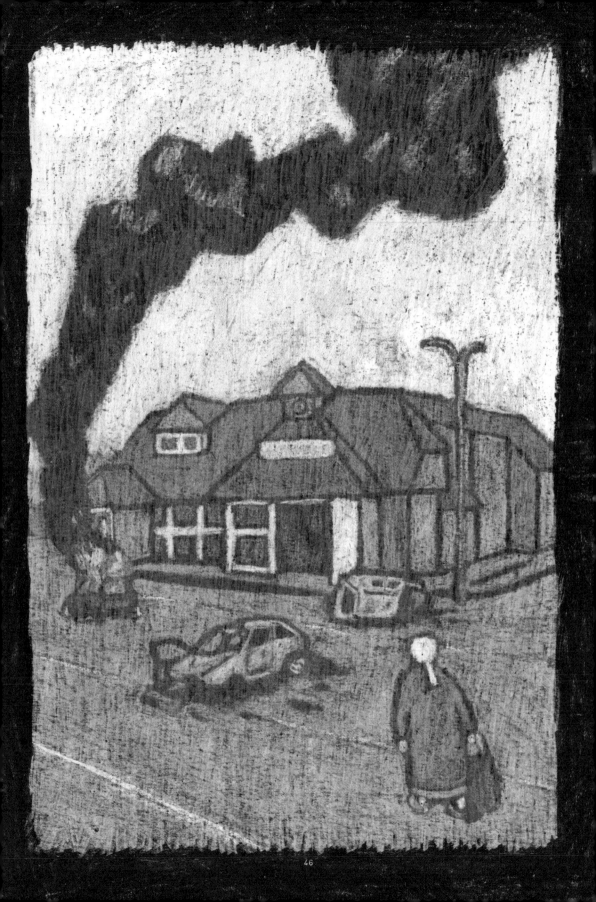

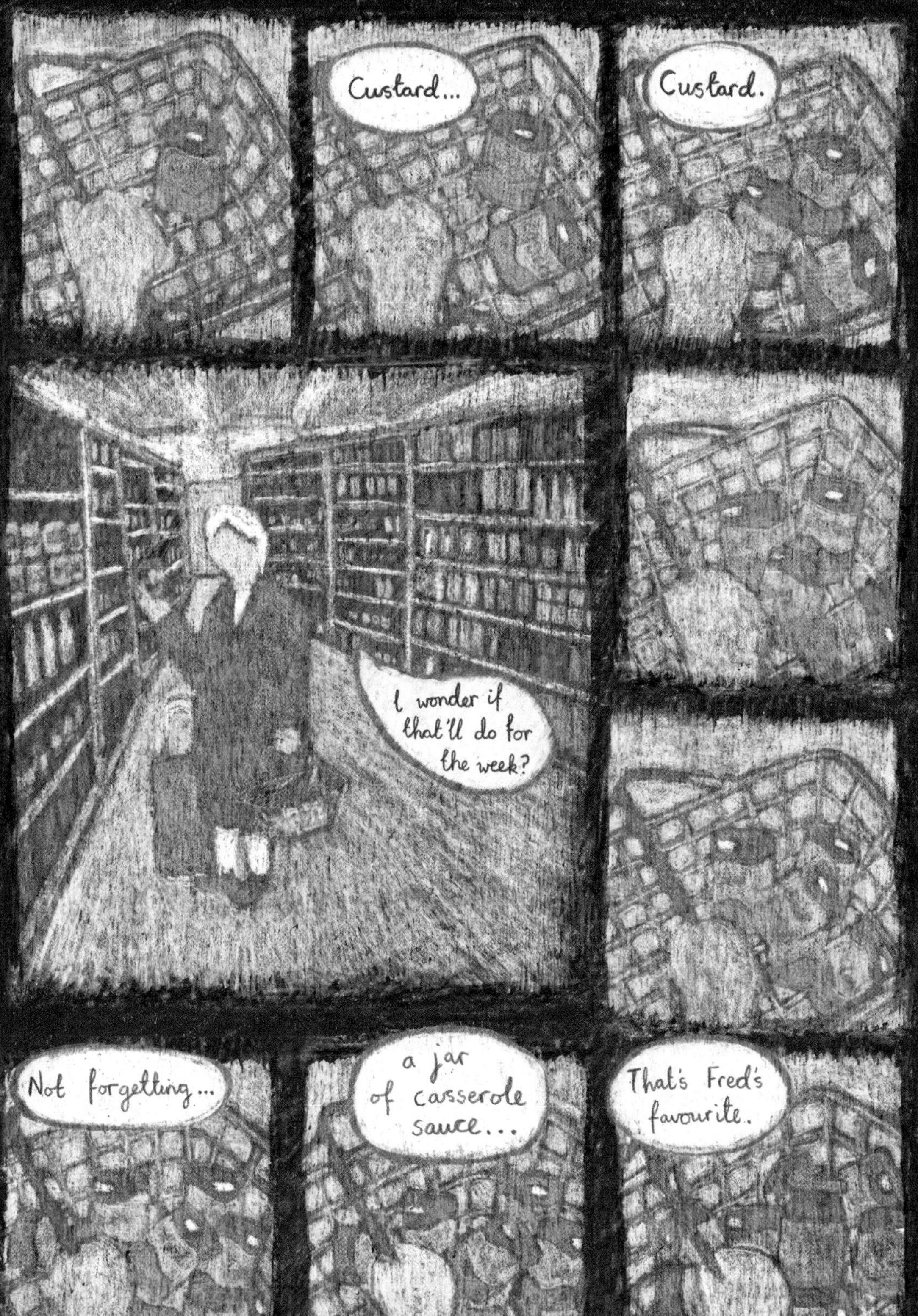
Custard...
Custard.
I wonder if that'll do for the week?
Not forgetting...
a jar of casserole sauce...
That's Fred's favourite.

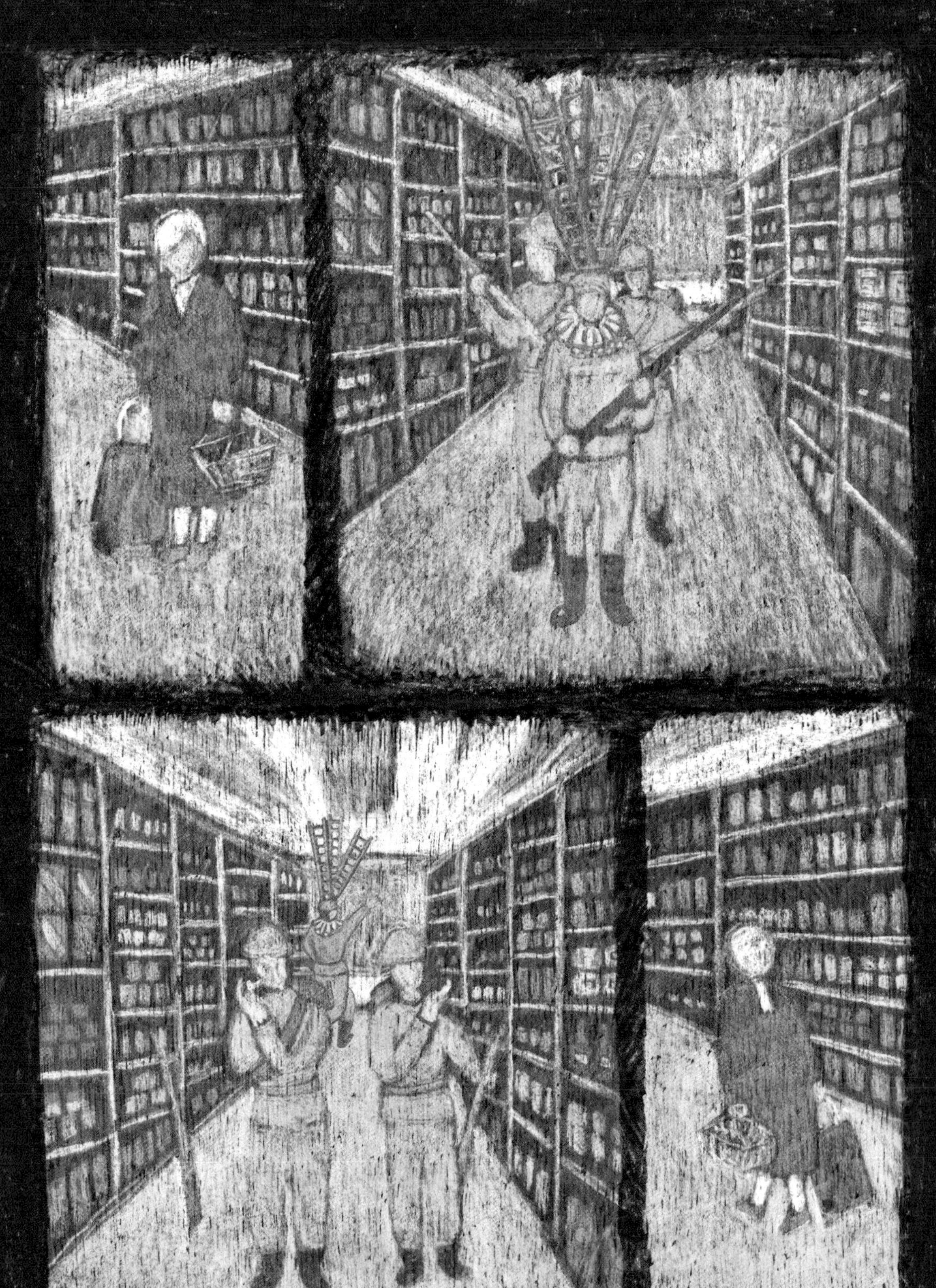

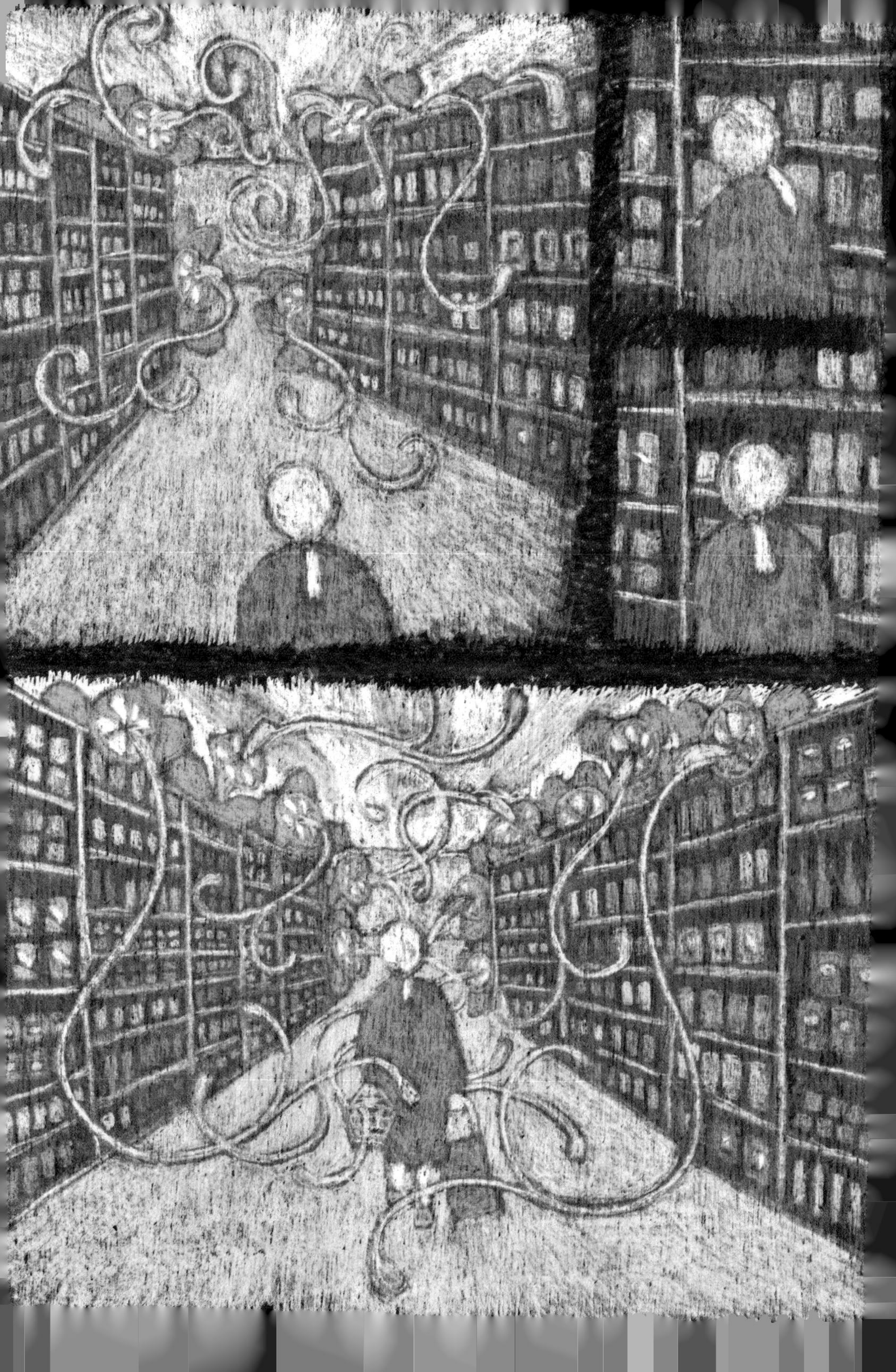

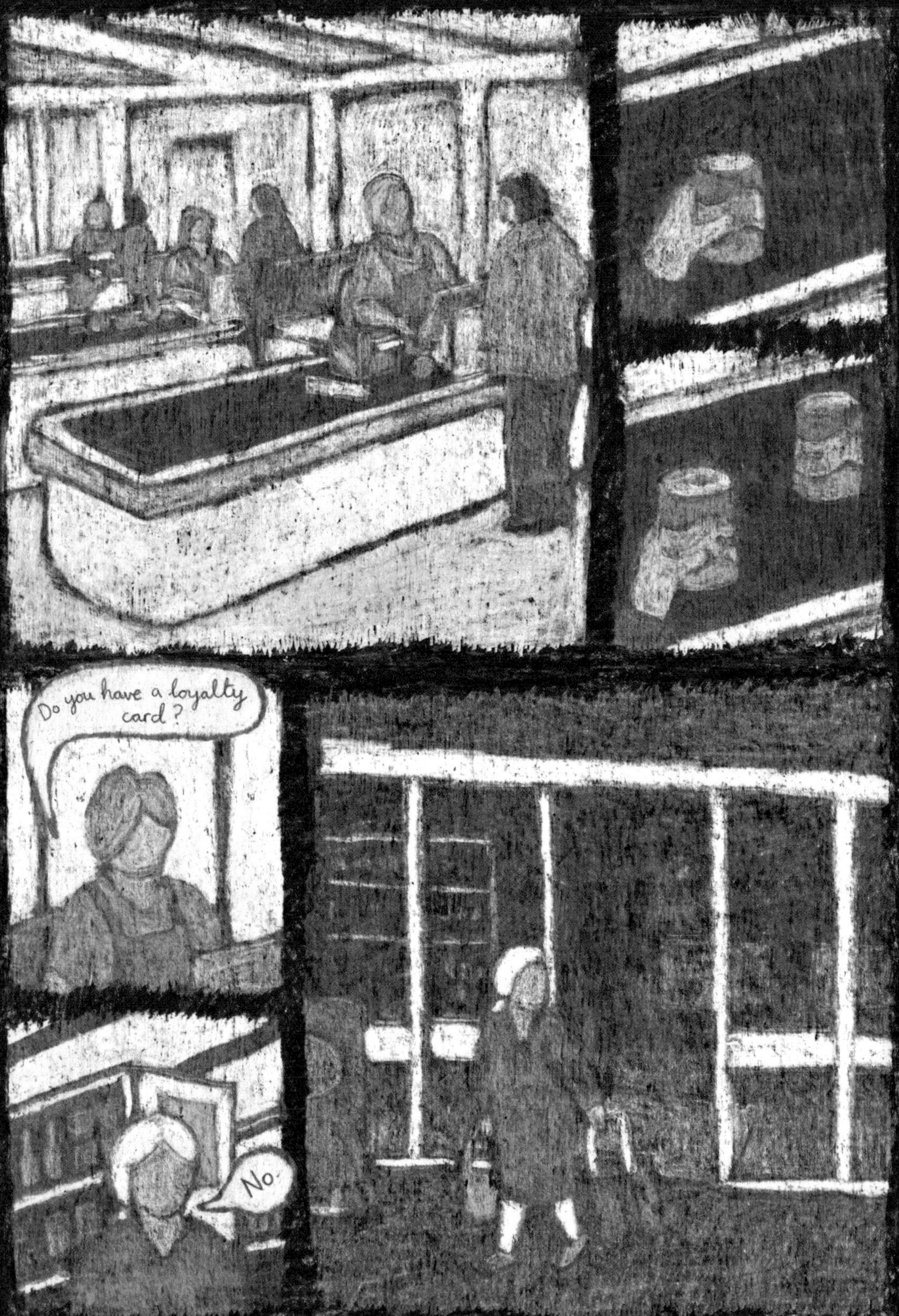
Do you have a loyalty card?
No.

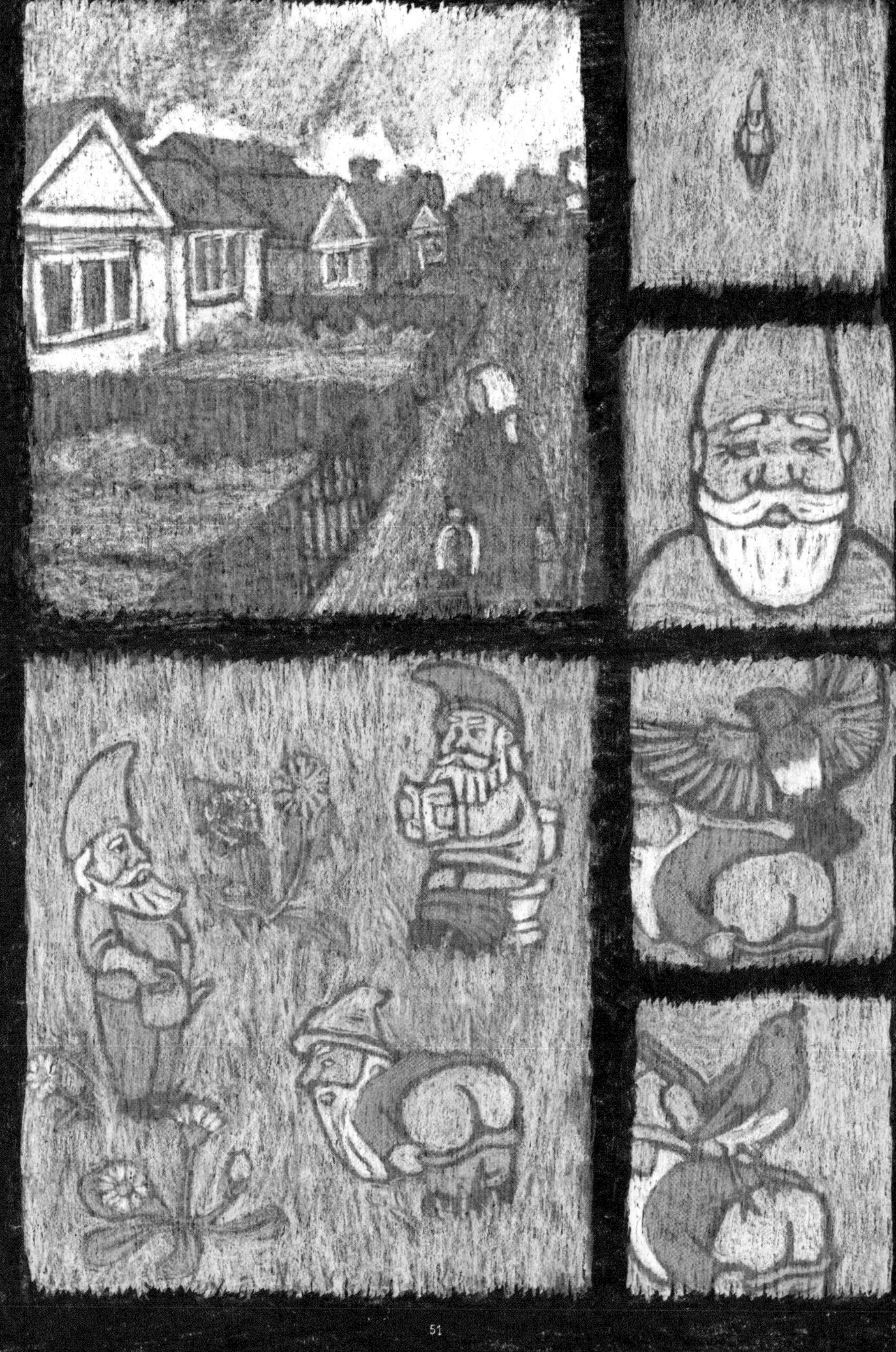

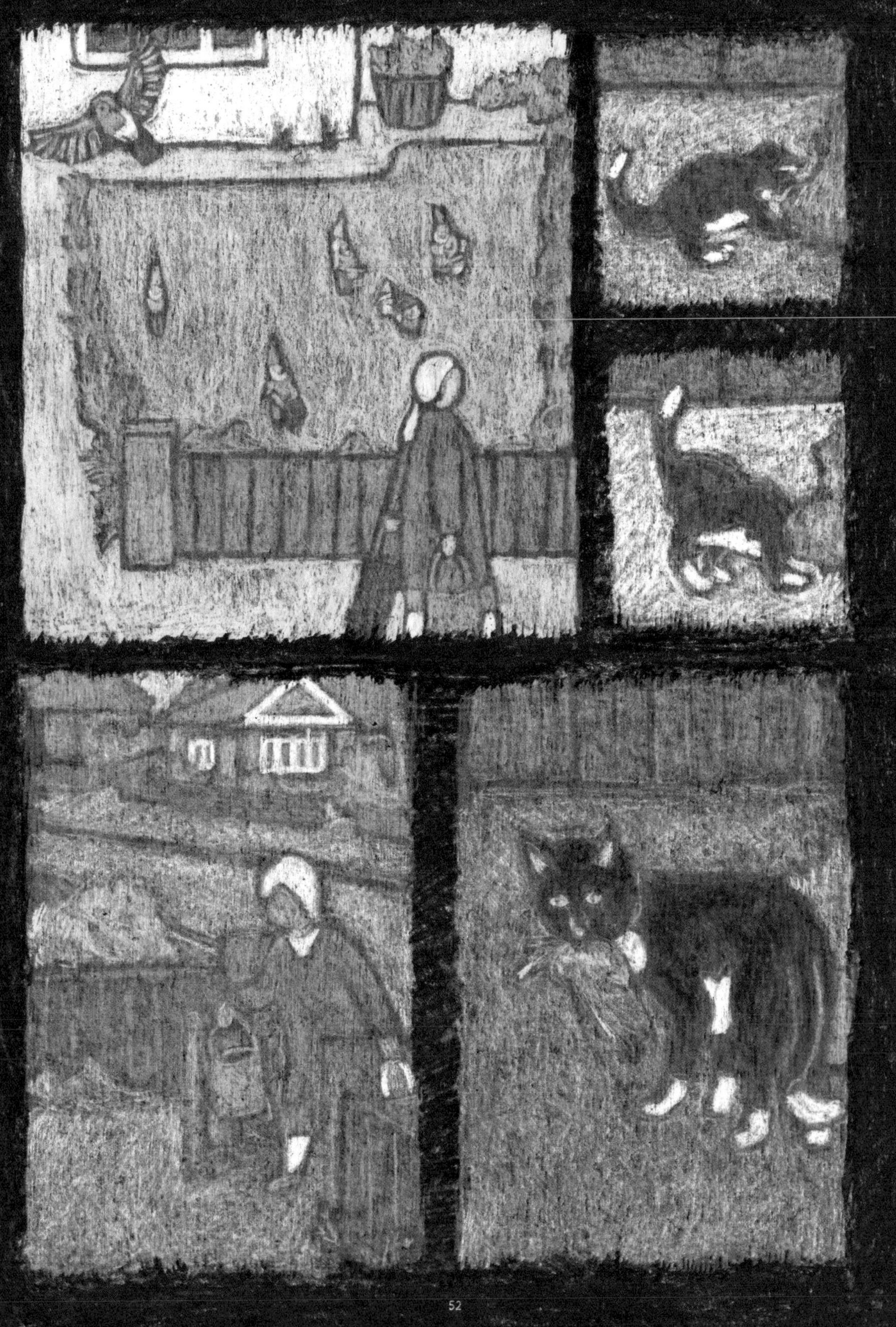

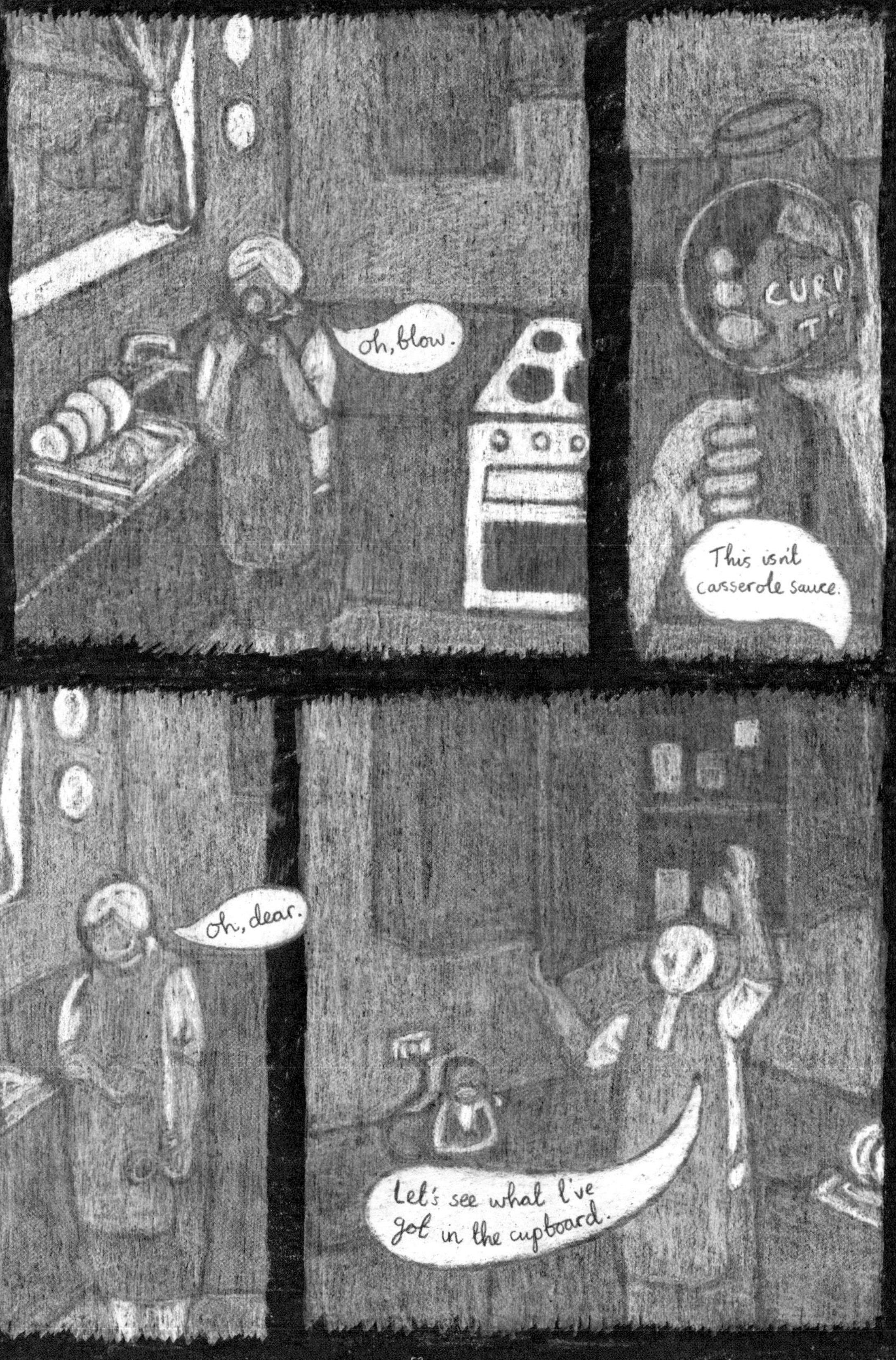
oh, blow.
CURR
This isn't casserole sauce.
oh, dear.
Let's see what I've got in the cupboard.

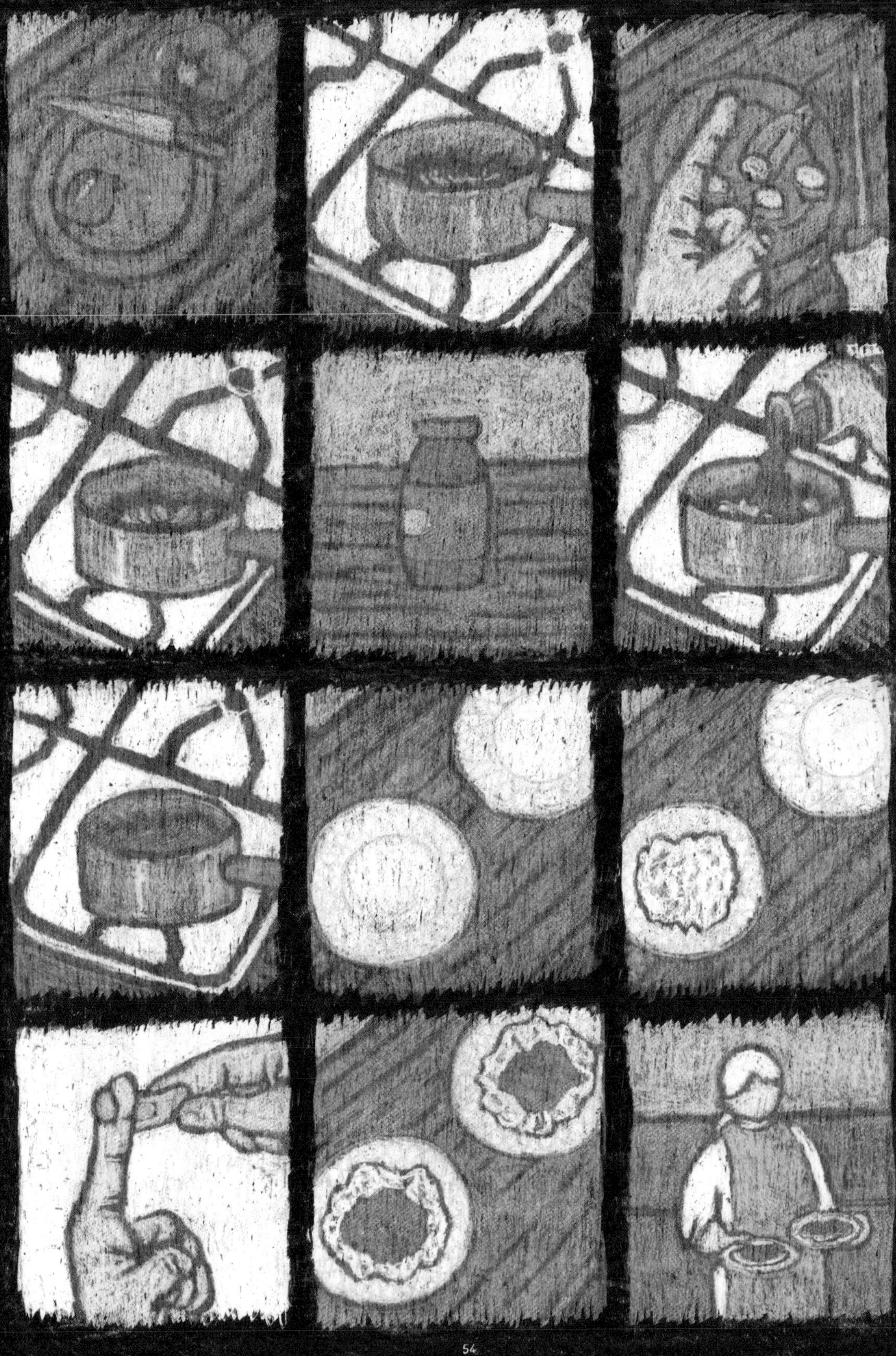

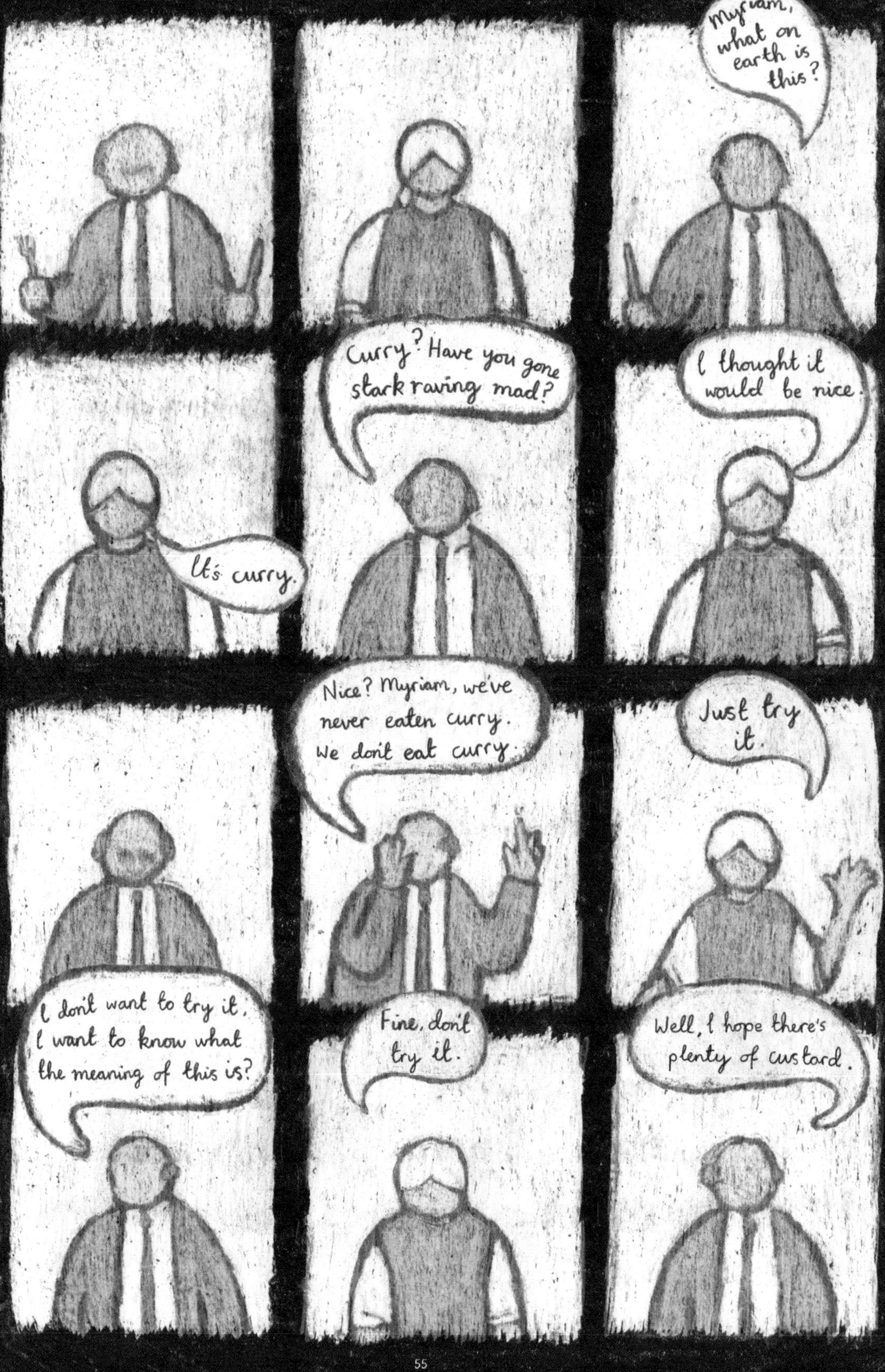
Myriam, what on earth is this?
It's curry.
Curry? Have you gone stark raving mad?
I thought it would be nice.
Nice? Myriam, we've never eaten curry. We don't eat curry.
Just try it.
I don't want to try it. I want to know what the meaning of this is?
Fine, don't try it.
Well, I hope there's plenty of custard.

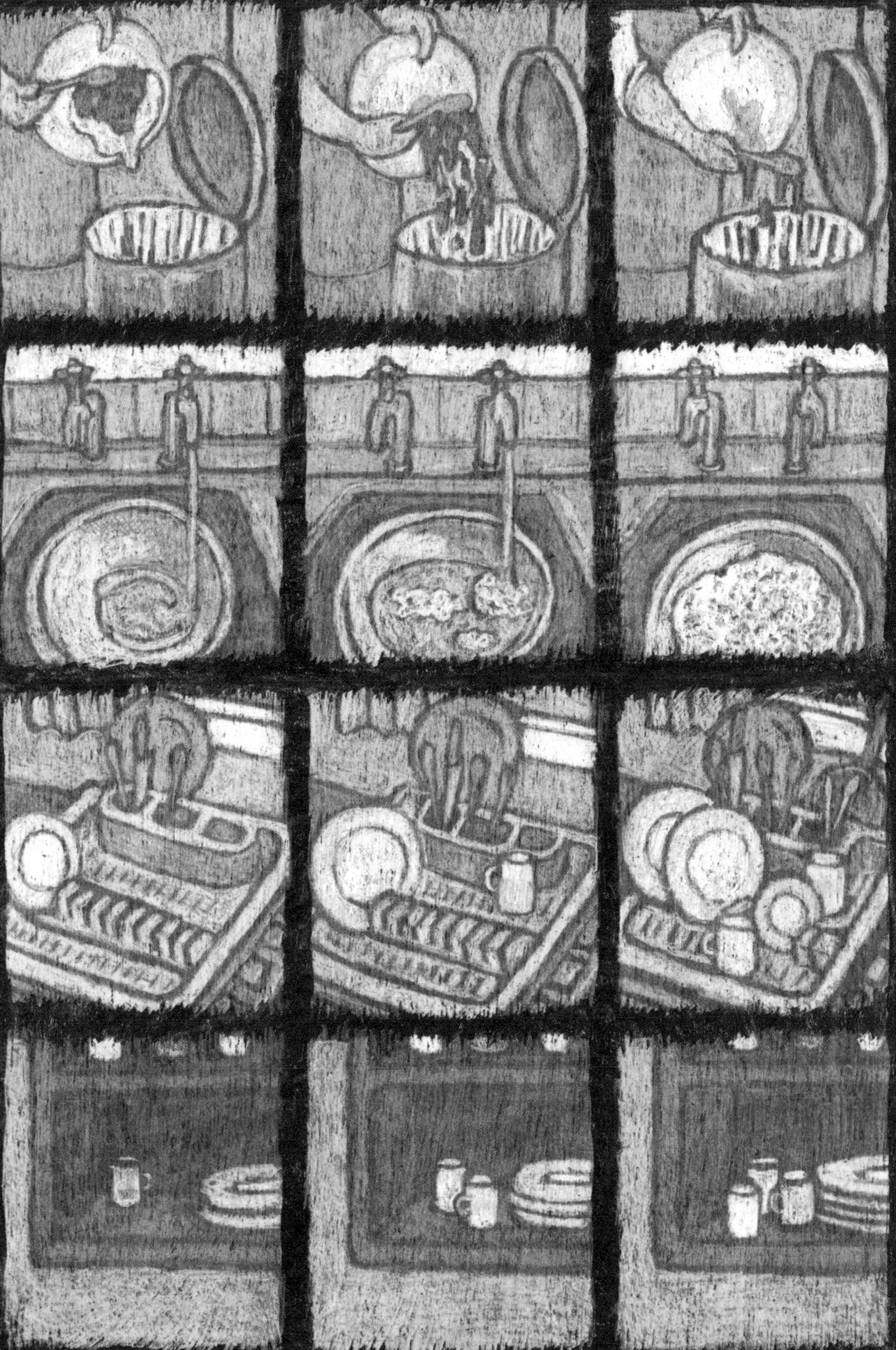

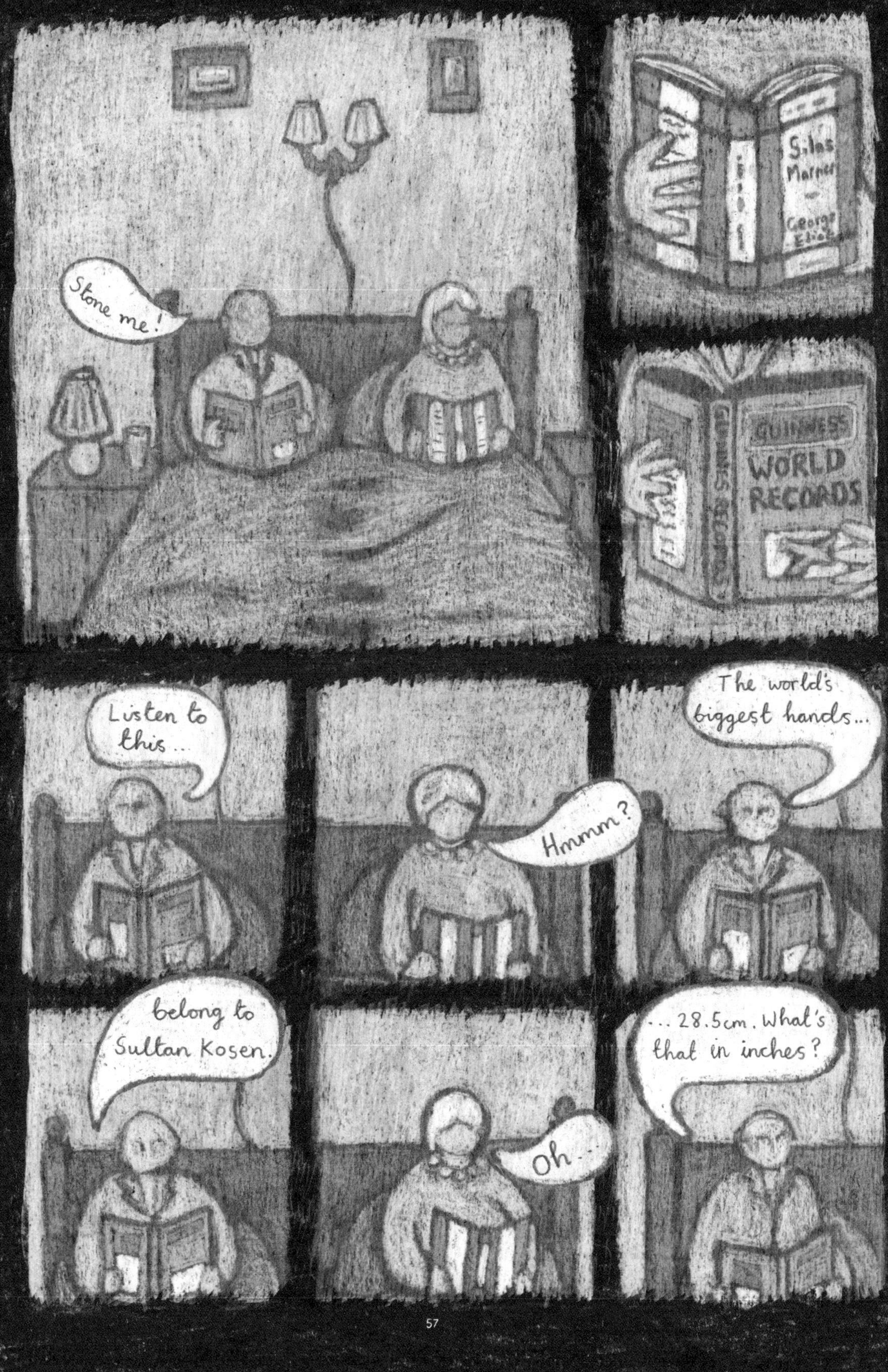
Stone me!
Silas Marner
George Eliot
GUINNESS WORLD RECORDS
Listen to this...
Hmmm?
The world's biggest hands...
belong to Sultan Kosen.
Oh...
...28.5cm. What's that in inches?

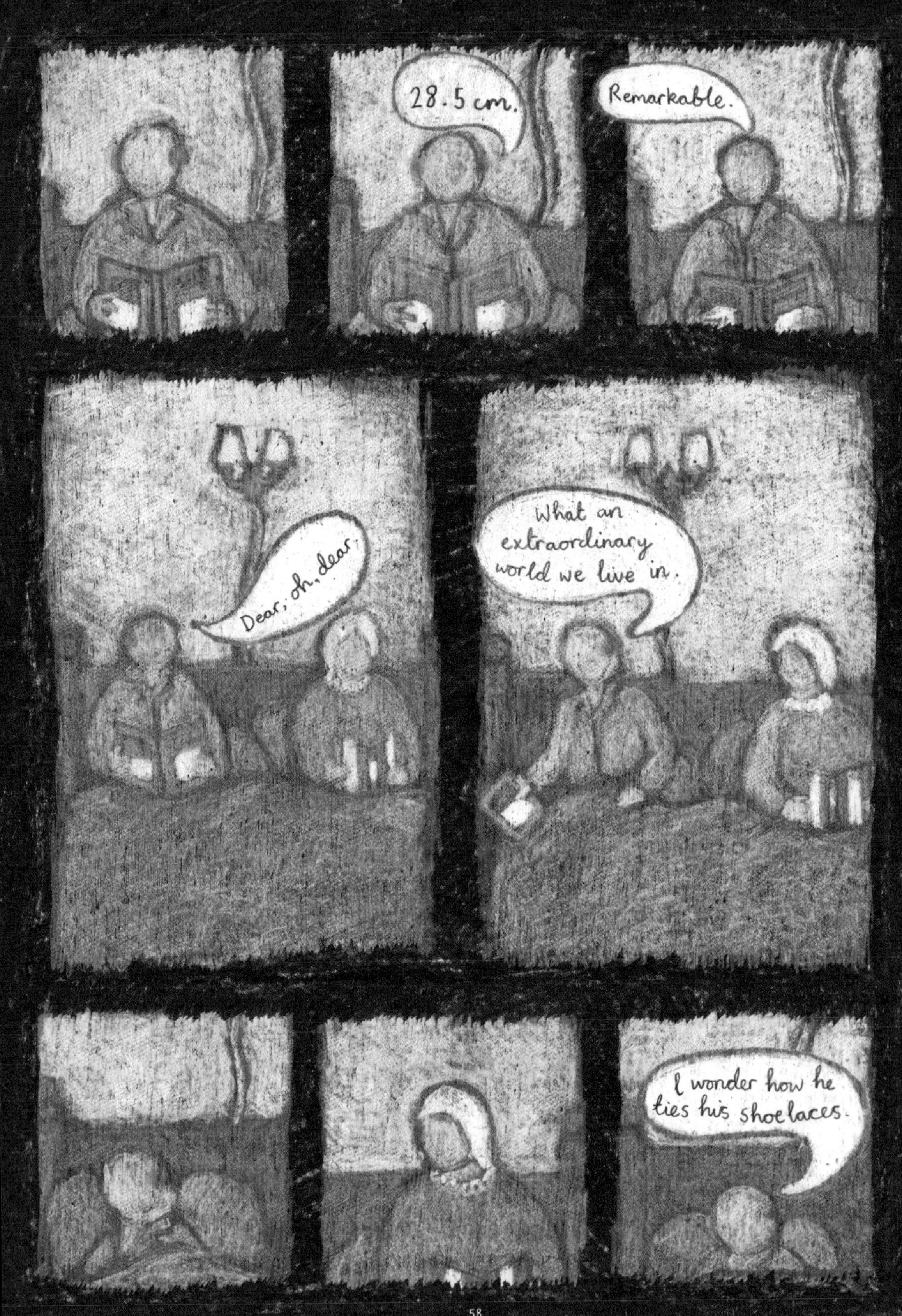
28.5 cm.
Remarkable.
Dear, oh, dear
What an extraordinary world we live in.
I wonder how he ties his shoelaces.

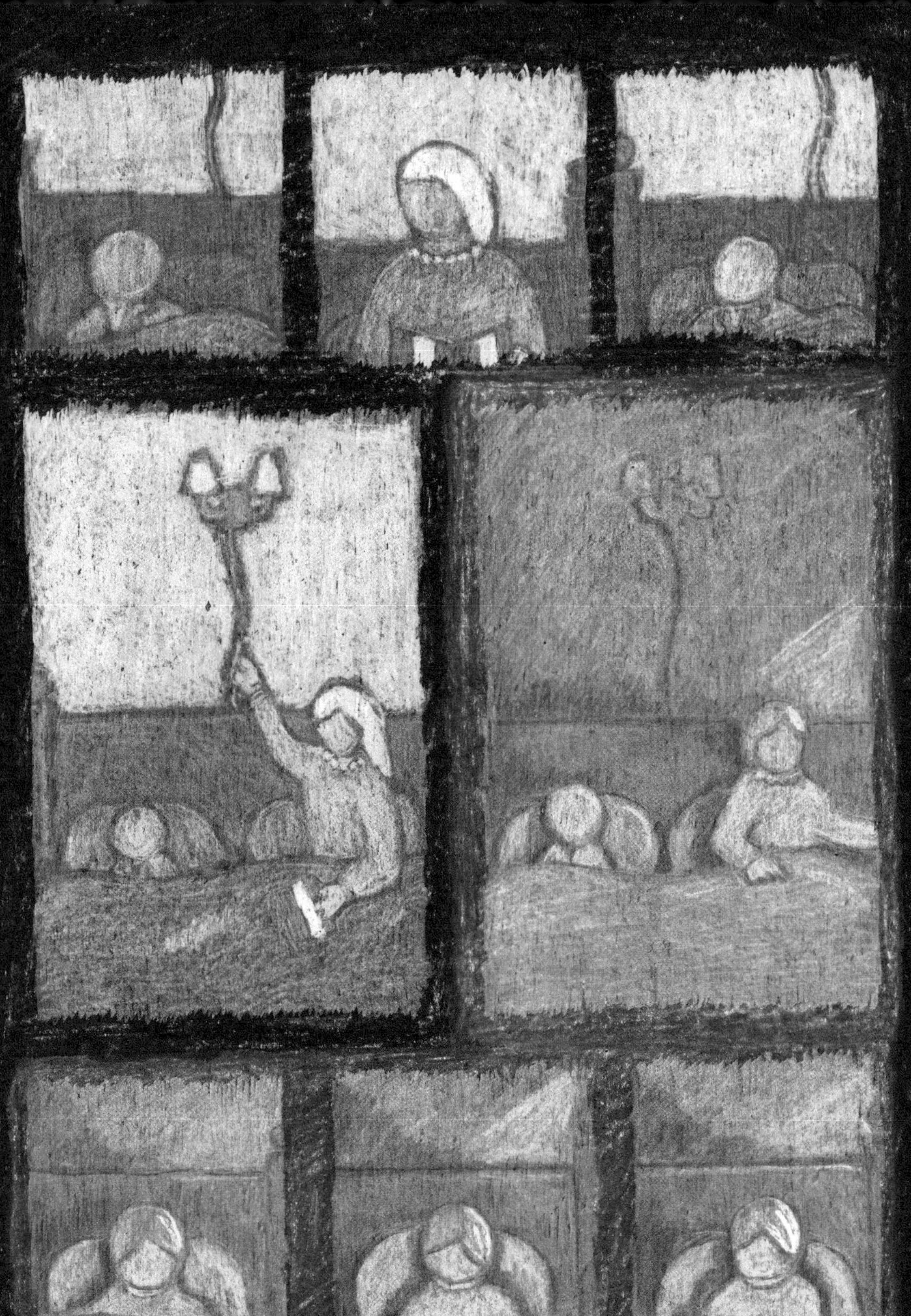

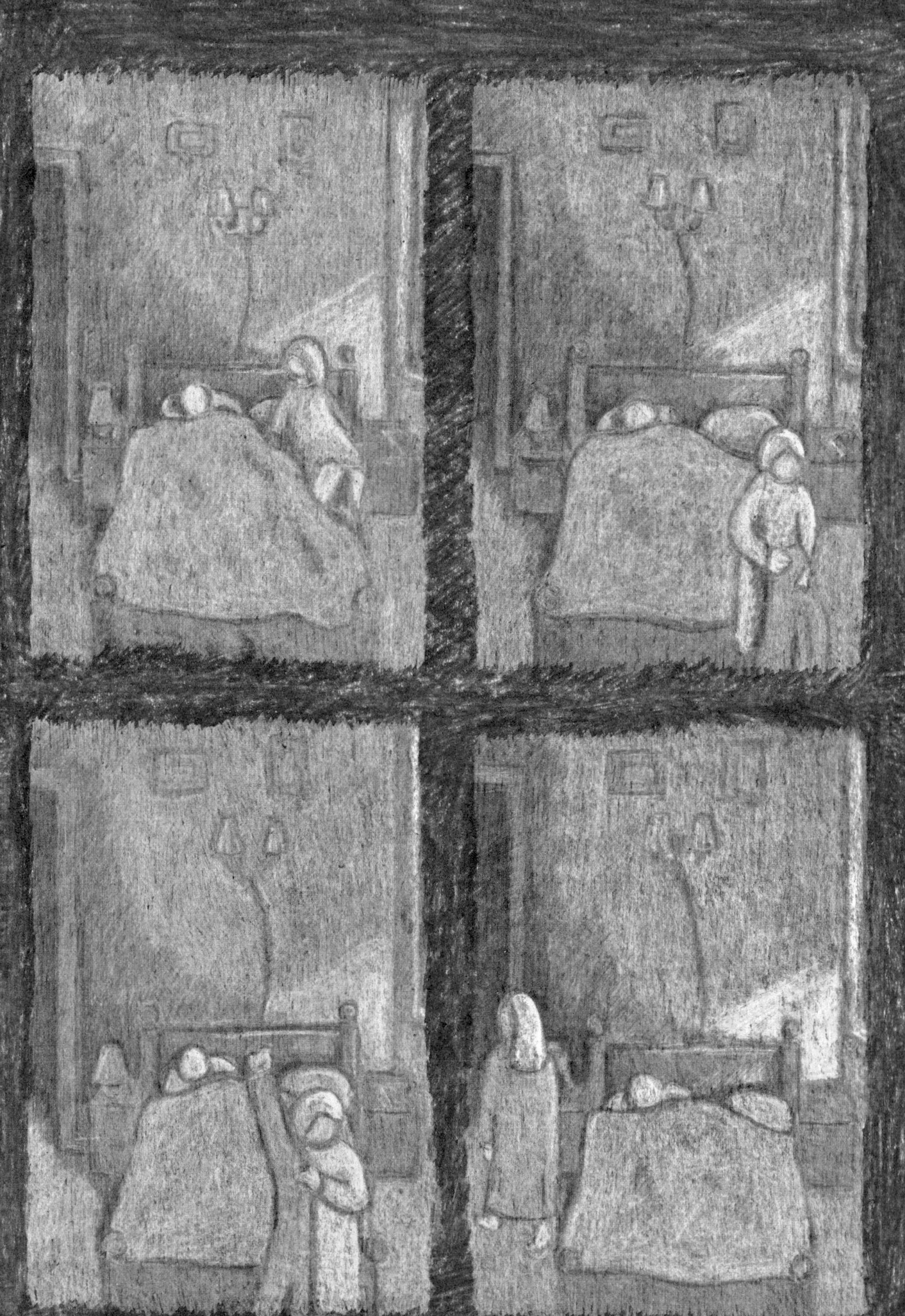

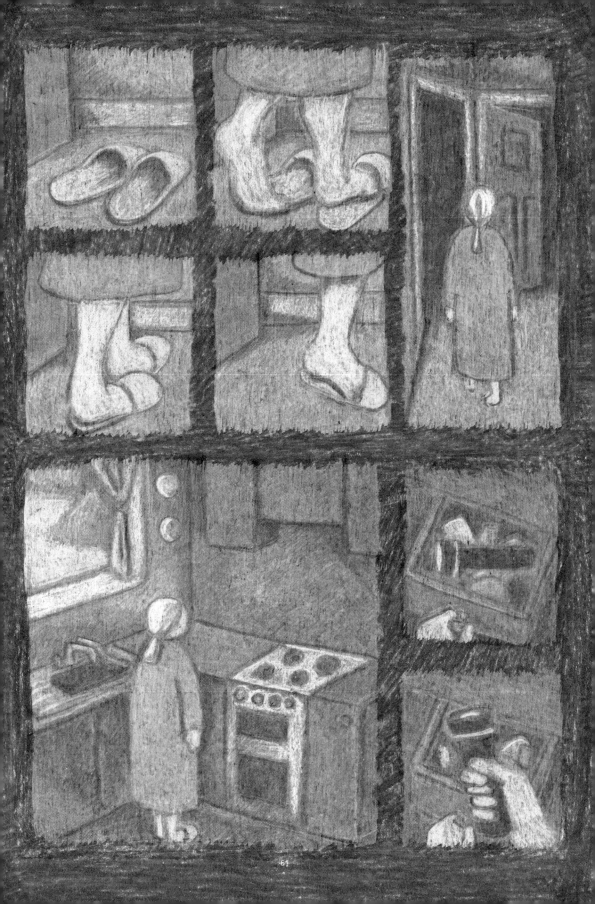

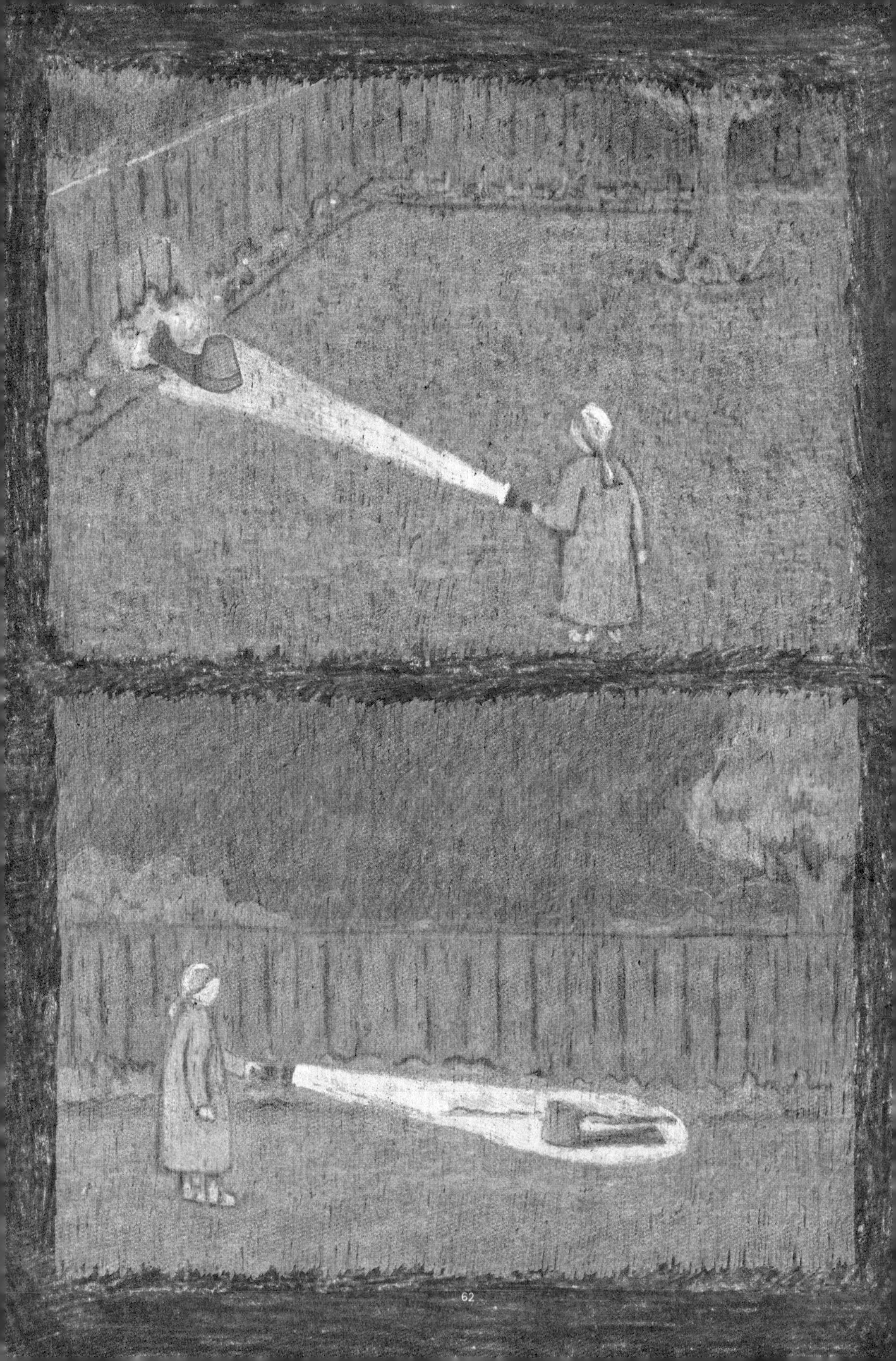

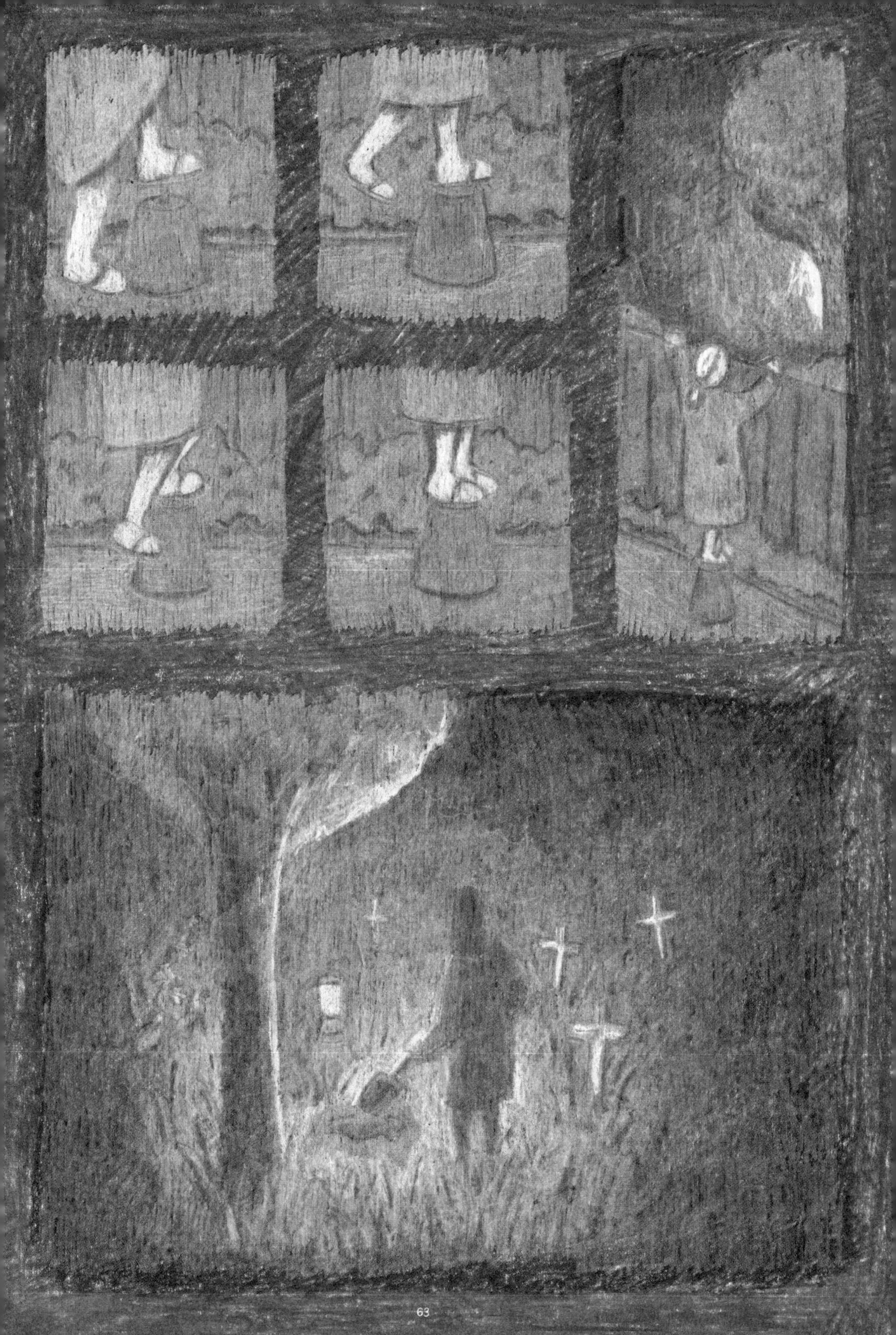

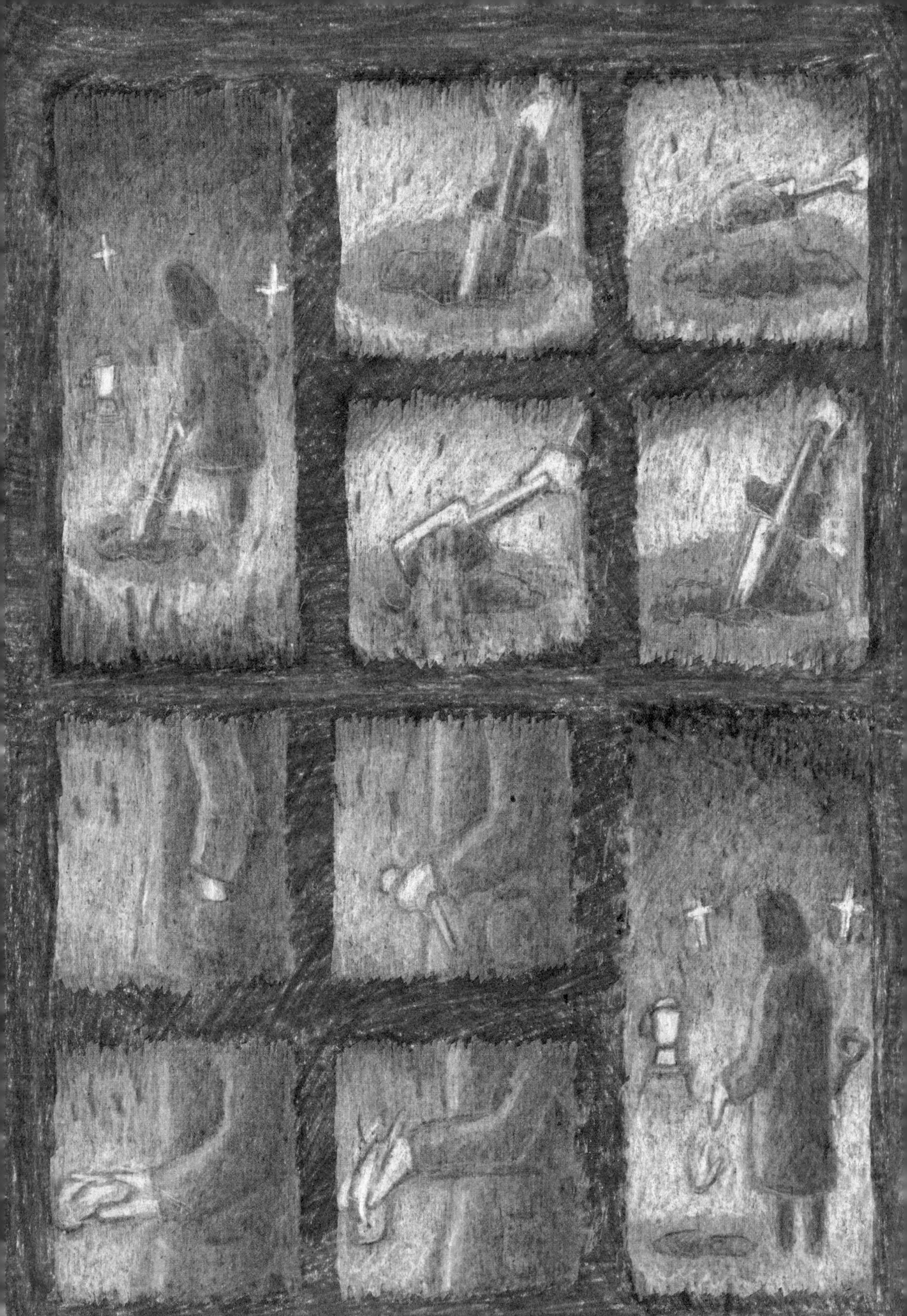

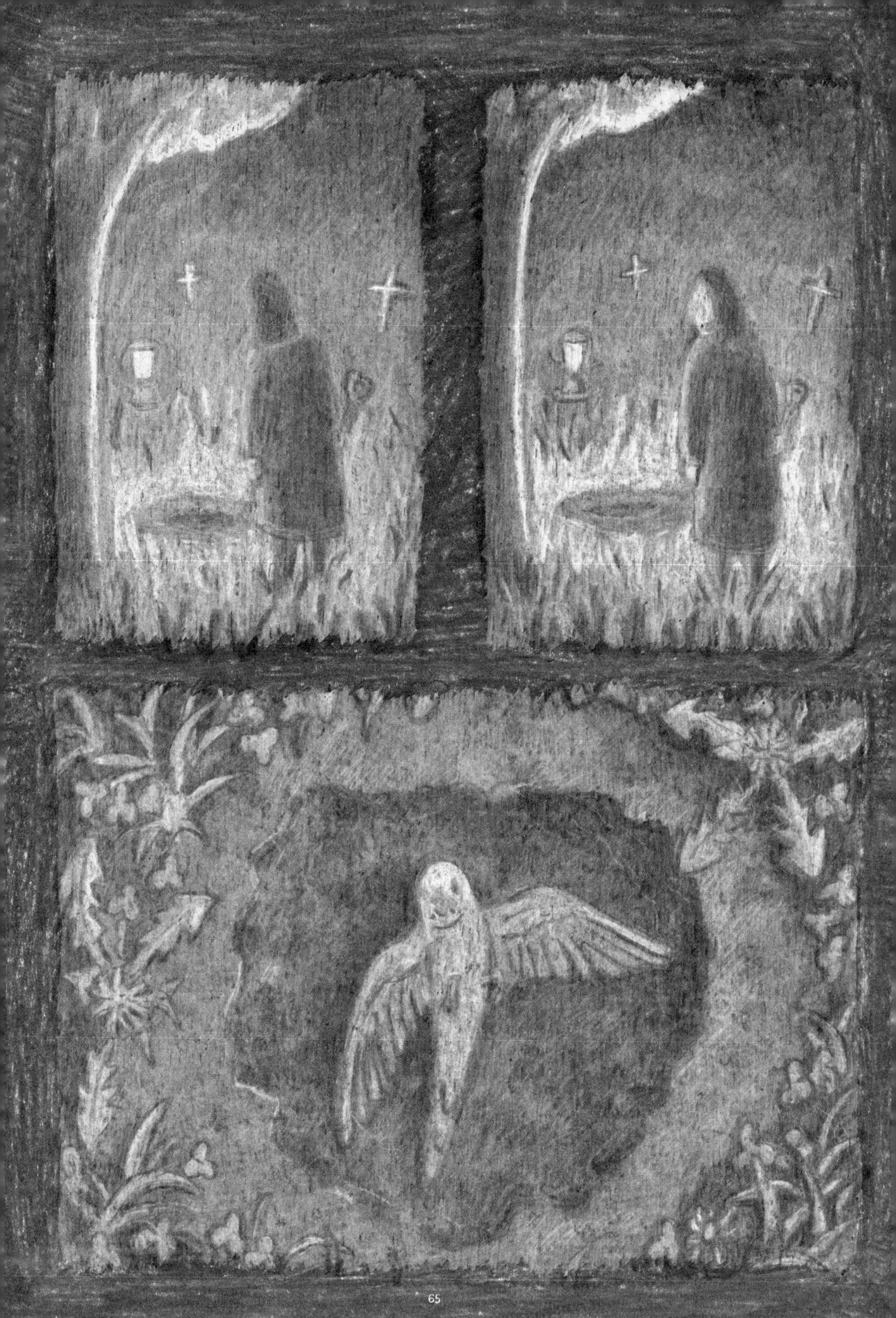

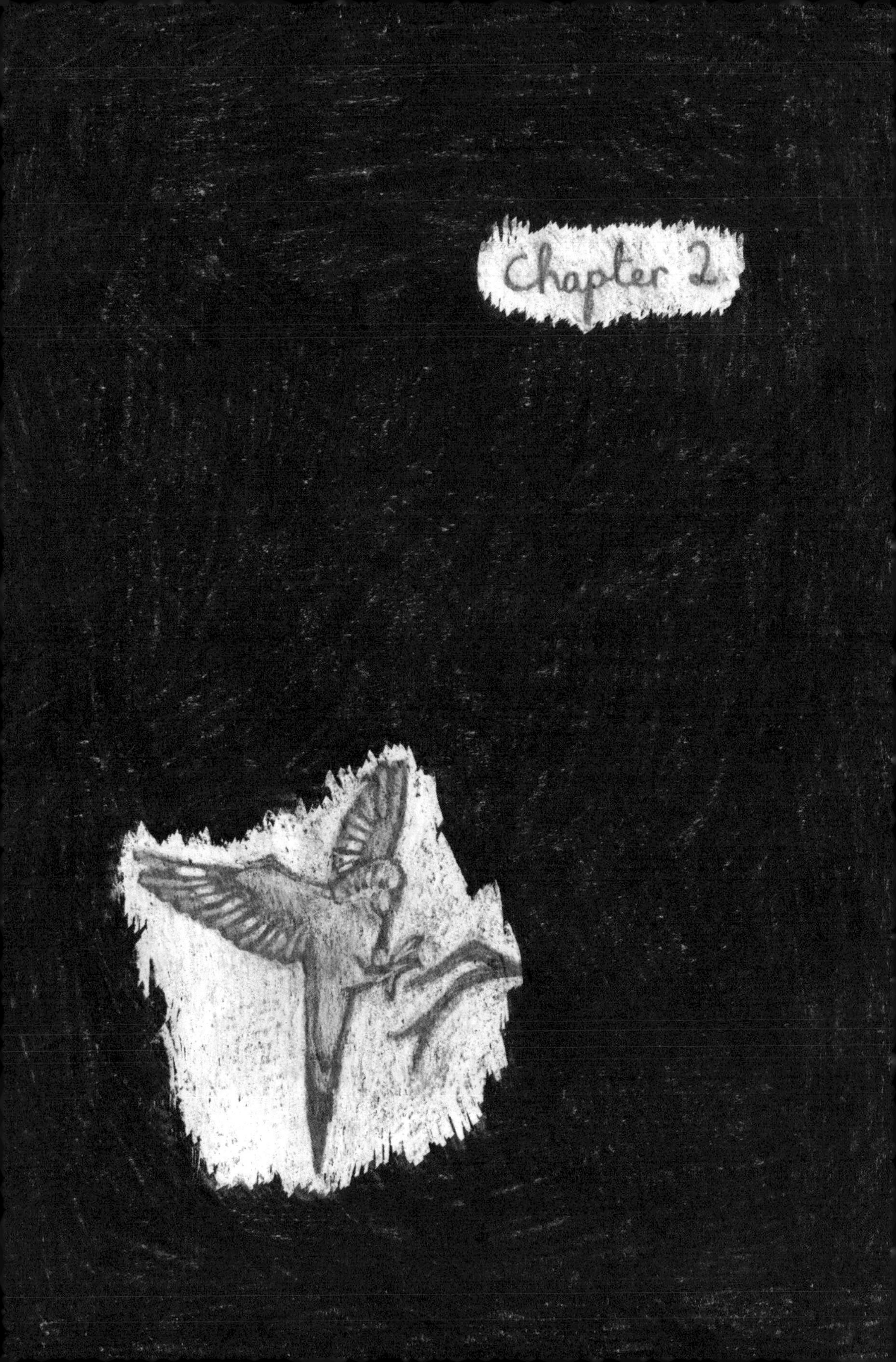
Chapter 2

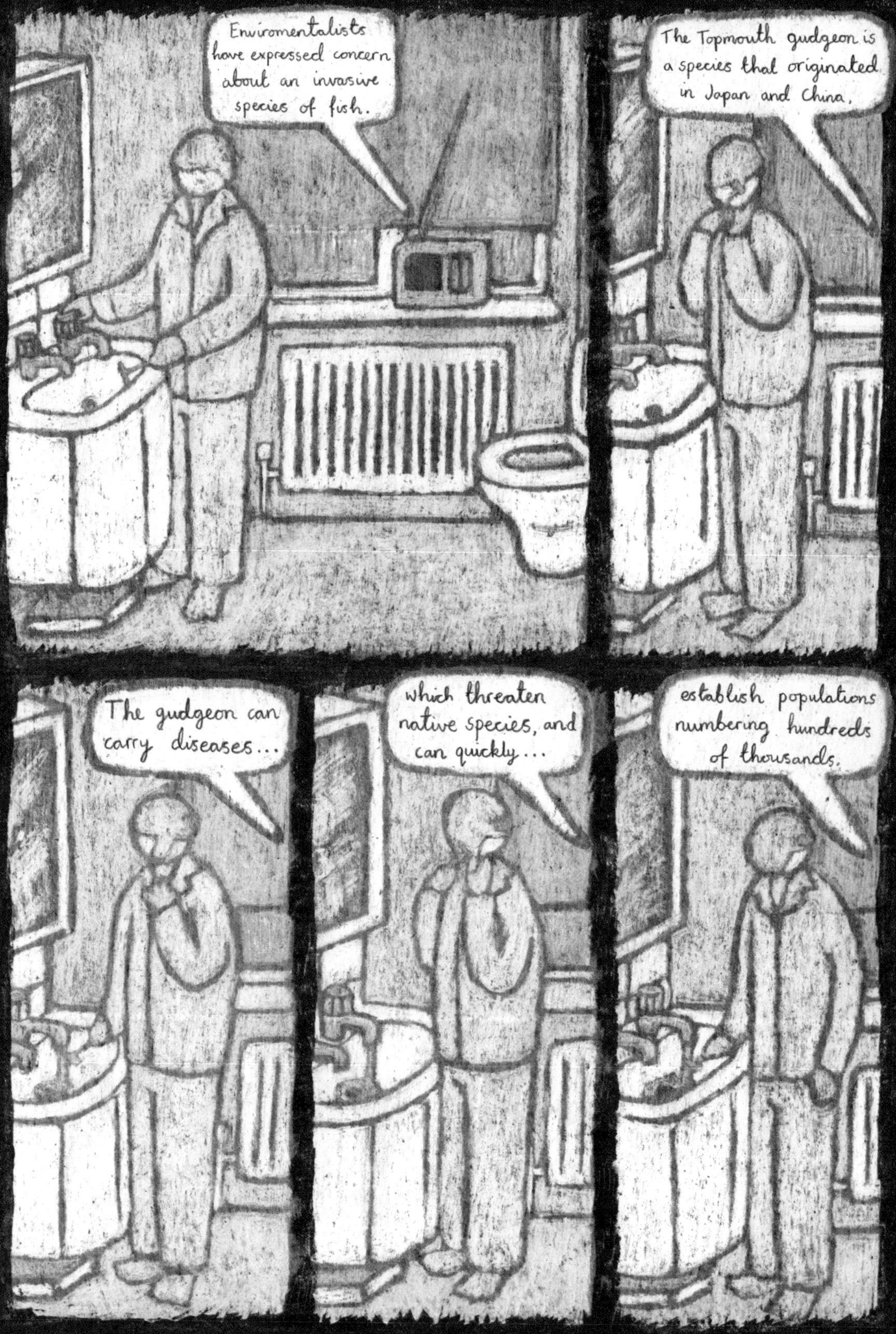
Enviromentalists have expressed concern about an invasive species of fish.
The Topmouth gudgeon is a species that originated in Japan and China,
The gudgeon can carry diseases...
which threaten native species, and can quickly...
establish populations numbering hundreds of thousands.

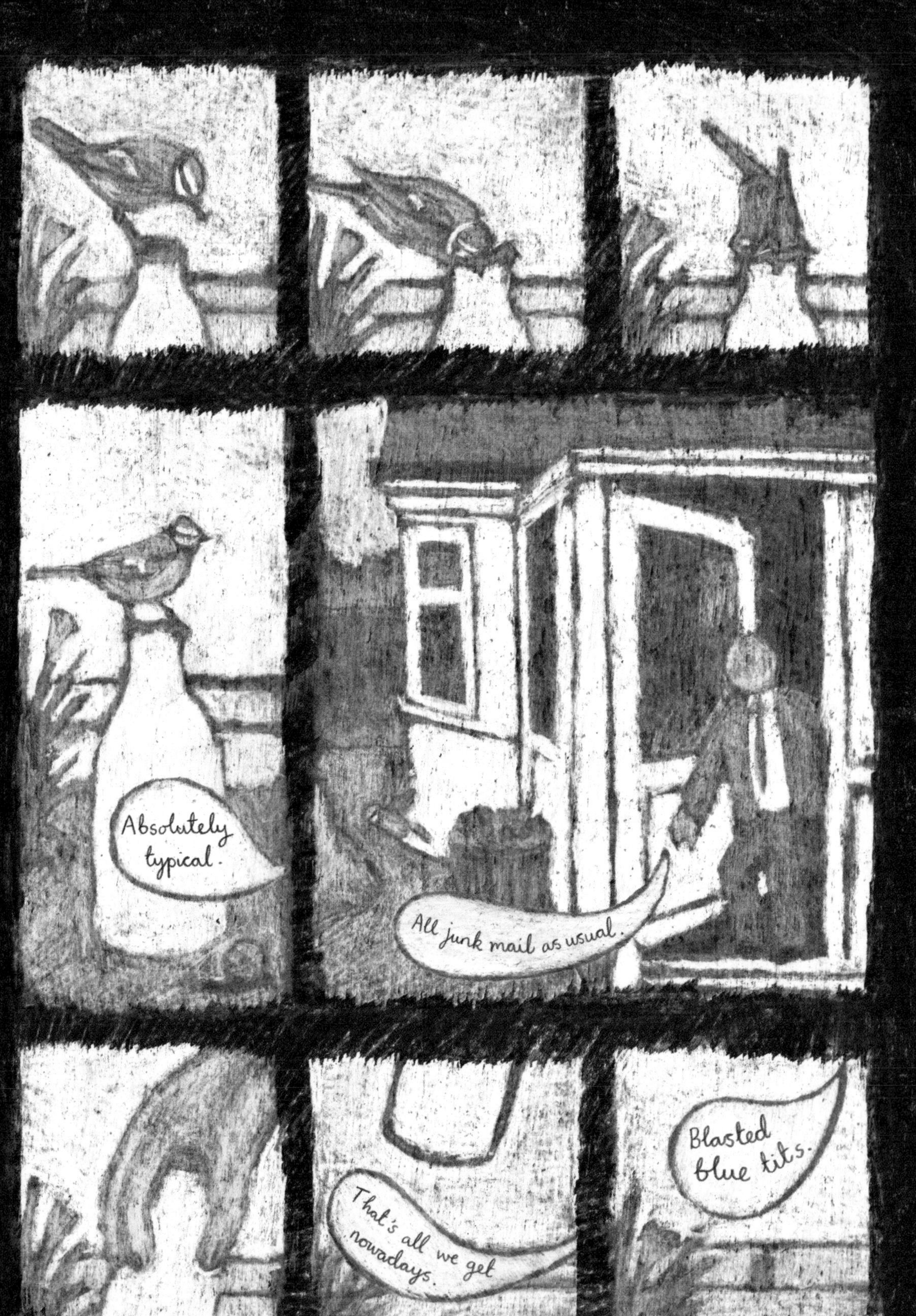
Absolutely typical.
All junk mail as usual.
That's all we get nowadays.
Blasted blue tits.

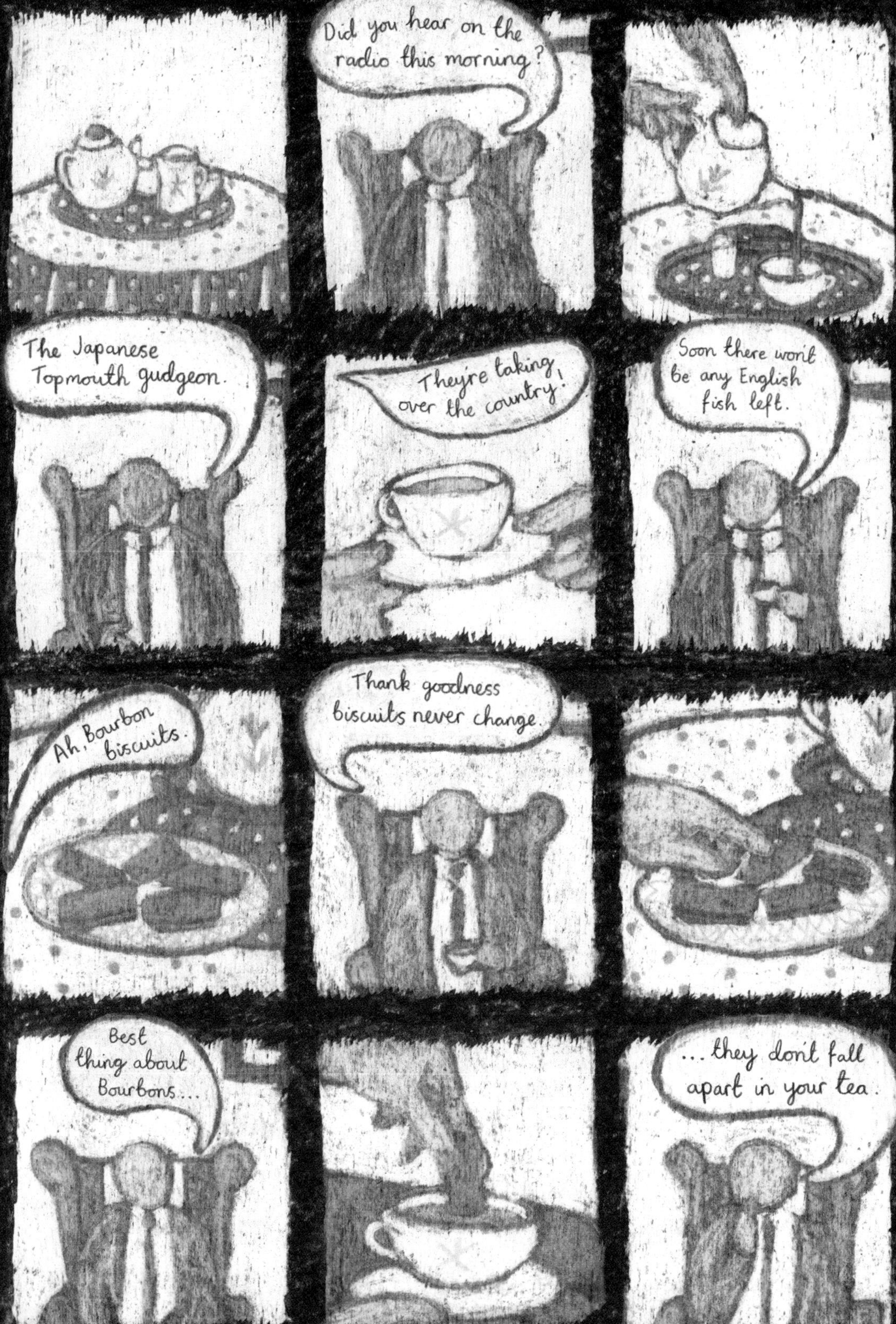
Did you hear on the radio this morning?
The Japanese Topmouth gudgeon.
They're taking over the country!
Soon there won't be any English fish left.
Ah, Bourbon biscuits.
Thank goodness biscuits never change.
Best thing about Bourbons....
...they don't fall apart in your tea.

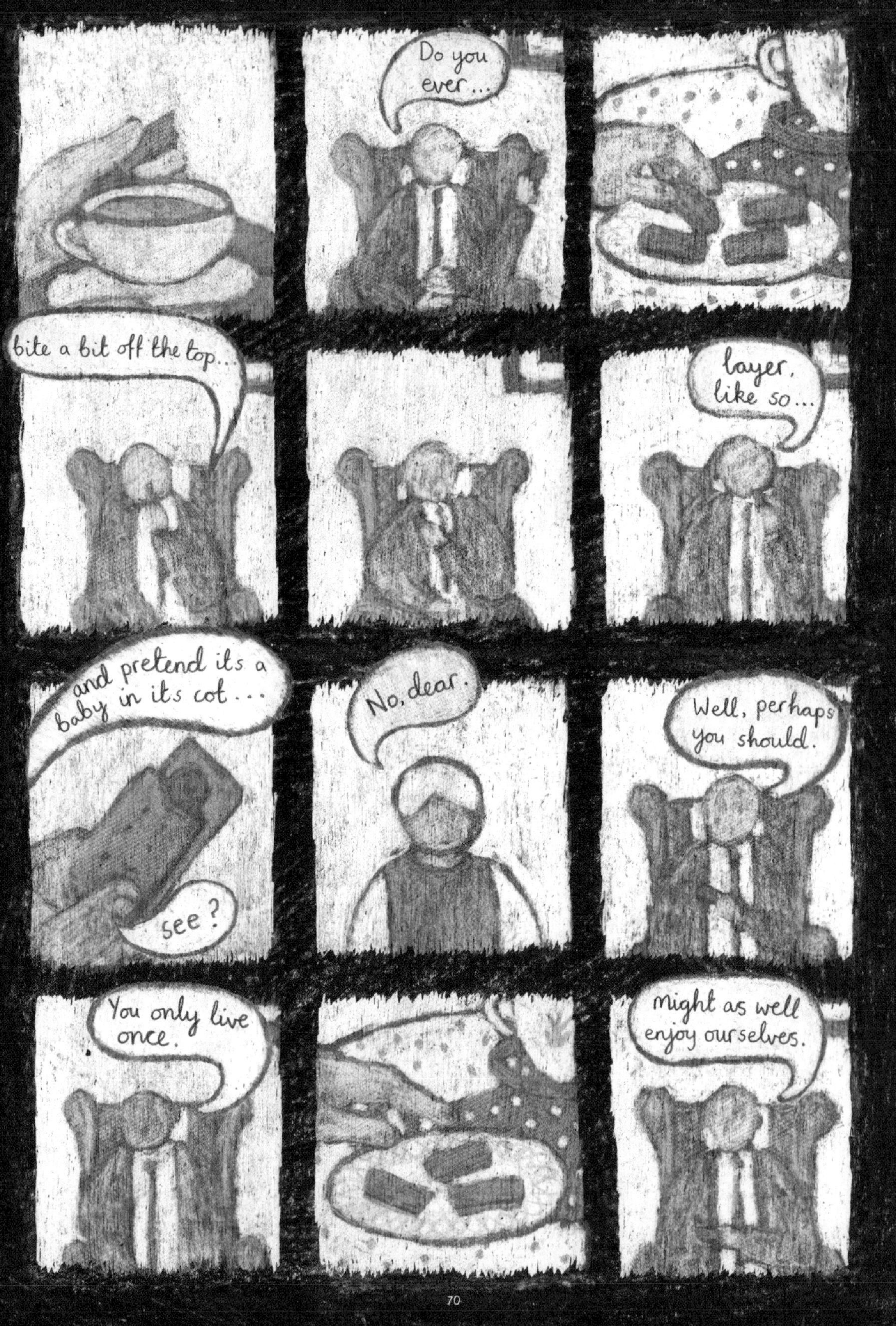
Do you ever...
bite a bit off the top...
layer, like so...
and pretend its a baby in its cot...
see?
No, dear.
Well, perhaps you should.
You only live once.
Might as well enjoy ourselves.

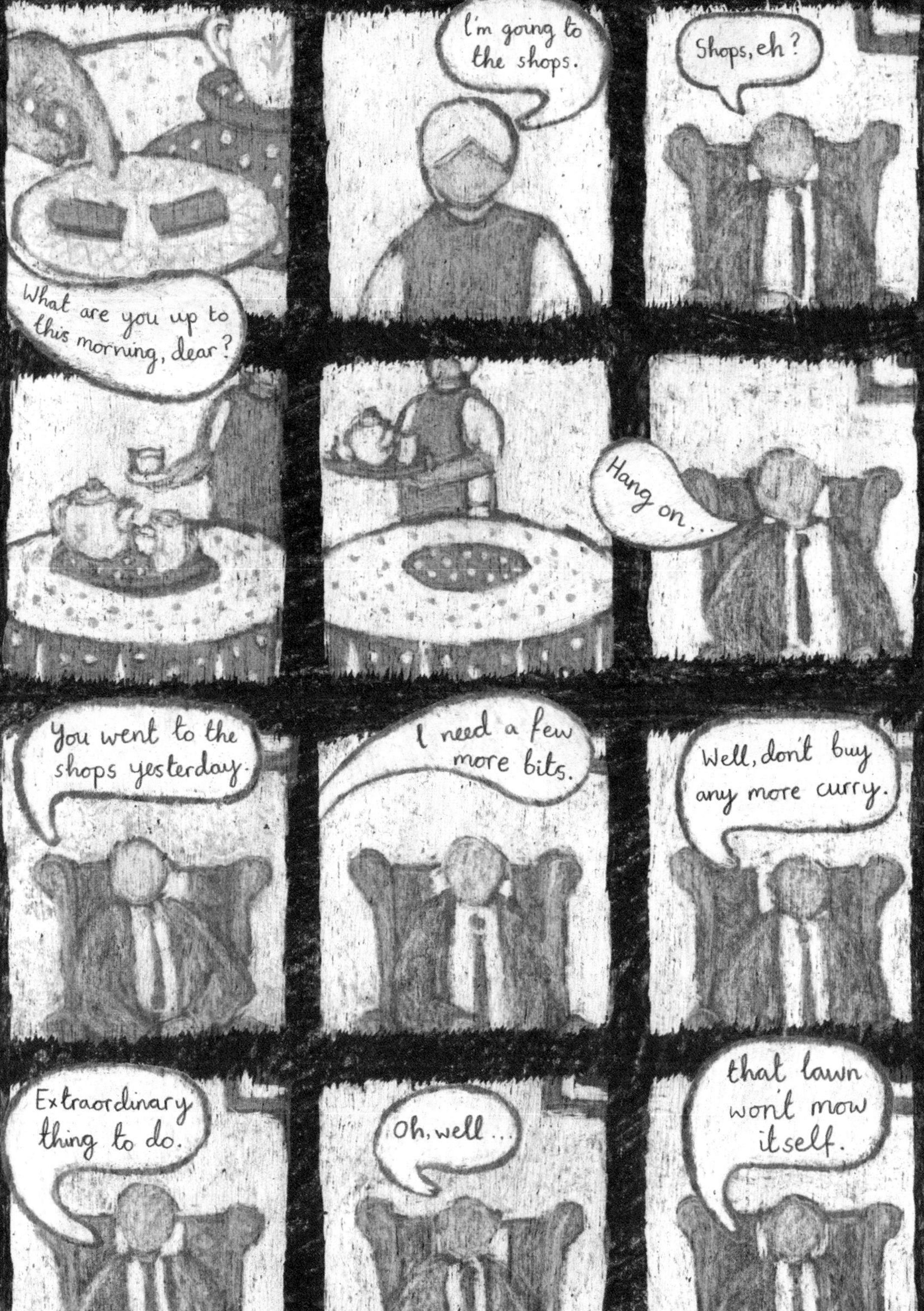
What are you up to this morning, dear?
I'm going to the shops.
Shops, eh?
Hang on...
You went to the shops yesterday.
I need a few more bits.
Well, don't buy any more curry.
Extraordinary thing to do.
Oh, well...
that lawn won't mow itself.

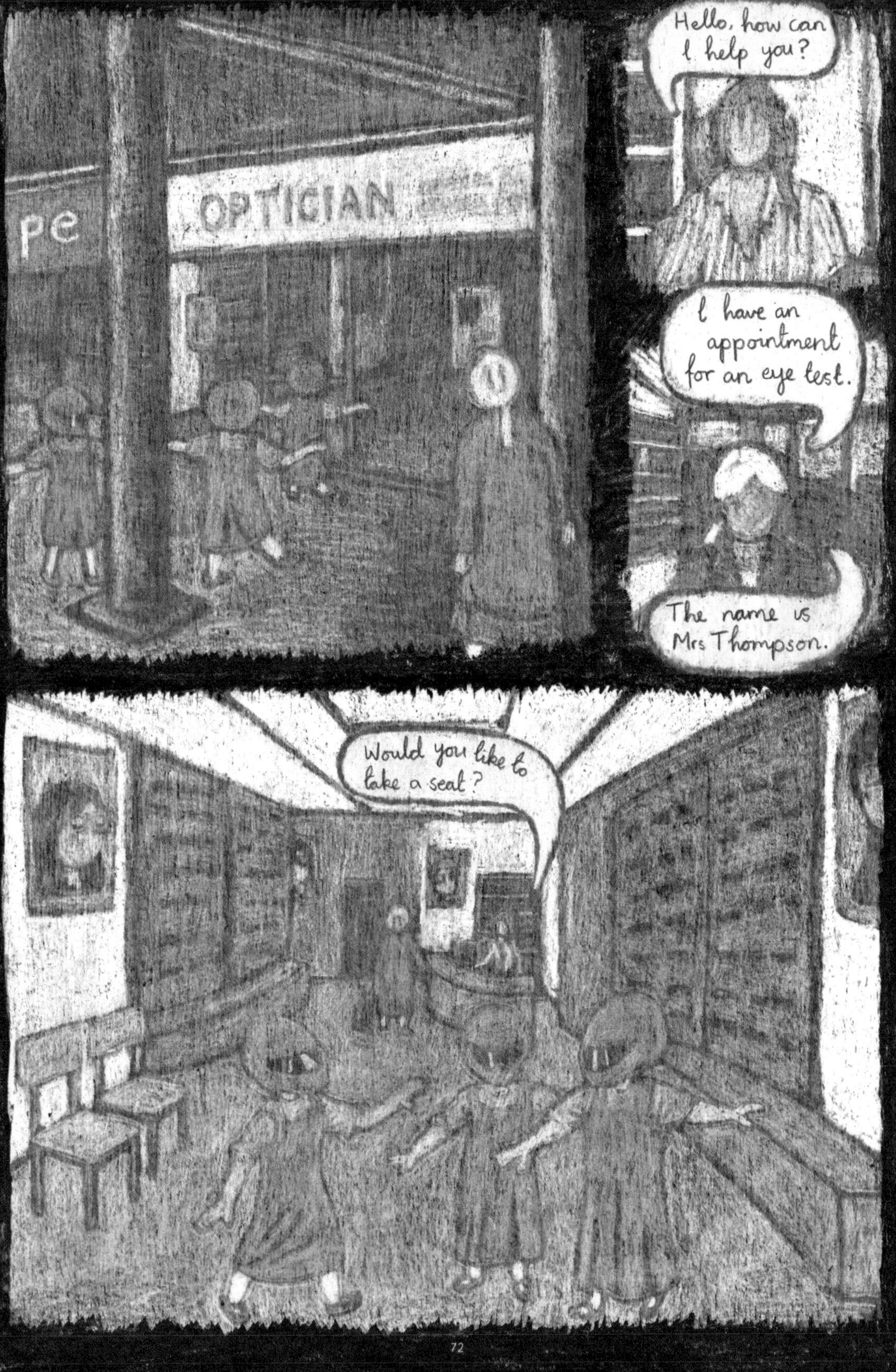
pe
OPTICIAN
Hello, how can I help you?
I have an appointment for an eye test.
The name is Mrs Thompson.
Would you like to take a seat?

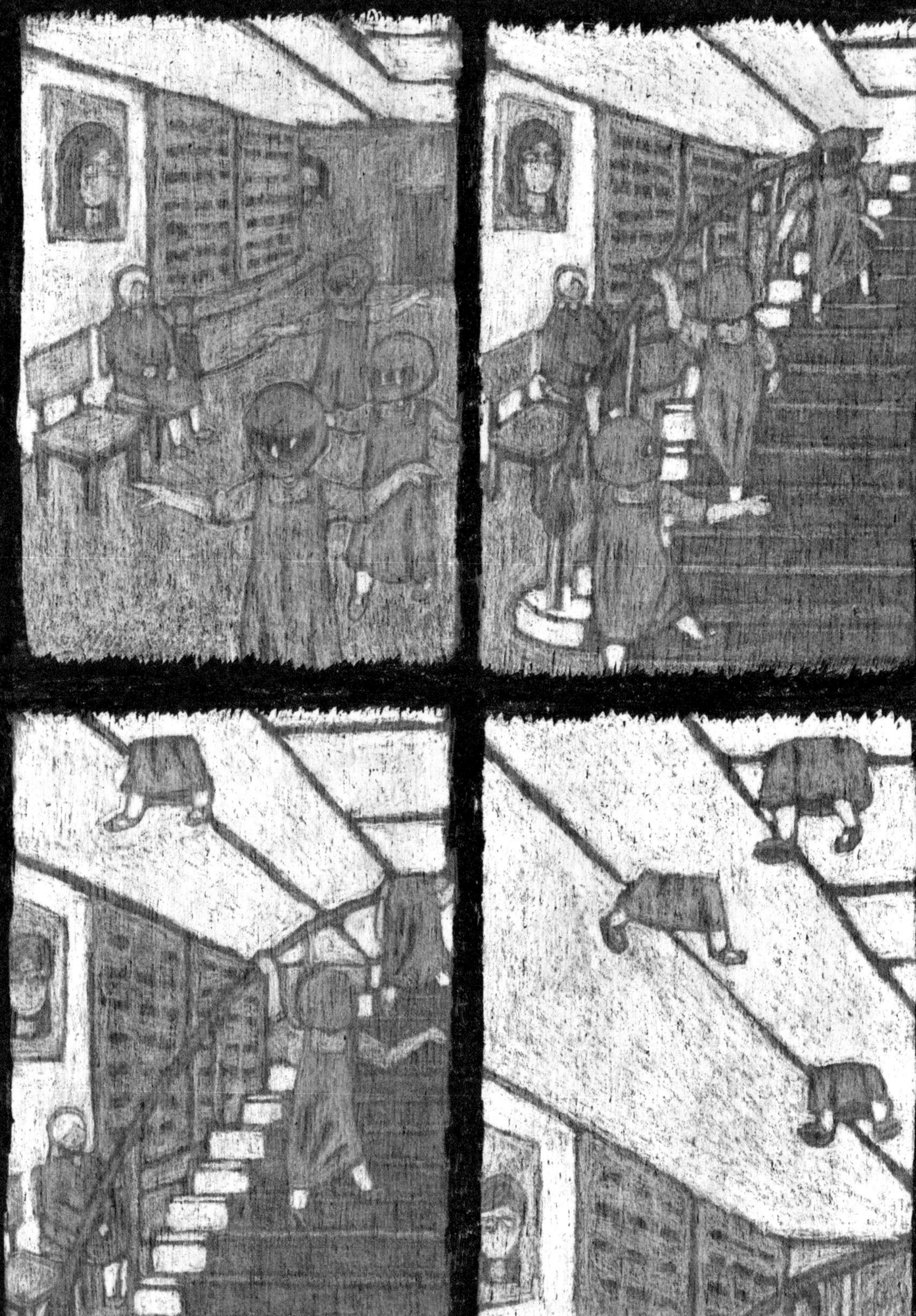

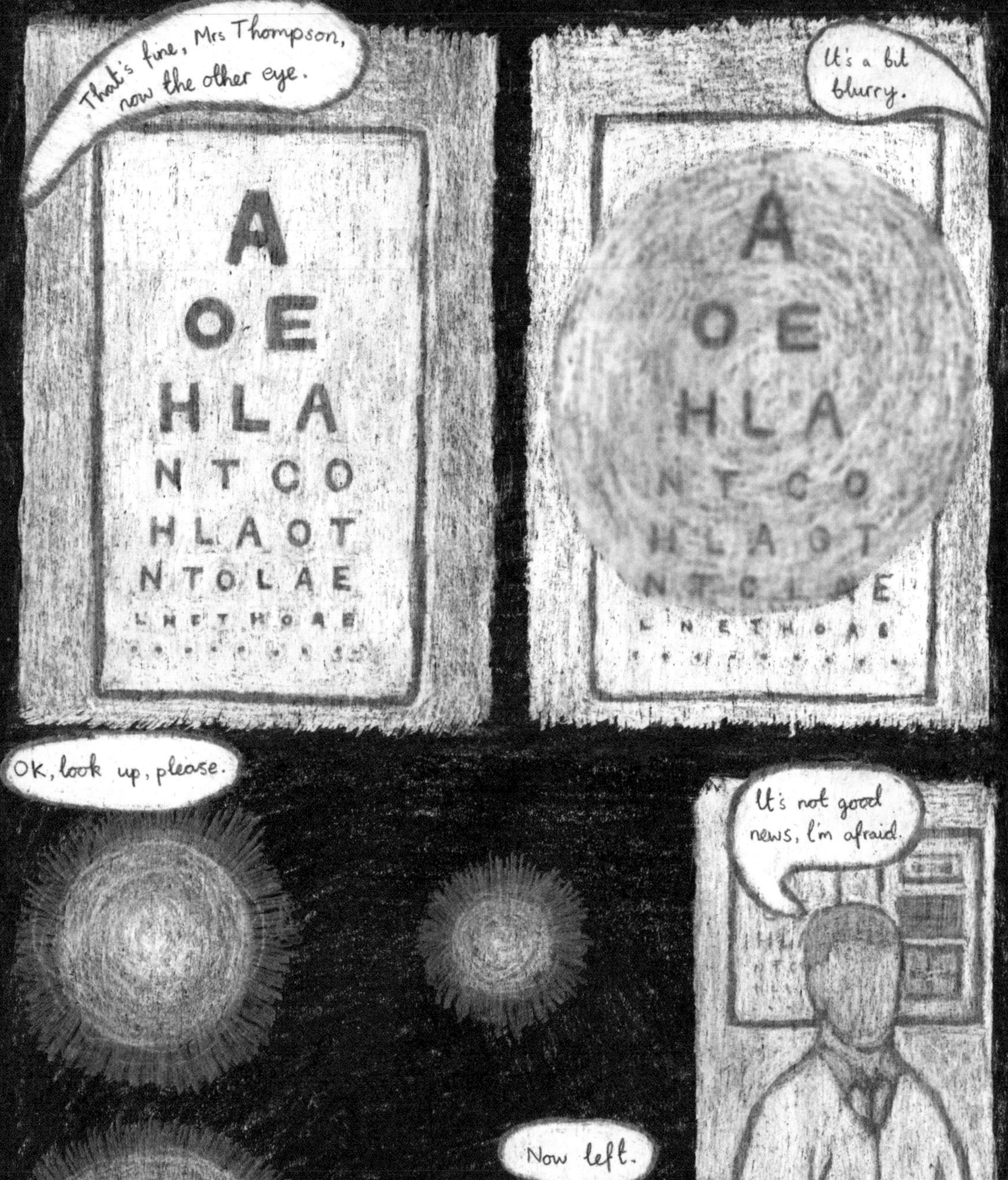
That's fine, Mrs Thompson, now the other eye.
It's a bit blurry.
OK, look up, please.
Now left.
It's not good news, I'm afraid.

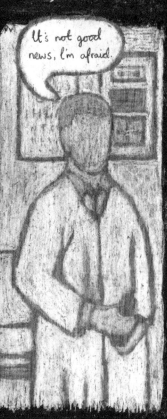

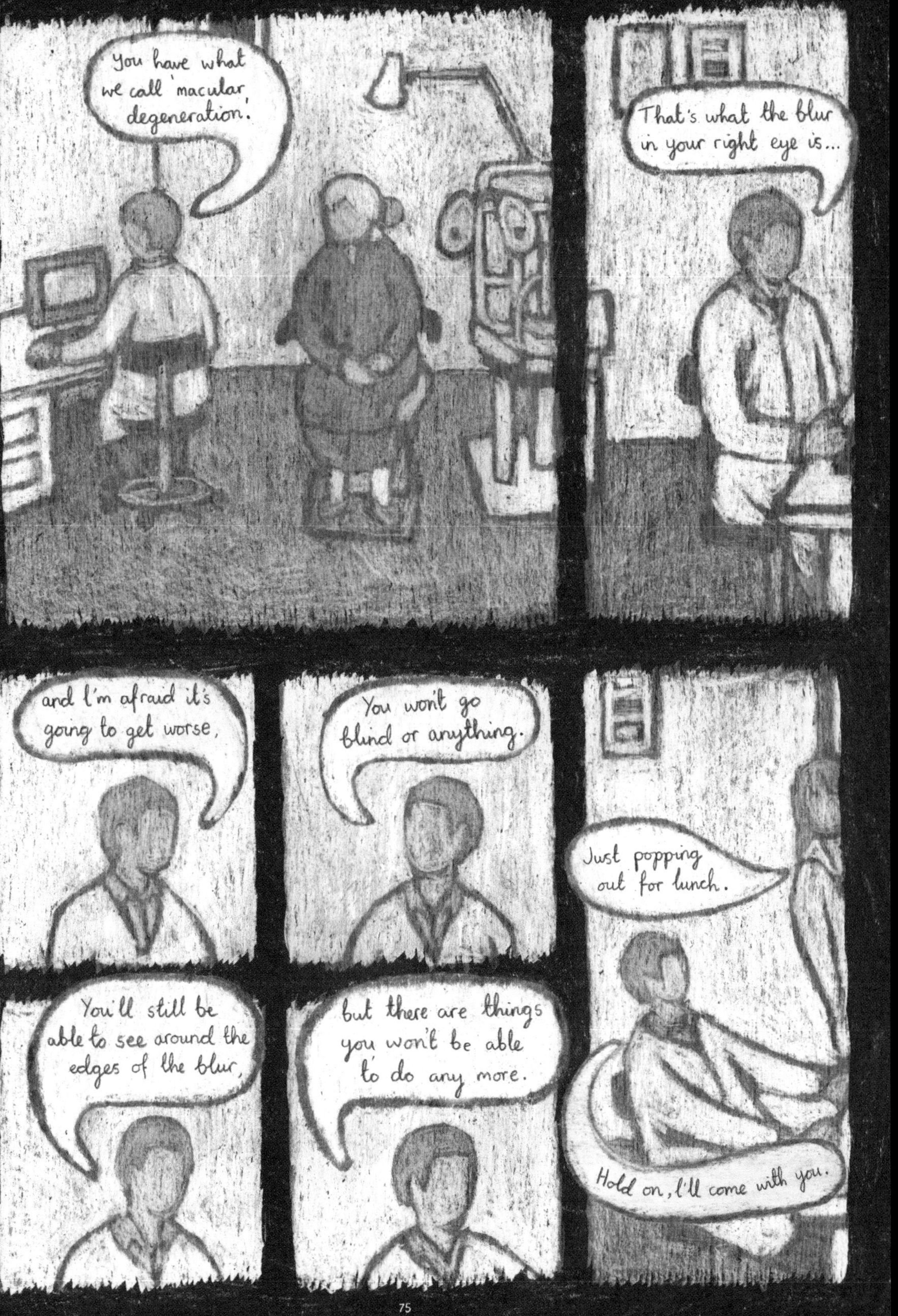
You have what we call 'macular degeneration.'
That's what the blur in your right eye is...
and I'm afraid it's going to get worse,
You won't go blind or anything.
You'll still be able to see around the edges of the blur,
but there are things you won't be able to do any more.
Just popping out for lunch.
Hold on, I'll come with you.

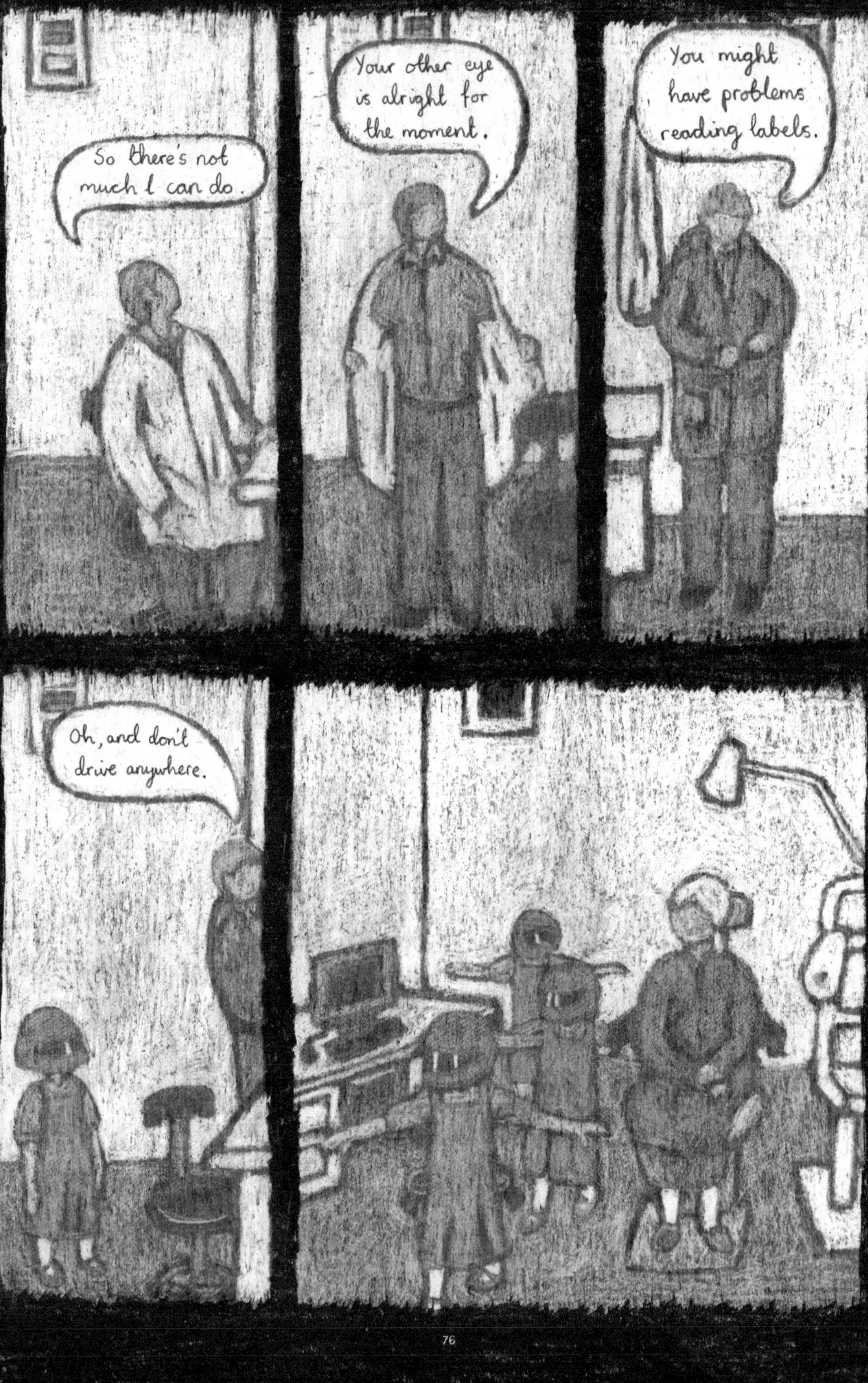
So there's not much I can do.
Your other eye is alright for the moment.
You might have problems reading labels.
Oh, and don't drive anywhere.

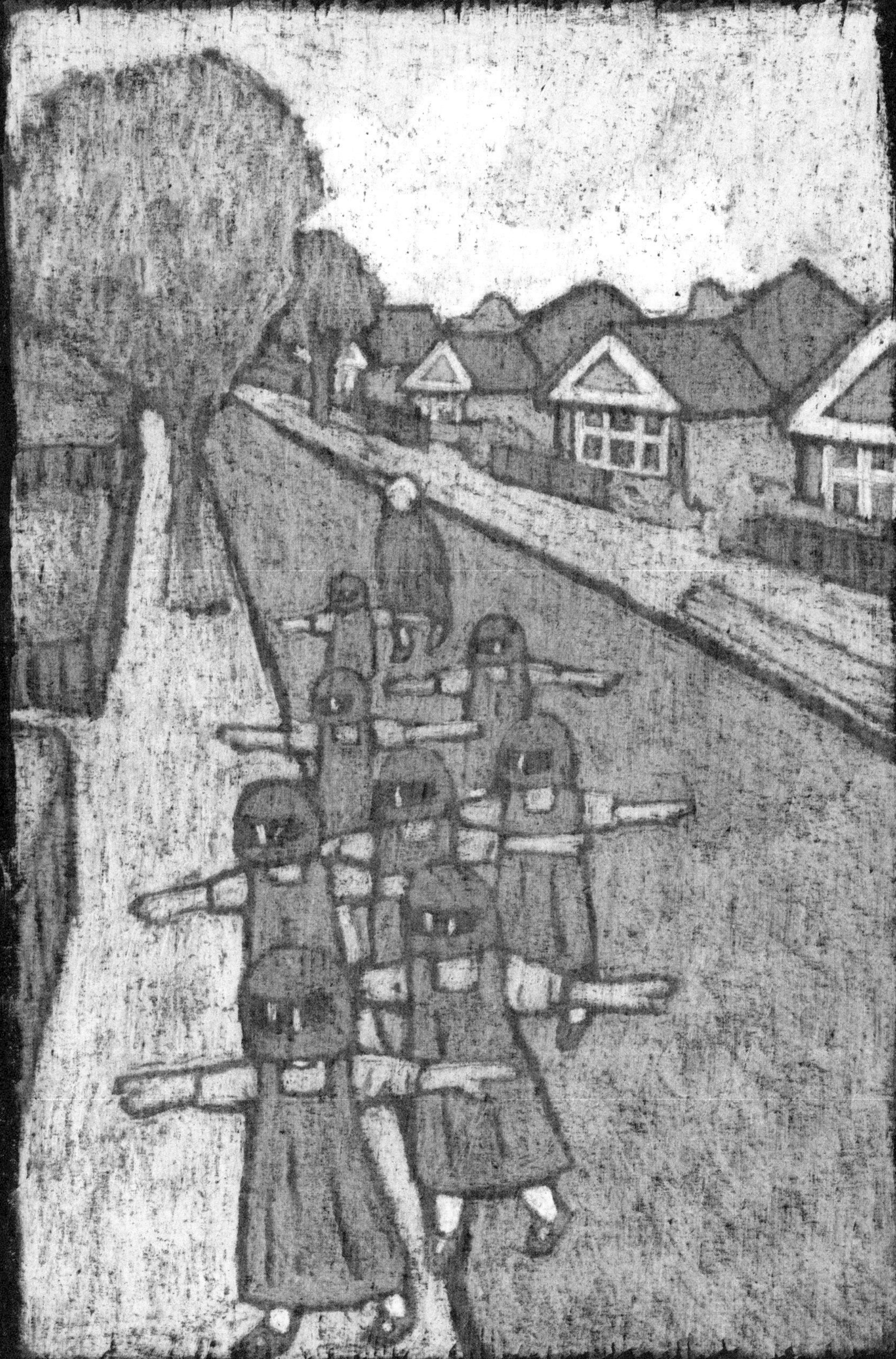

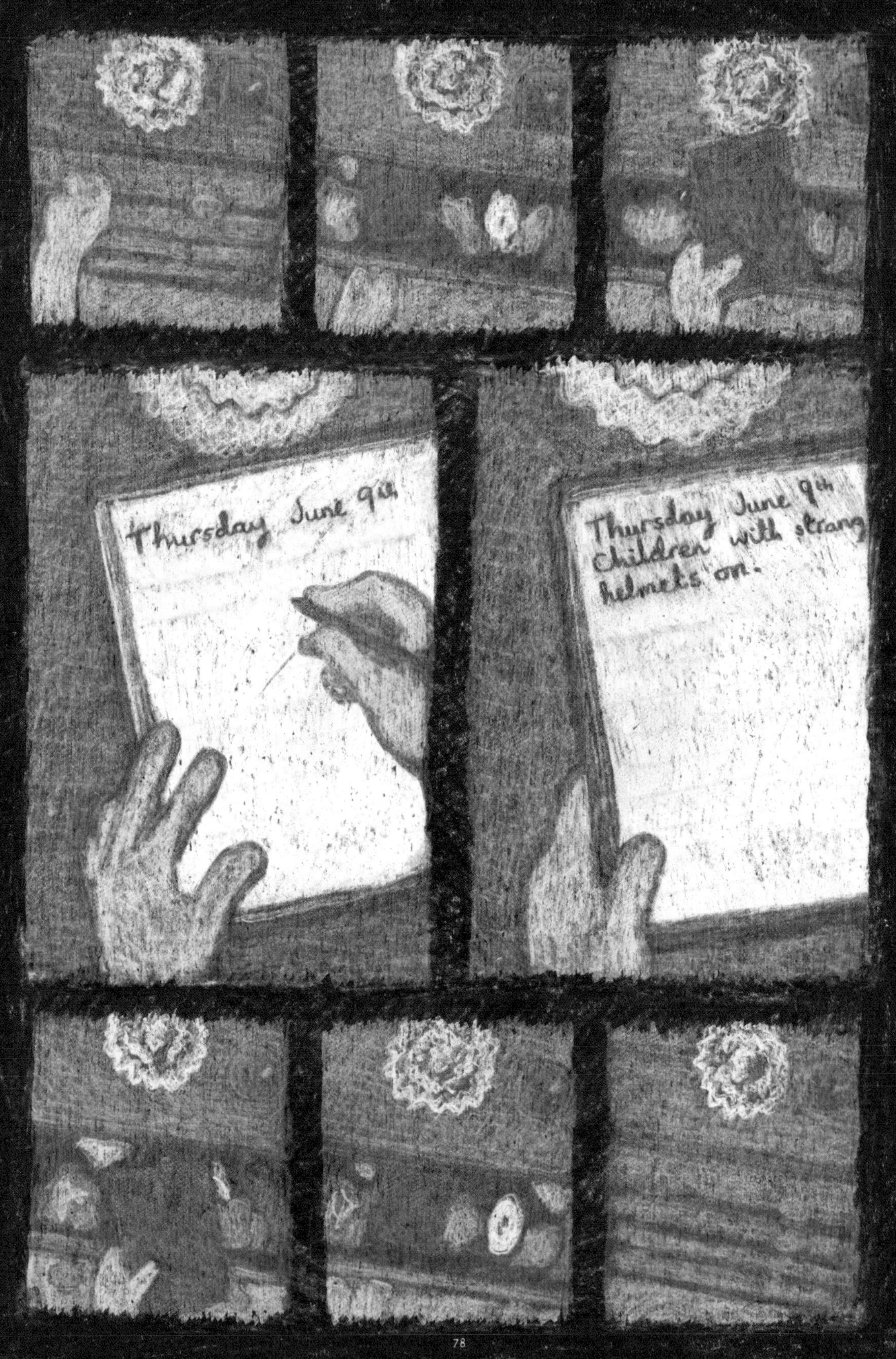

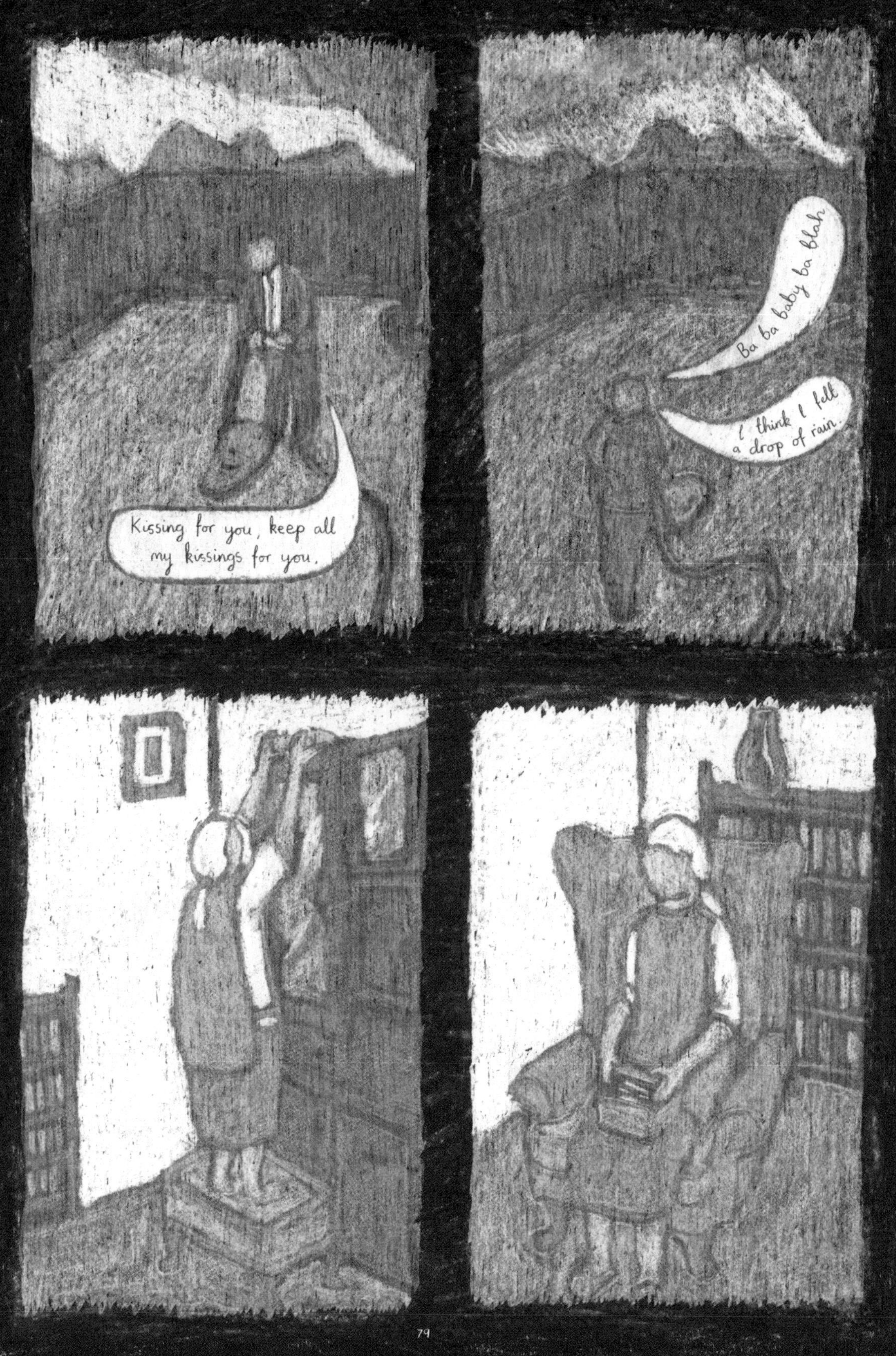
Kissing for you, keep all my kissings for you.
Ba ba baby ba blah
I think I felt a drop of rain.

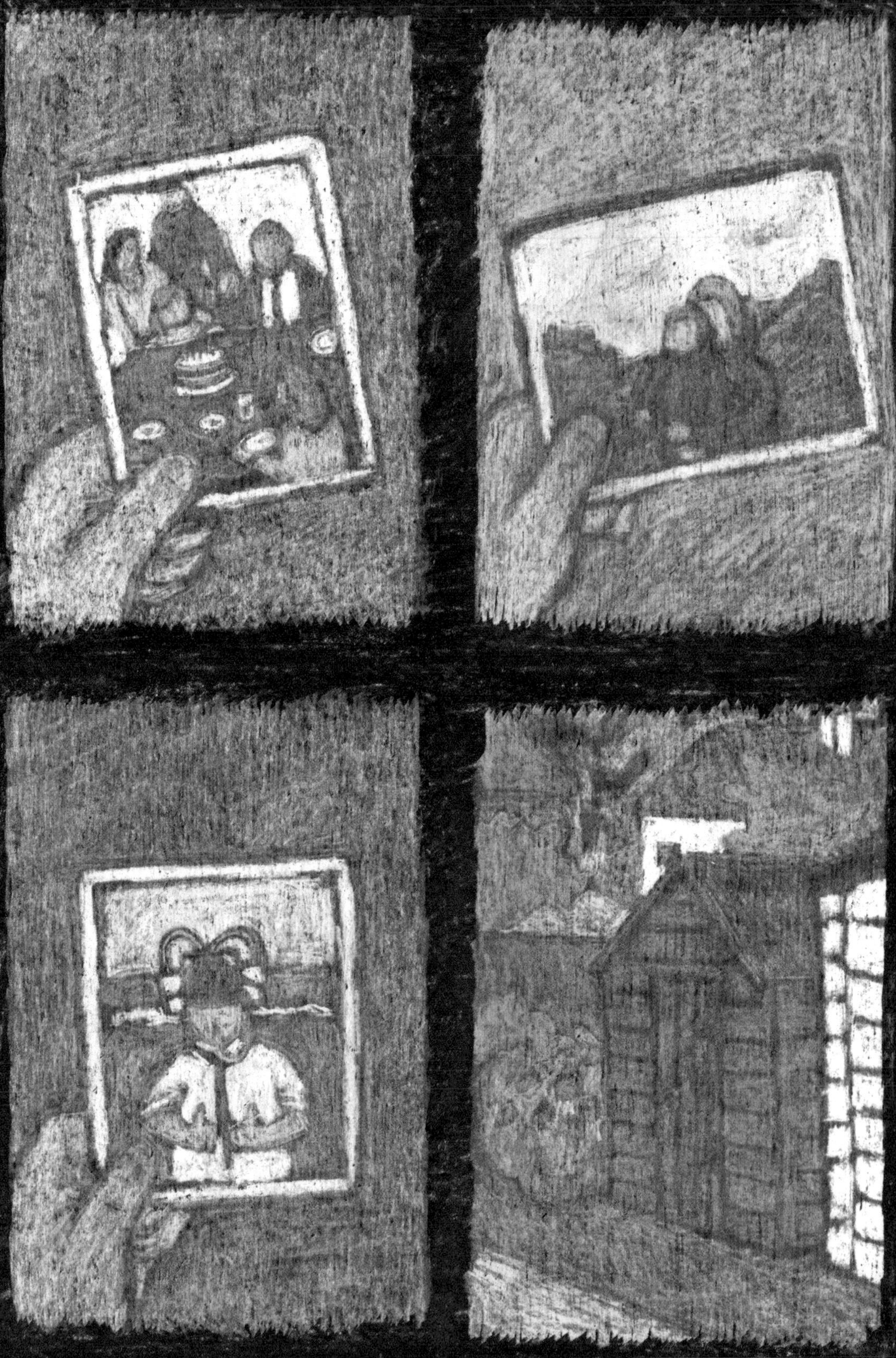

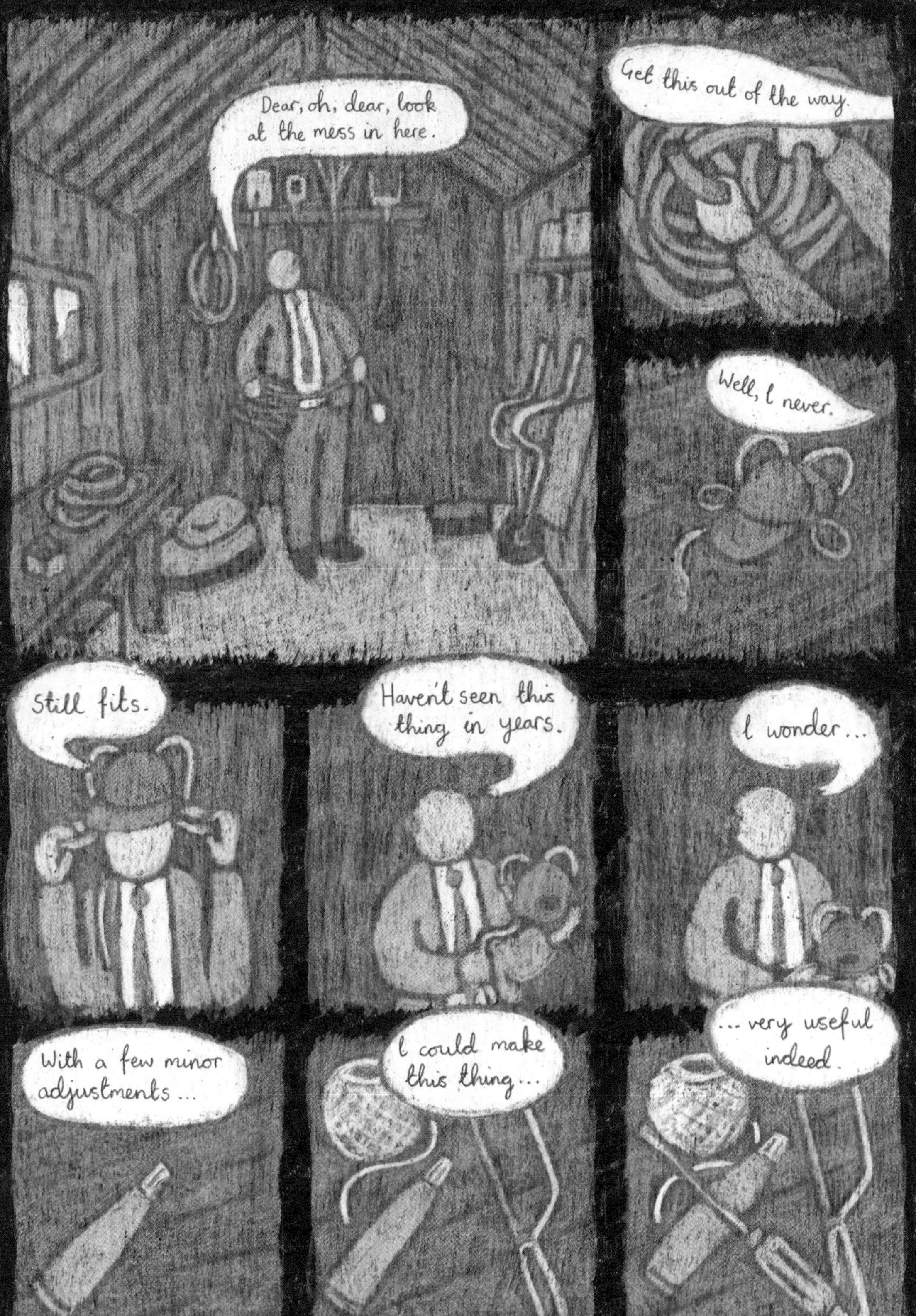
Dear, oh, dear, look at the mess in here.
Get this out of the way.
Well, I never.
Still fits.
Haven't seen this thing in years.
I wonder...
With a few minor adjustments...
I could make this thing...
... very useful indeed.

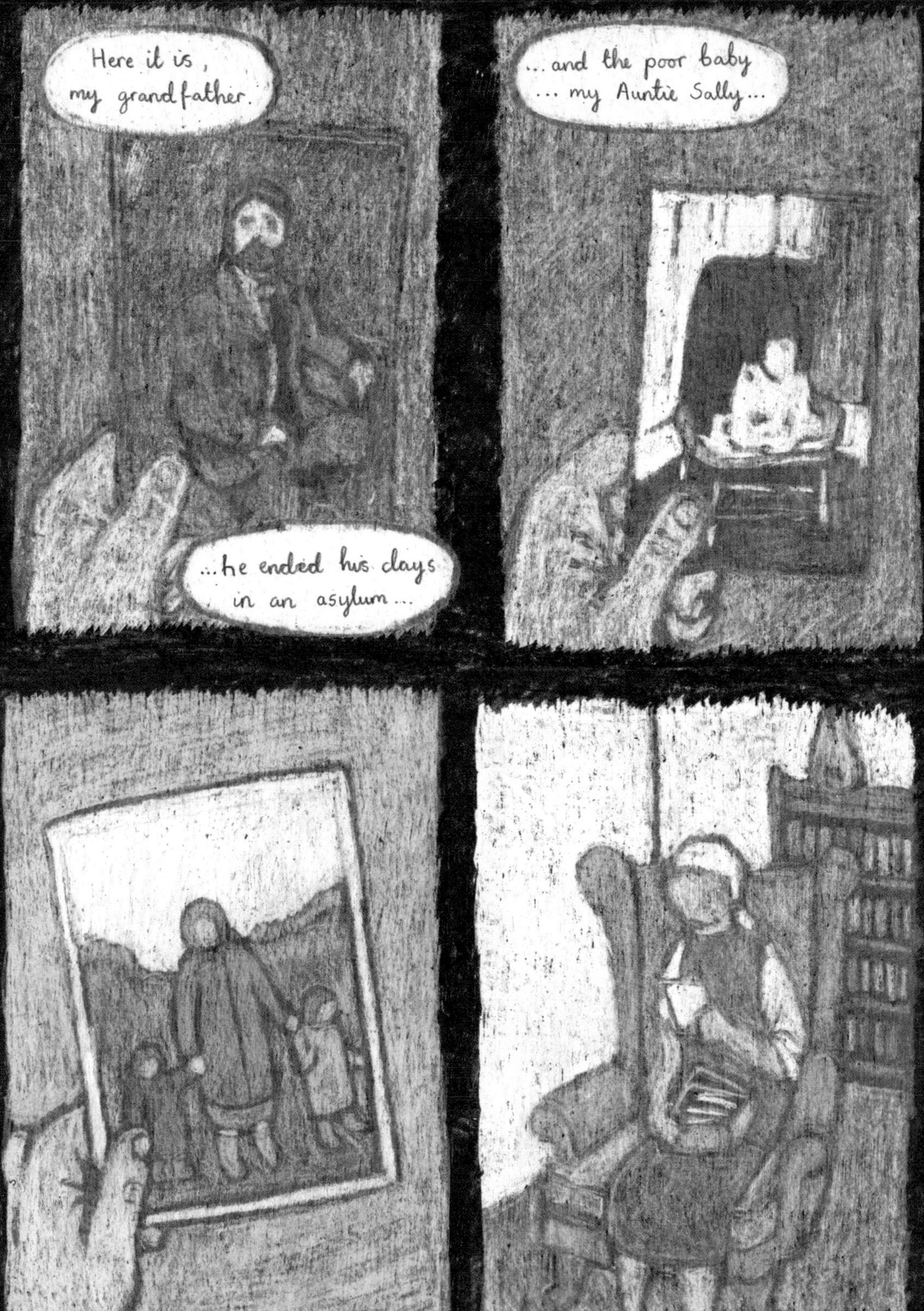
Here it is, my grandfather.
...he ended his days in an asylum...
...and the poor baby ... my Auntie Sally...

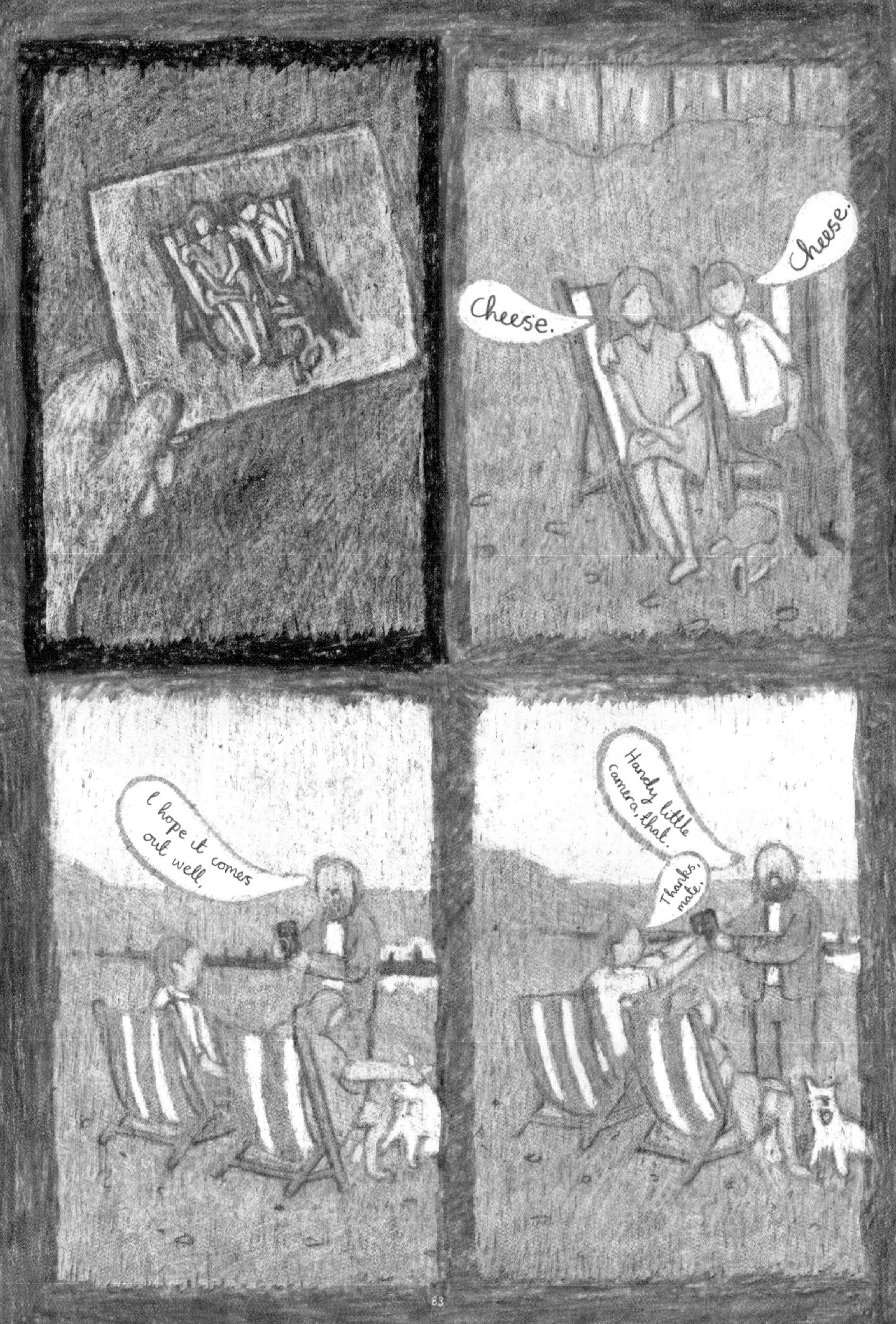
Cheese.
Cheese.
I hope it comes out well.
Handy little camera, that.
Thanks, mate.

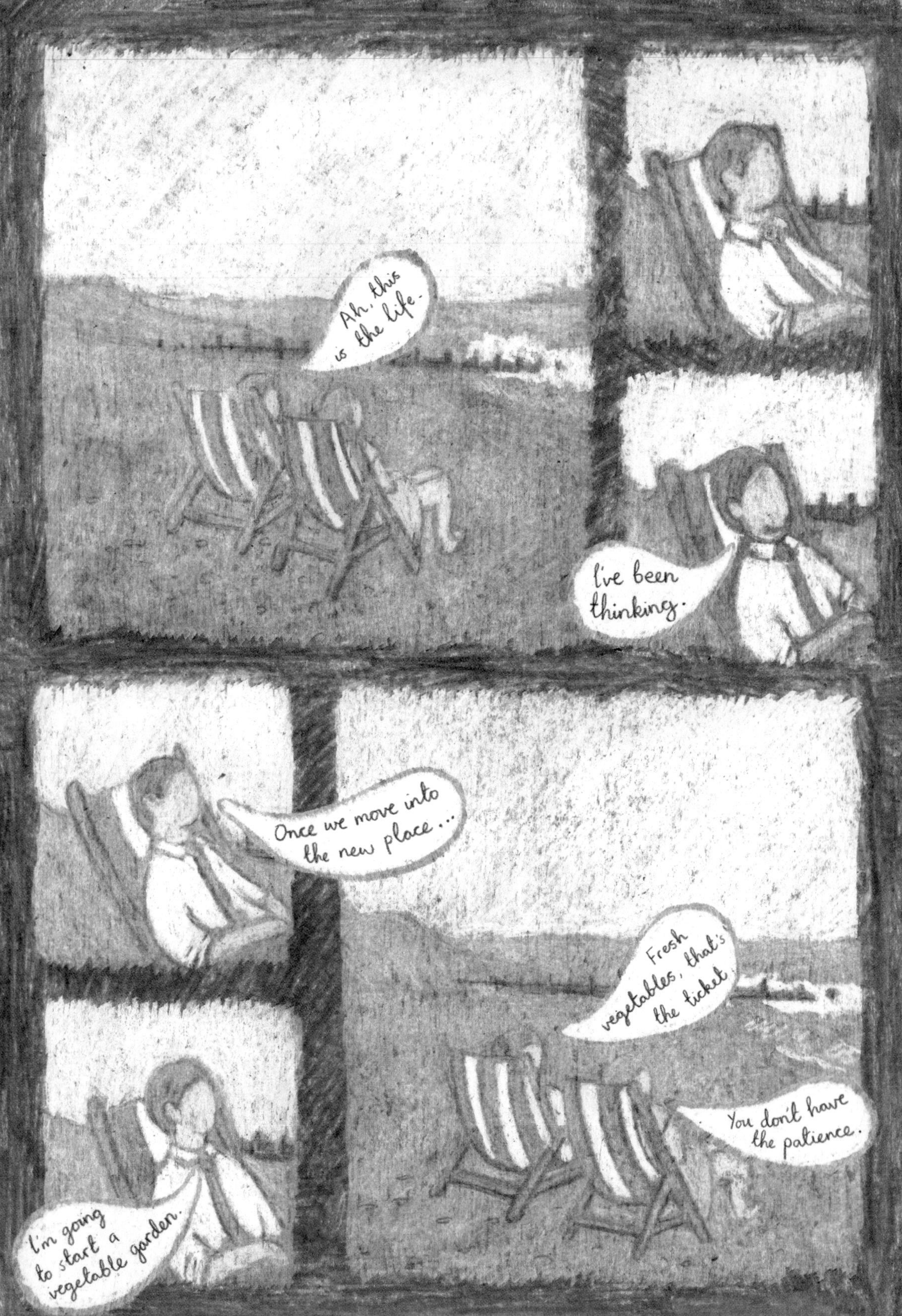
Ah, this is the life.
I've been thinking.
Once we move into the new place ...
I'm going to start a vegetable garden.
Fresh vegetables, that's the ticket.
You don't have the patience.

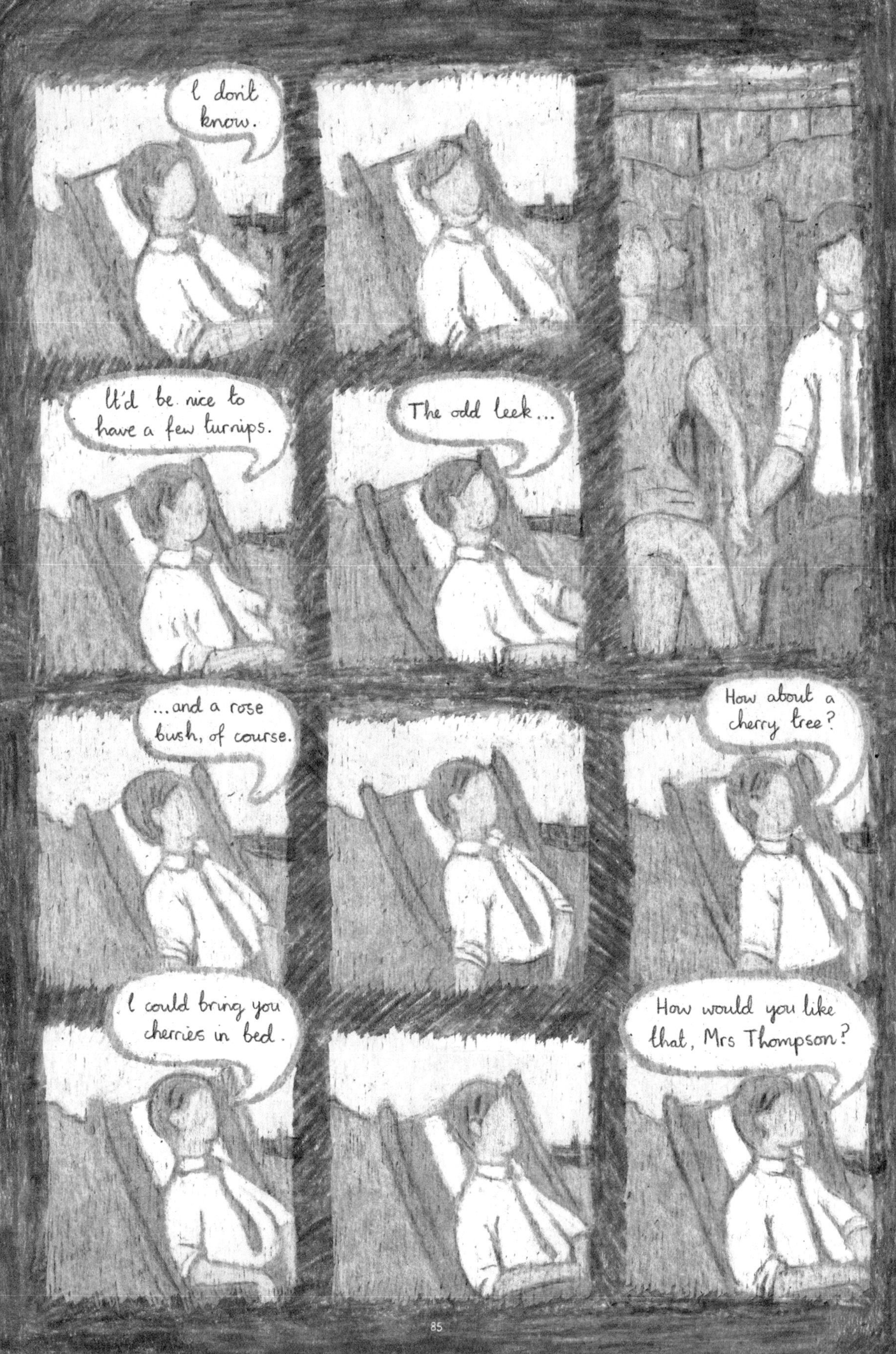
I don't know.
It'd be nice to have a few turnips.
The odd leek...
...and a rose bush, of course.
How about a cherry tree?
I could bring you cherries in bed.
How would you like that, Mrs Thompson?

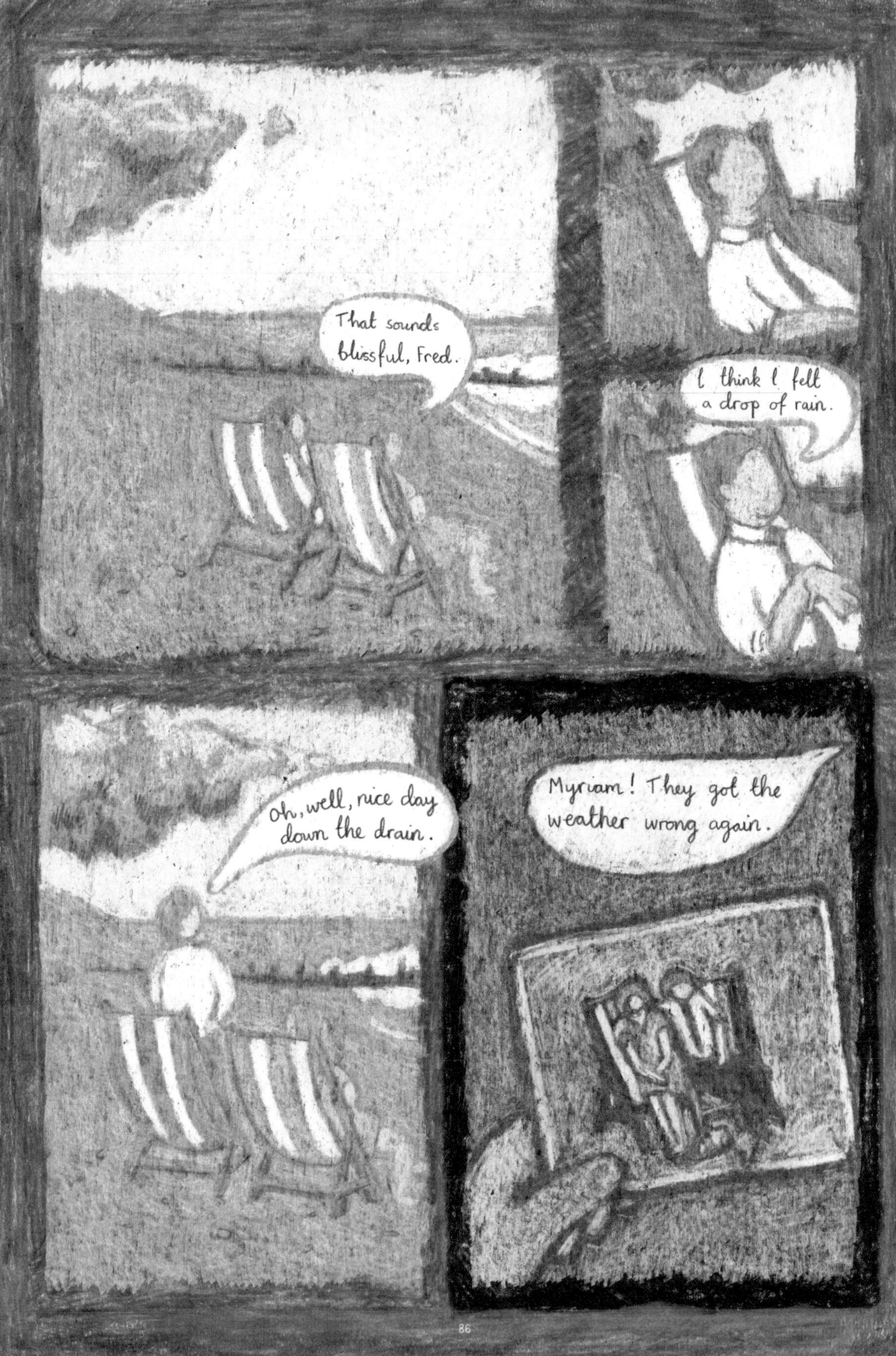
That sounds blissful, Fred.
I think I felt a drop of rain.
Oh, well, nice day down the drain.
Myriam! They got the weather wrong again.

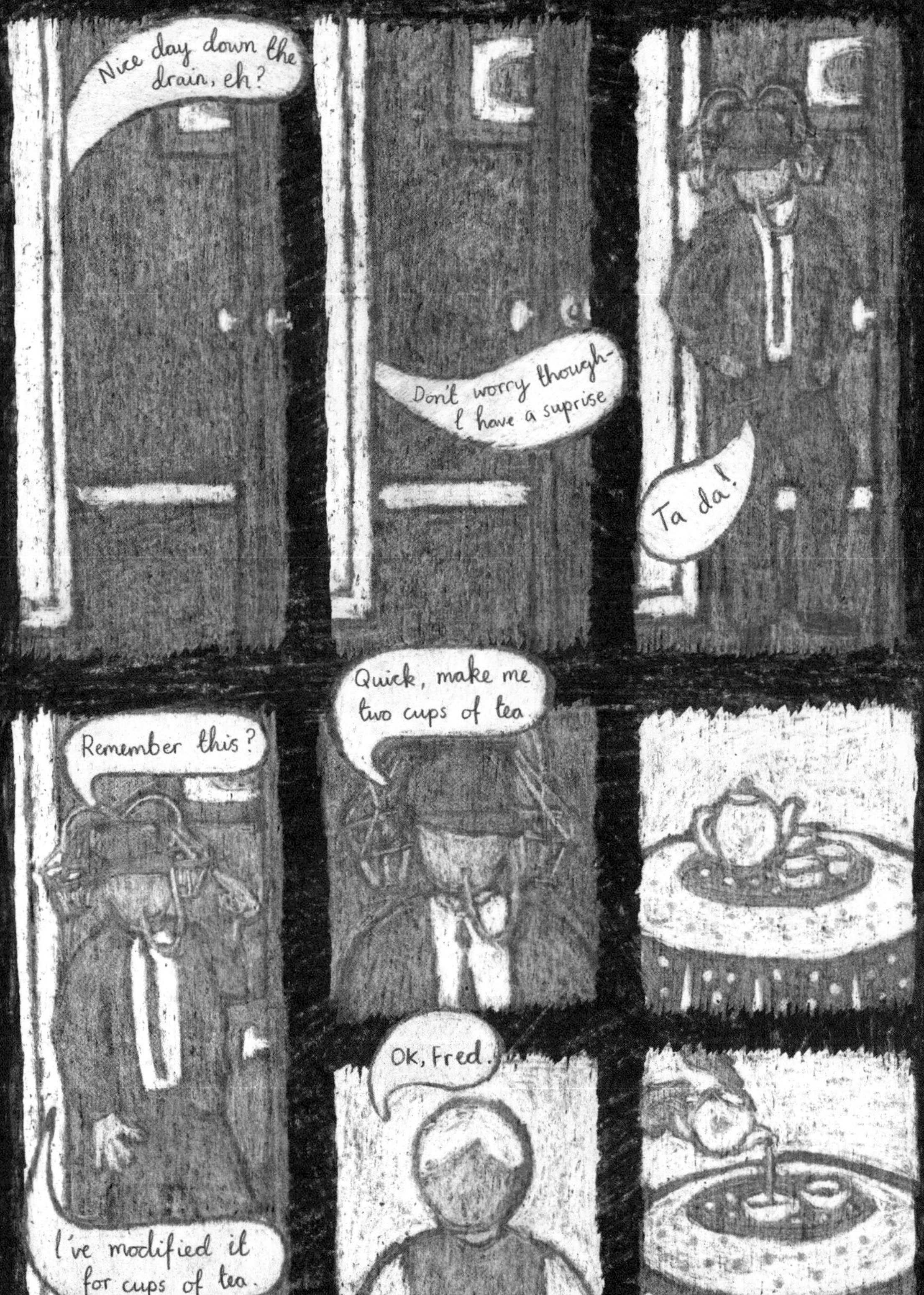
Nice day down the drain, eh?
Don't worry though- I have a suprise
Ta da!
Remember this?
I've modified it for cups of tea.
Quick, make me two cups of tea.
Ok, Fred.

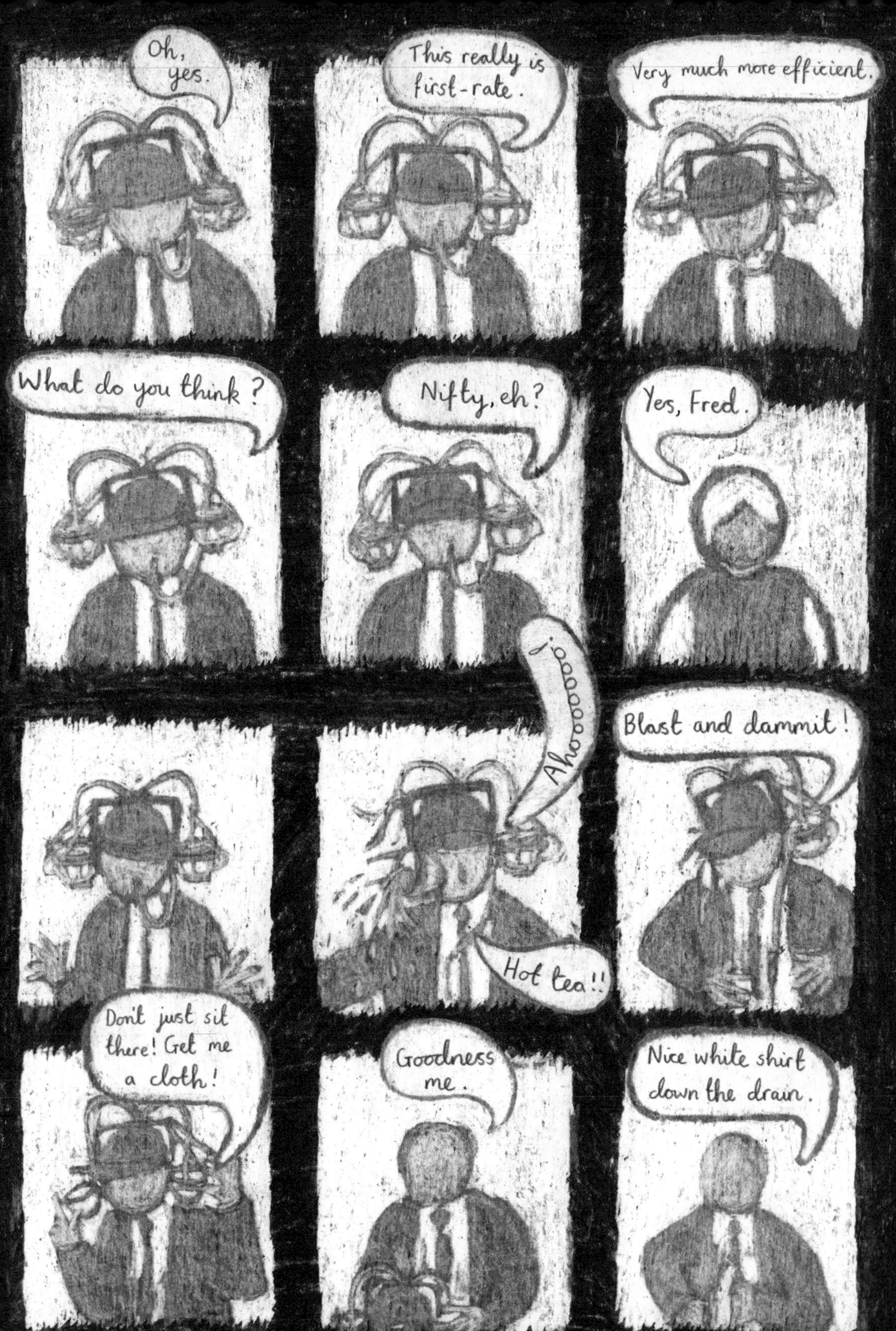
Oh, yes.
This really is first-rate.
Very much more efficient.
What do you think?
Nifty, eh?
Yes, Fred.
Ahooooooo!
Hot tea!!
Blast and dammit!
Don't just sit there! Get me a cloth!
Goodness me.
Nice white shirt down the drain.

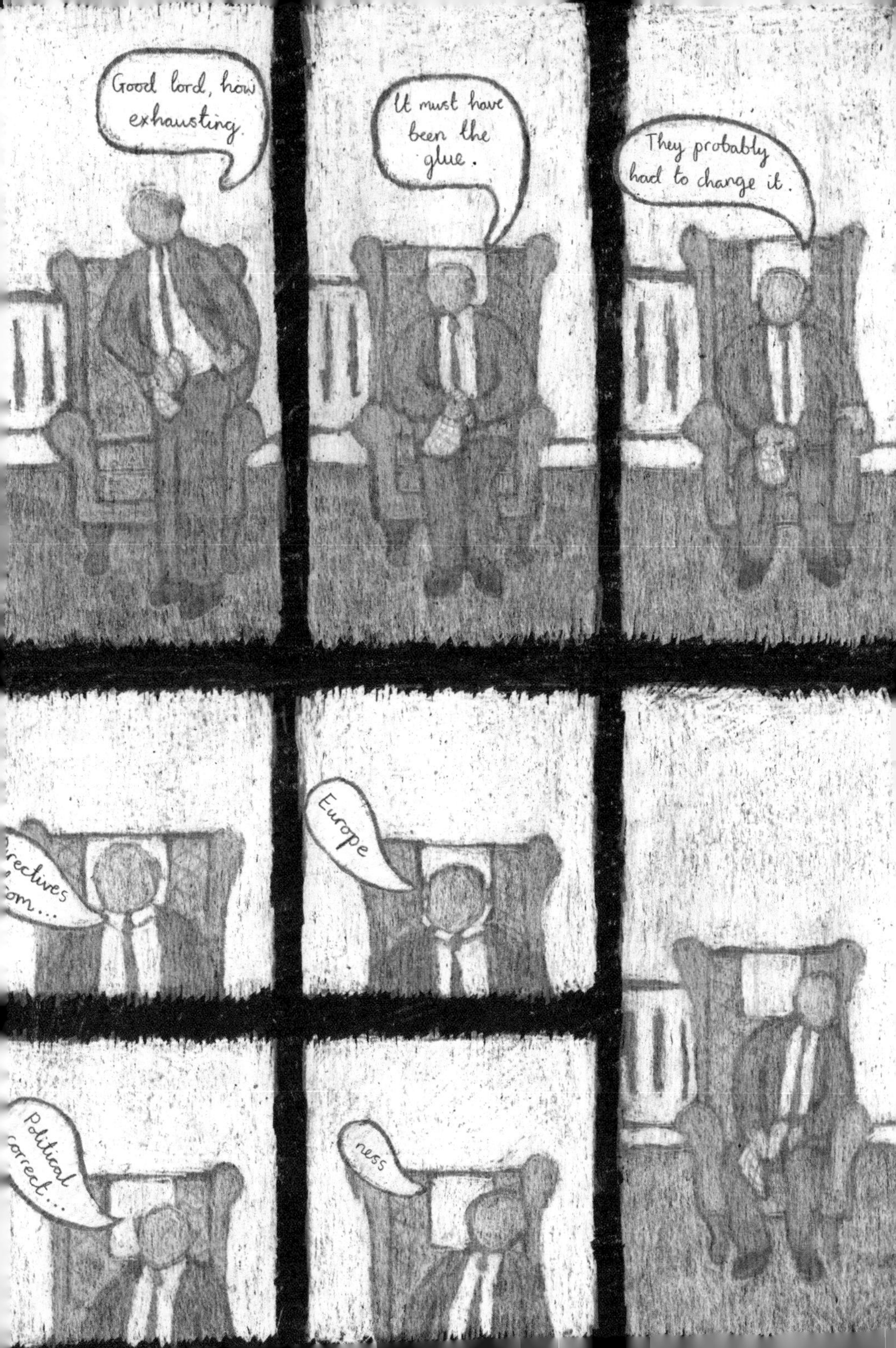
Good lord, how exhausting.
It must have been the glue.
They probably had to change it.
rectives
om…
Europe
Political
correct…
ness

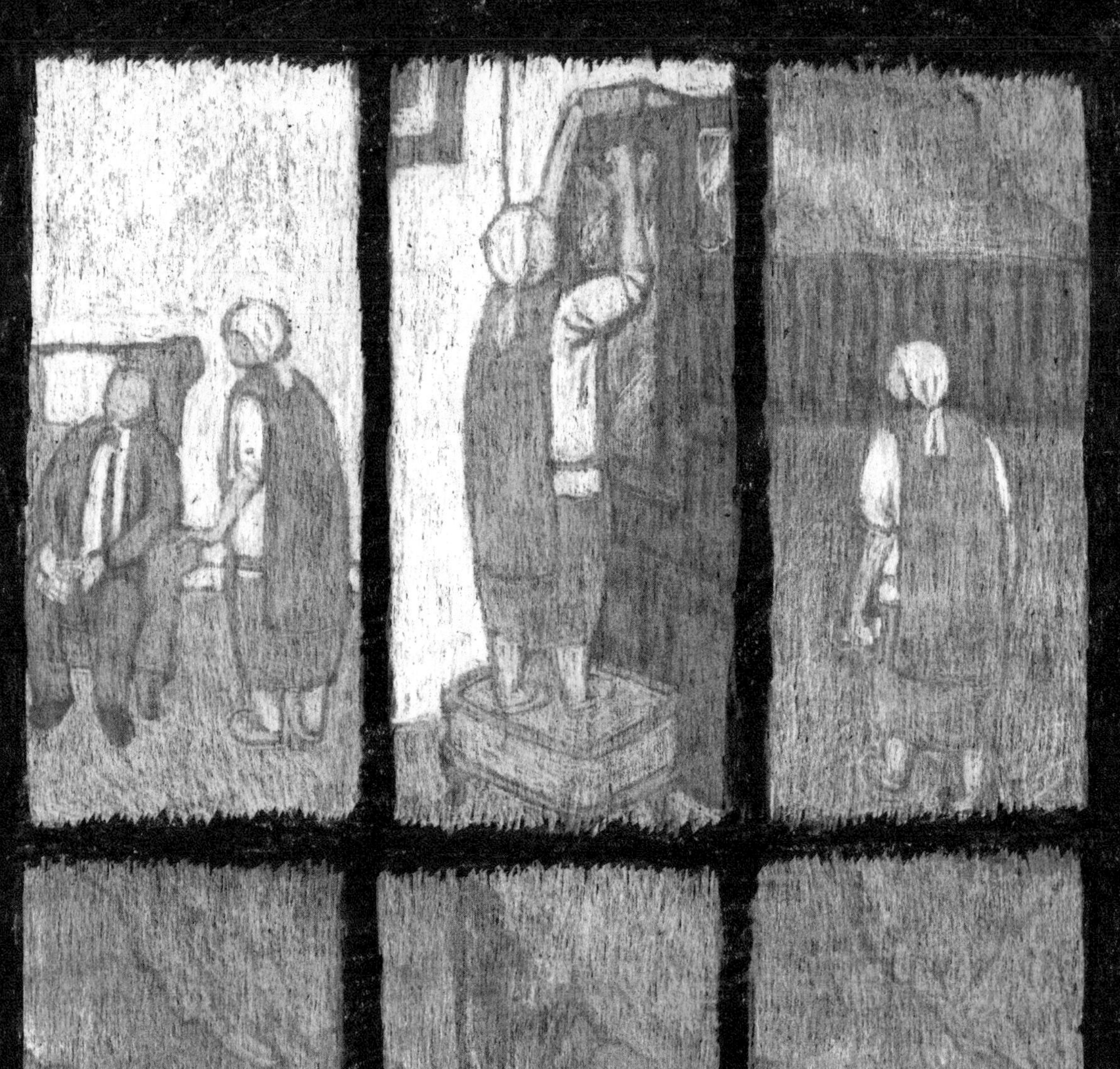

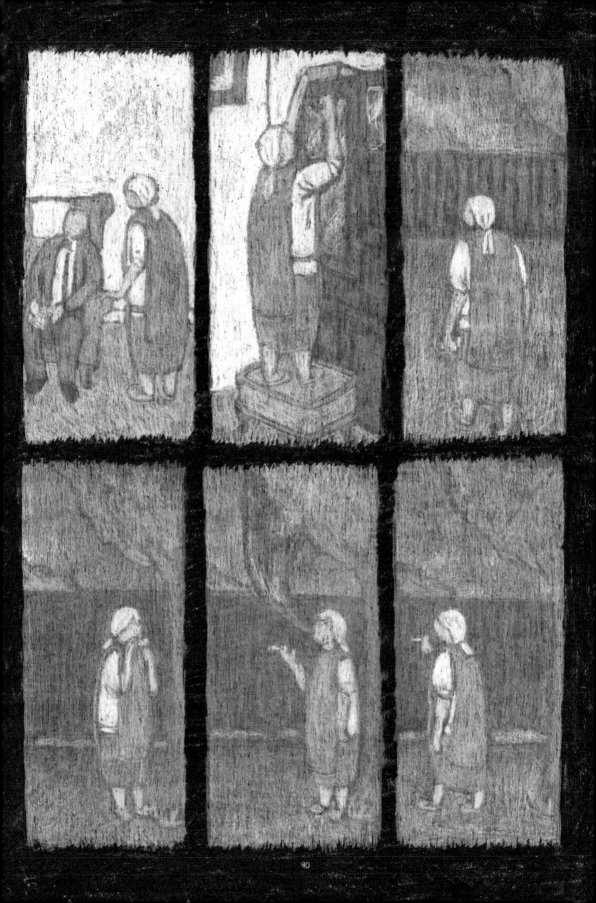

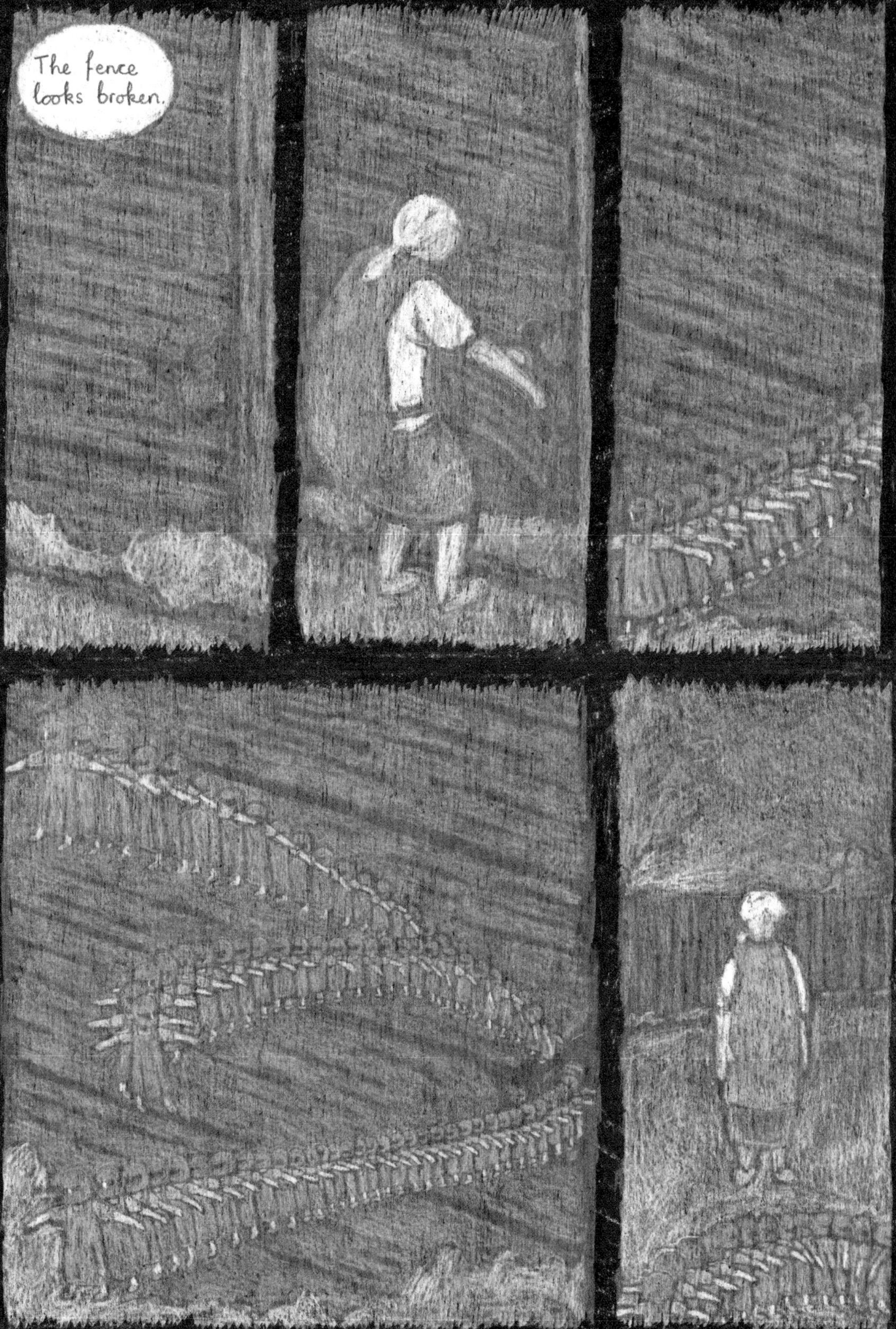
The fence looks broken.

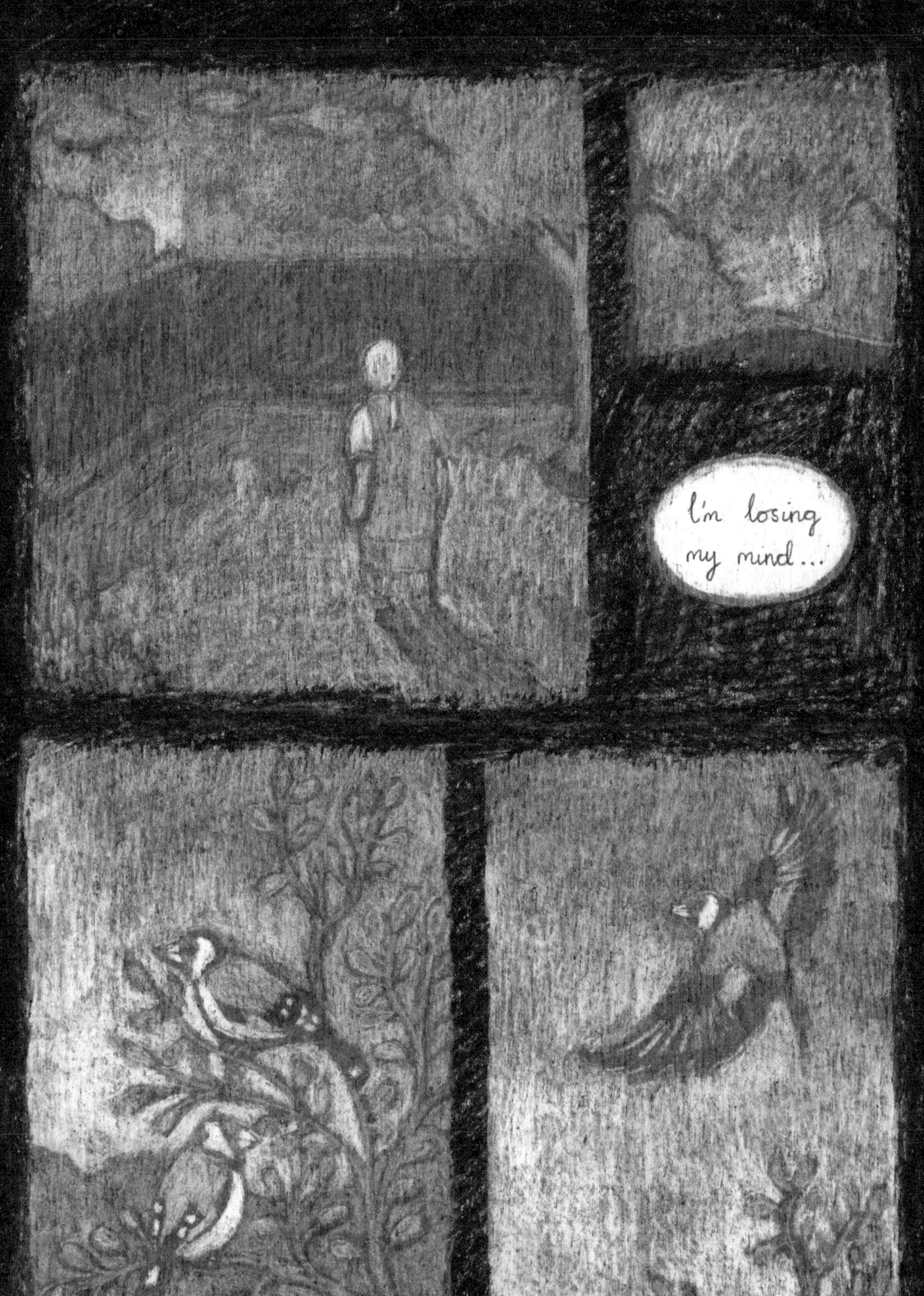
I'm losing my mind...

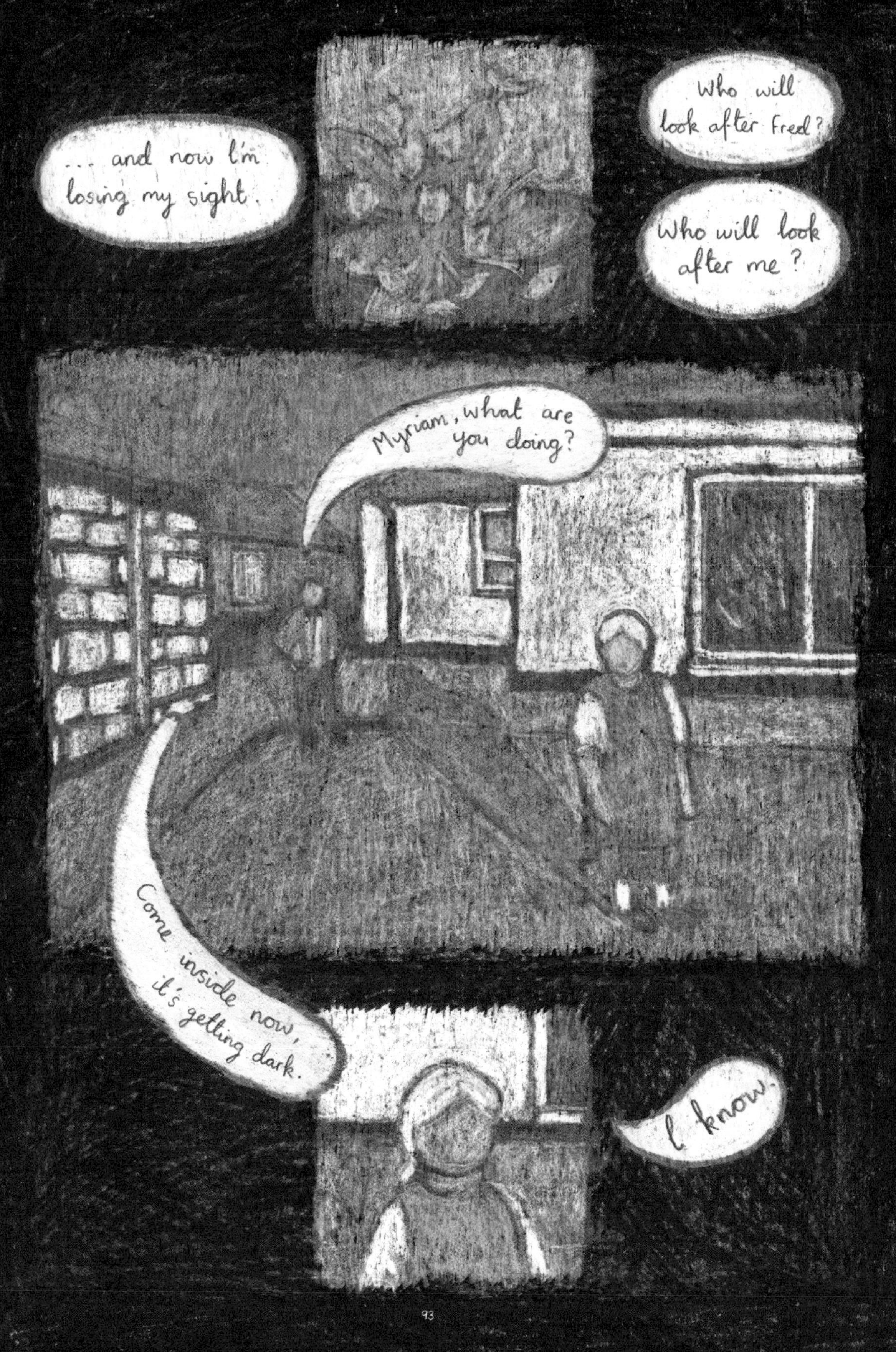
... and now I'm losing my sight.
Who will look after Fred?
Who will look after me?
Myriam, what are you doing?
Come inside now, it's getting dark.
I know.

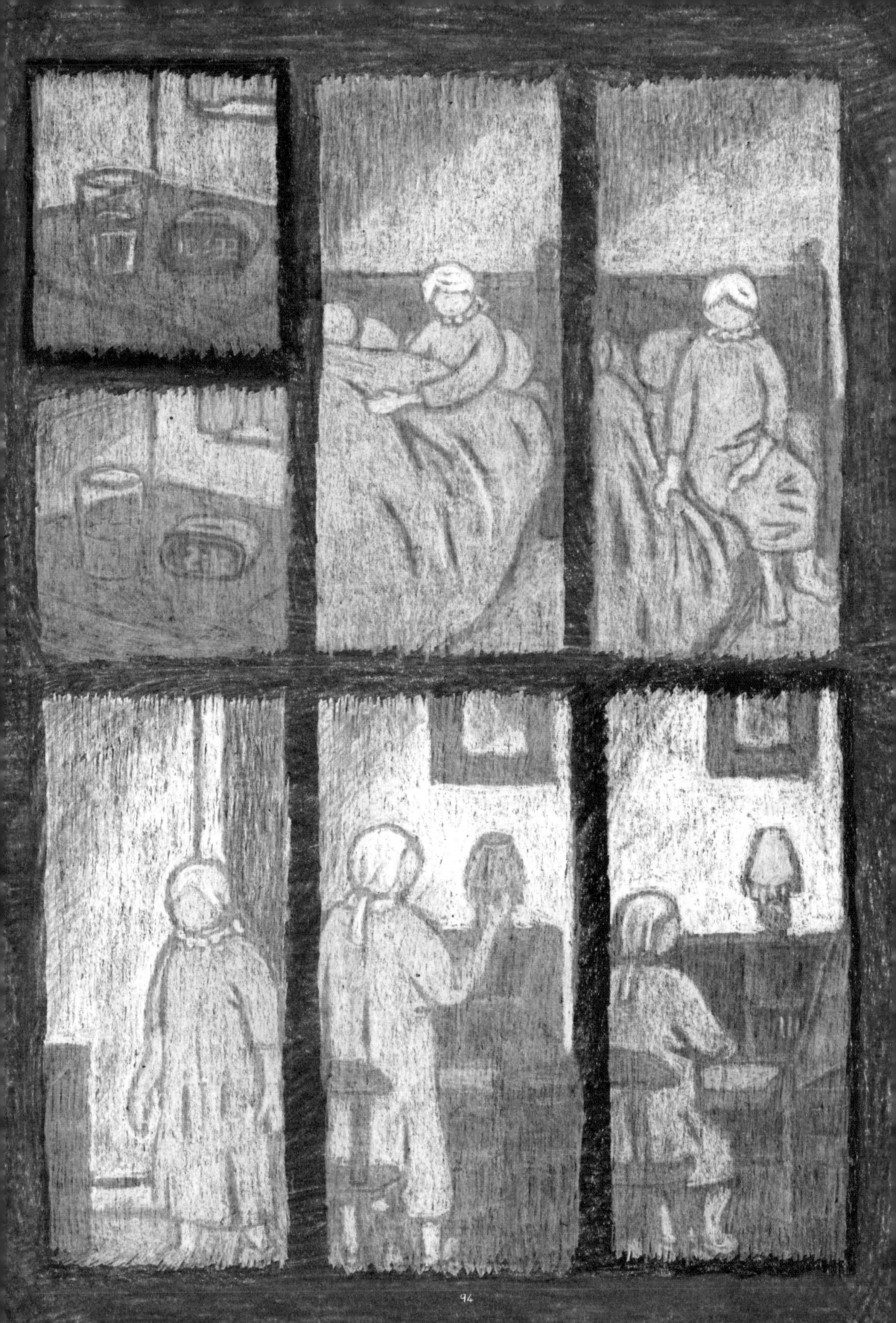

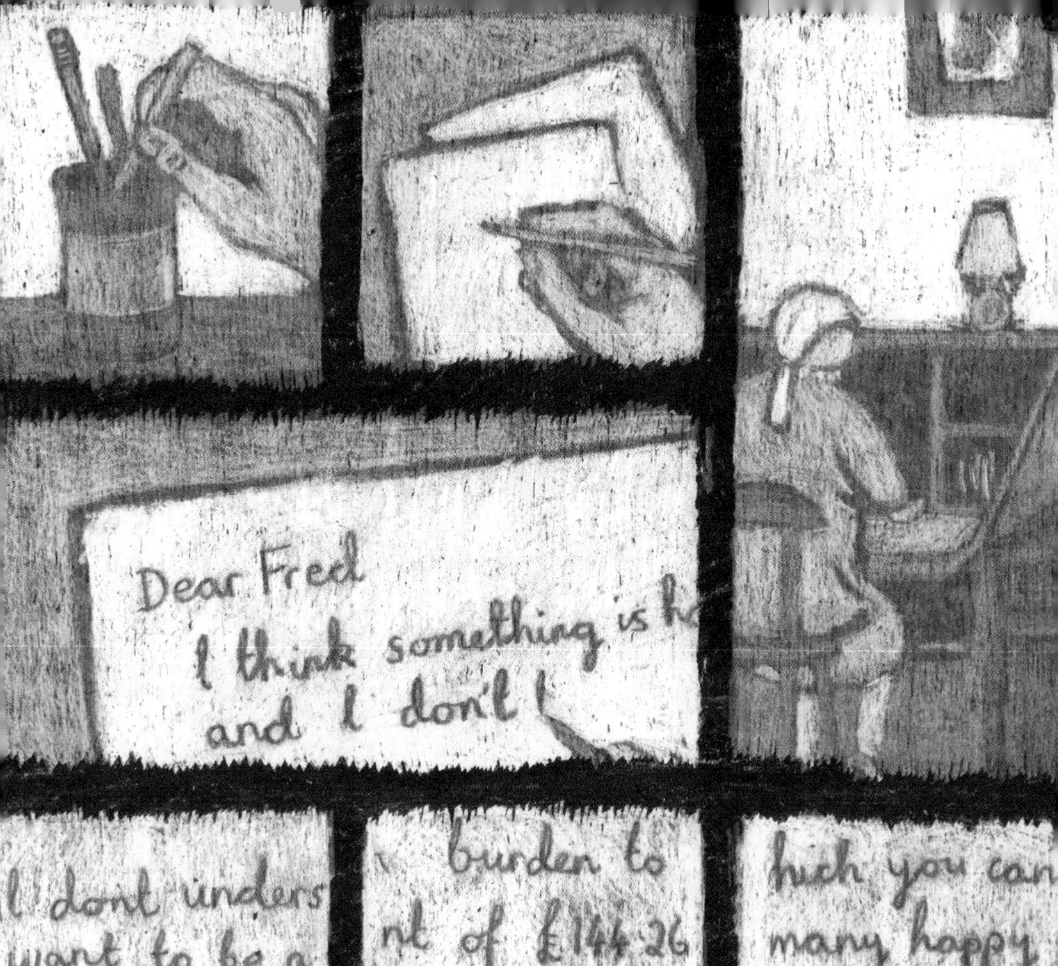
Dear Fred
I think something is h
and I don't
I dont unders
want to be a
post office a
burden to
nt of £144.26
we have had
hich you can
many happy
can use
an use to
happy
very nice

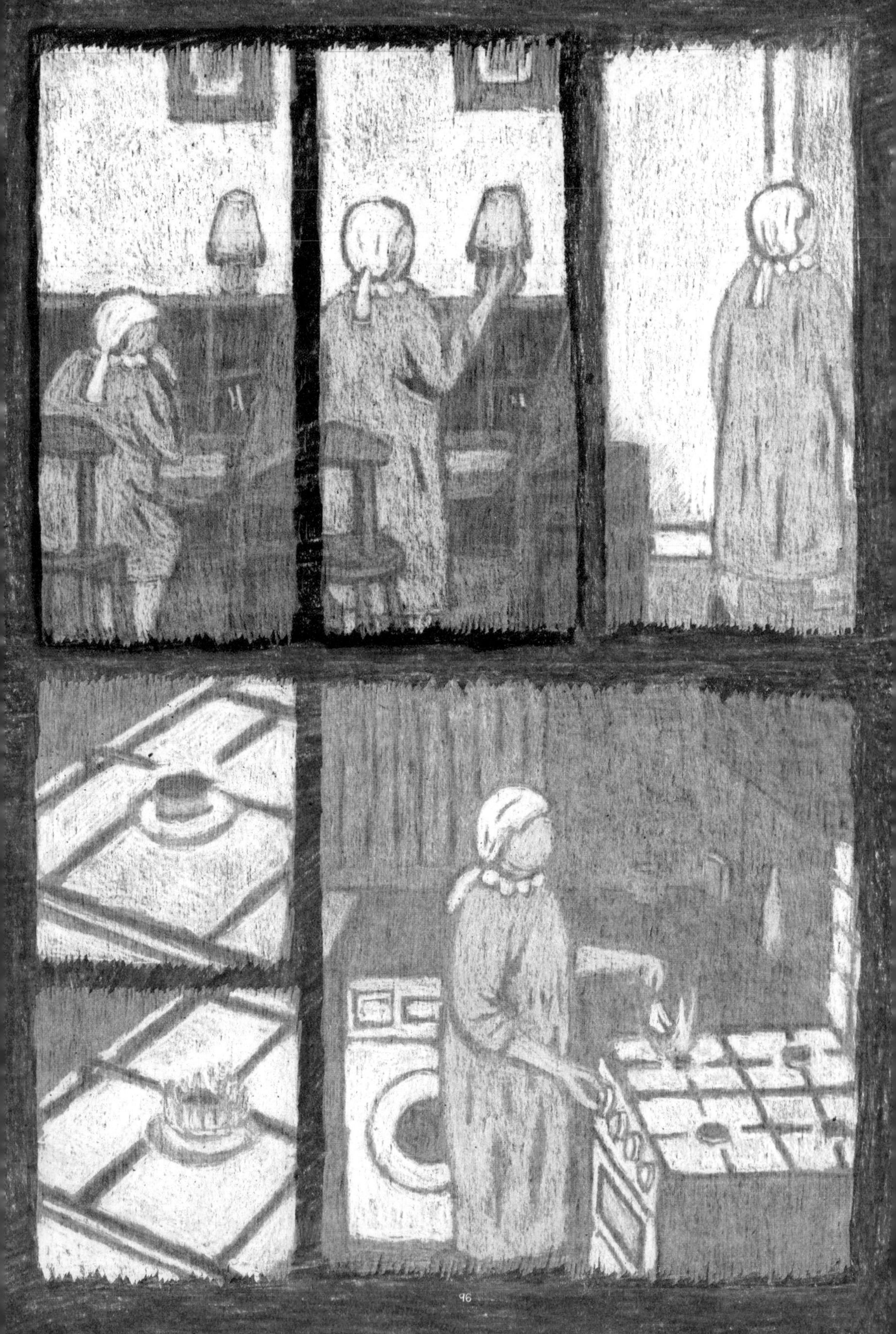

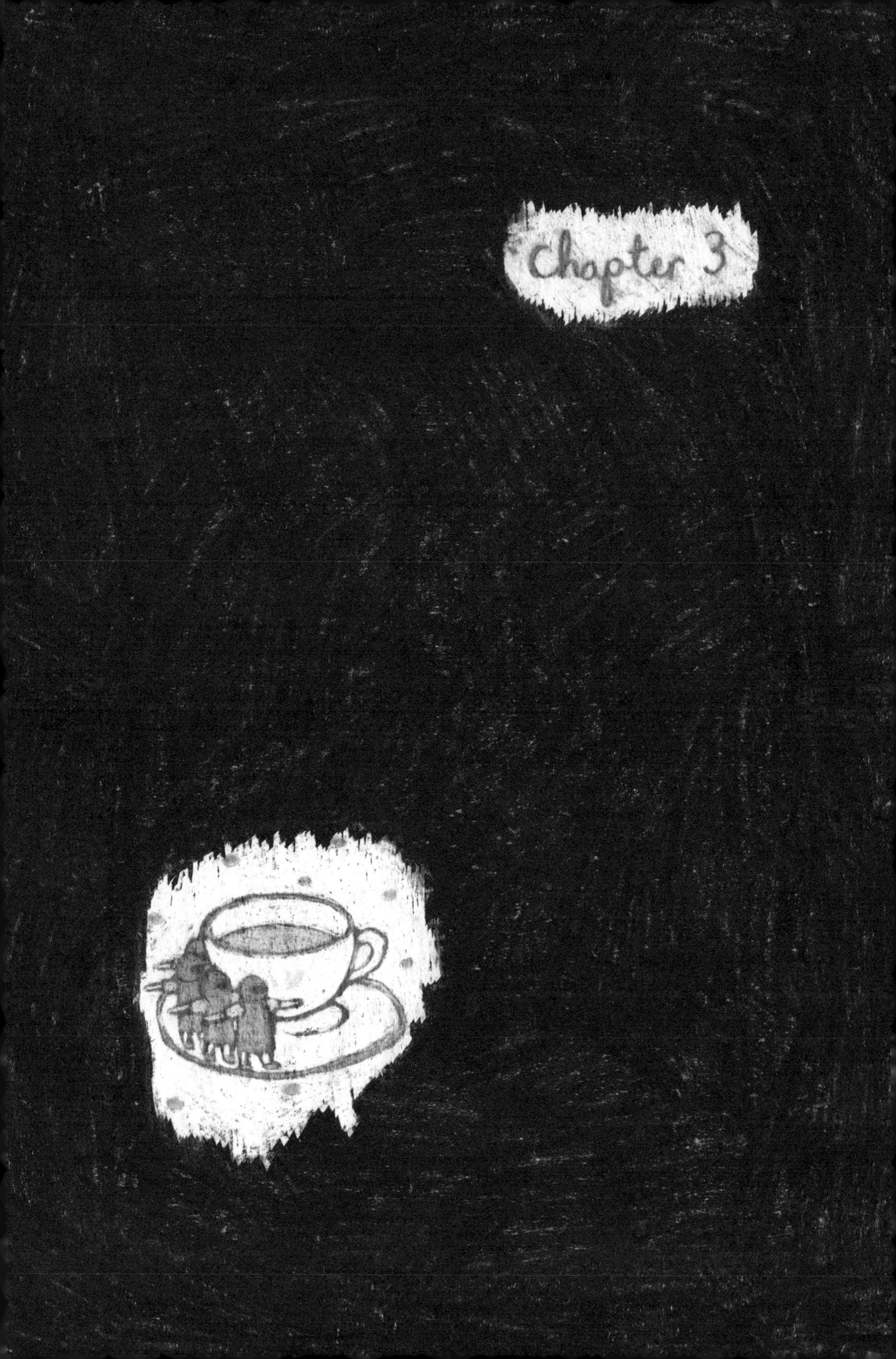
Chapter 3

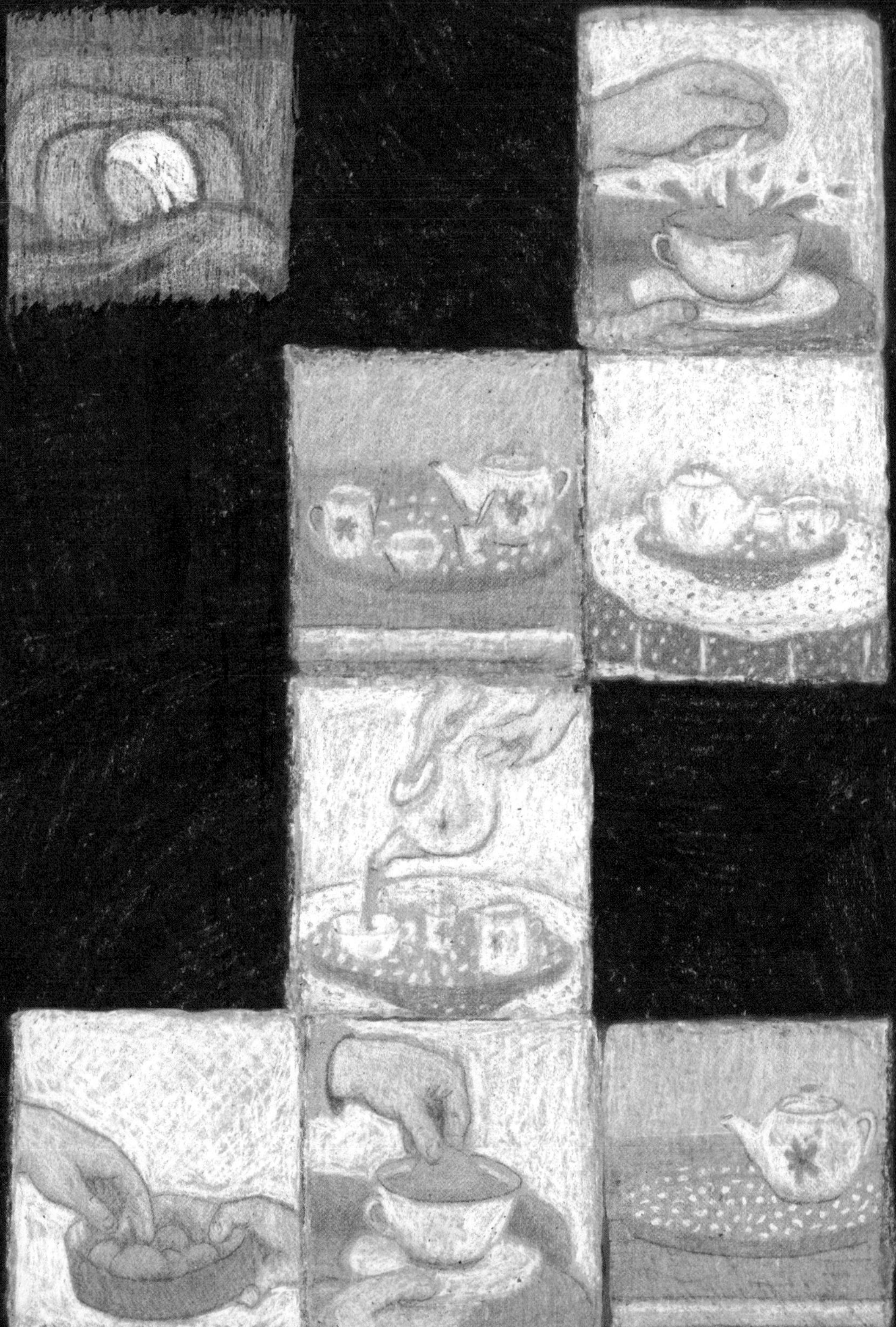

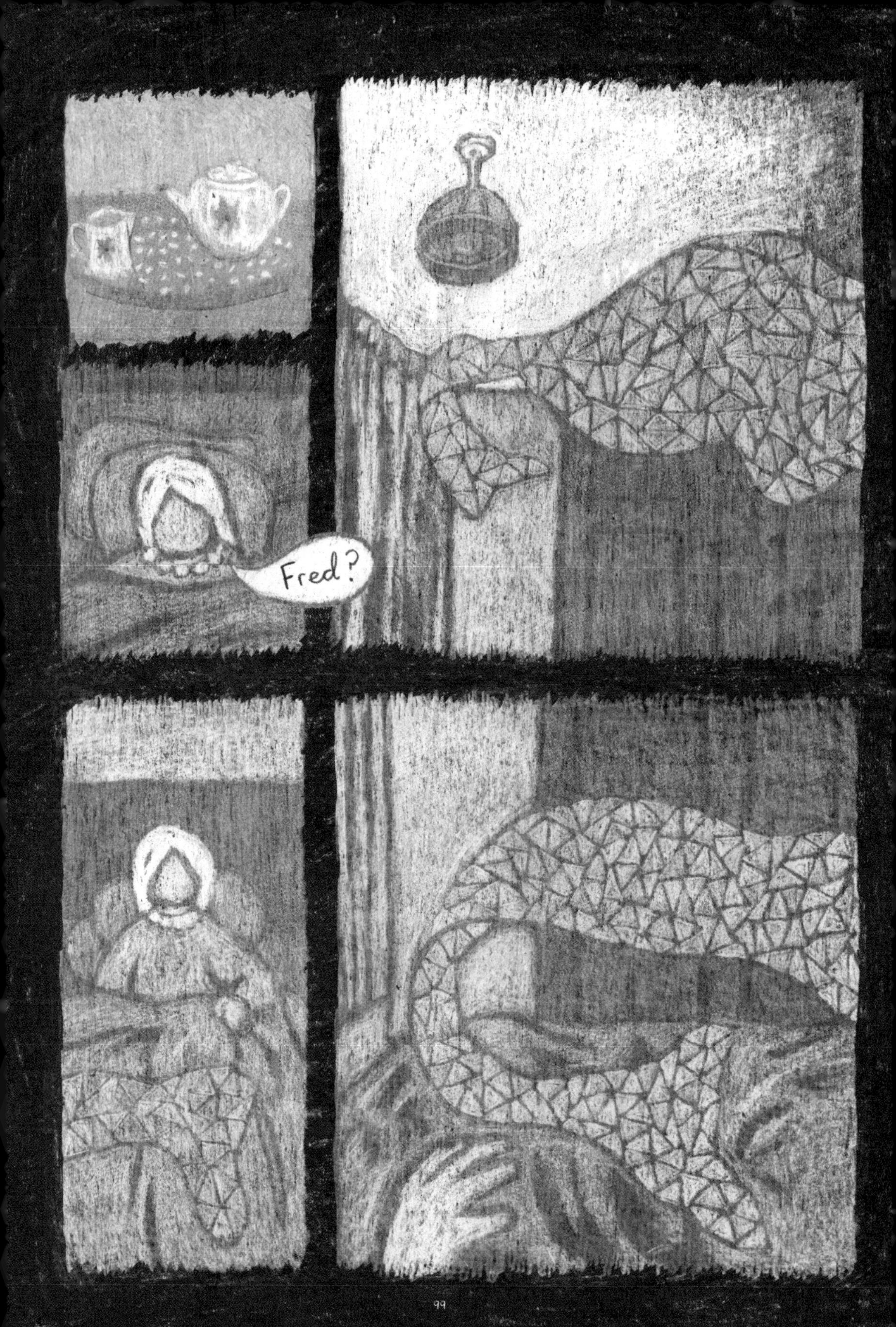
Fred?

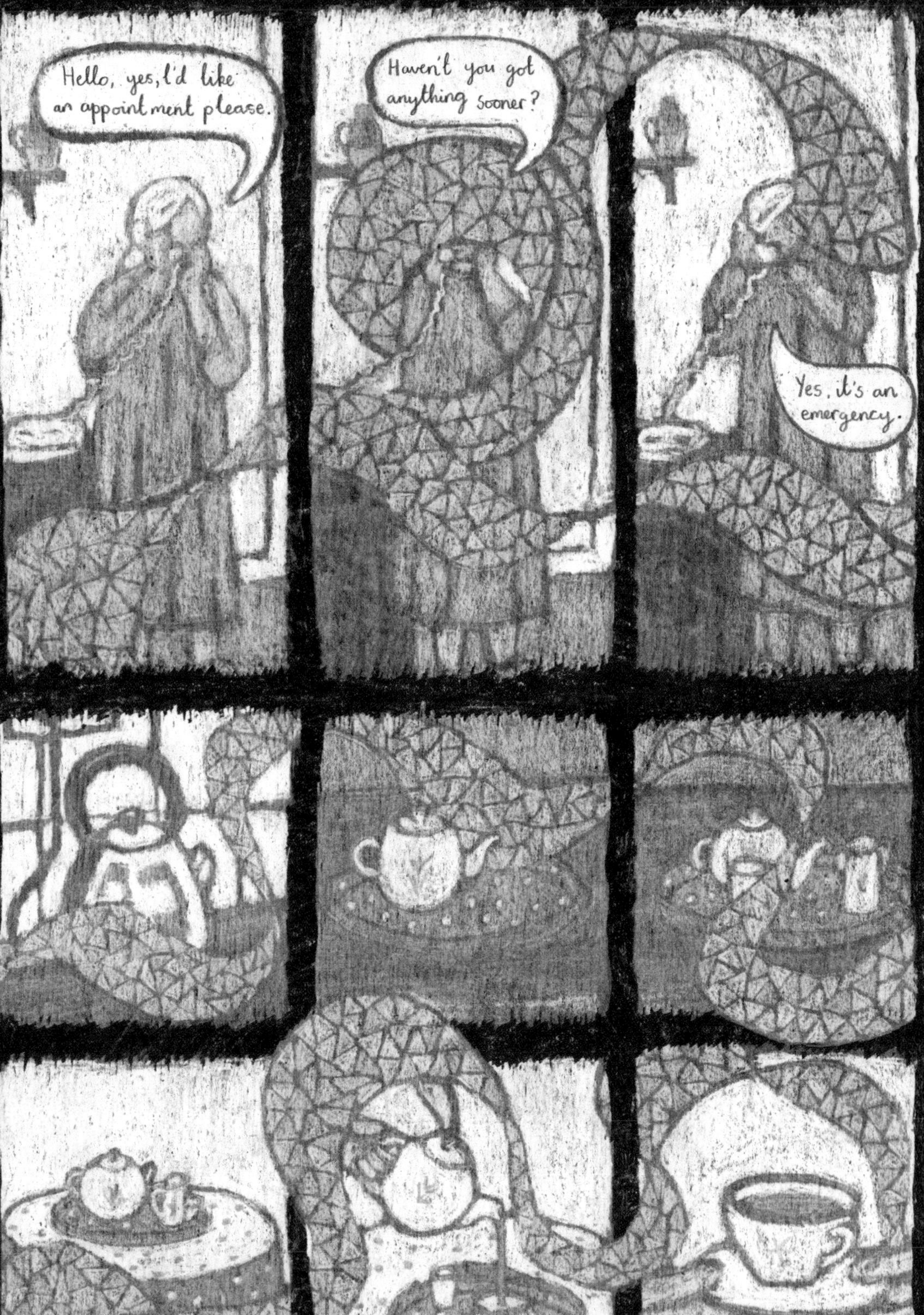
Hello, yes, I'd like an appointment please.
Haven't you got anything sooner?
Yes, it's an emergency.

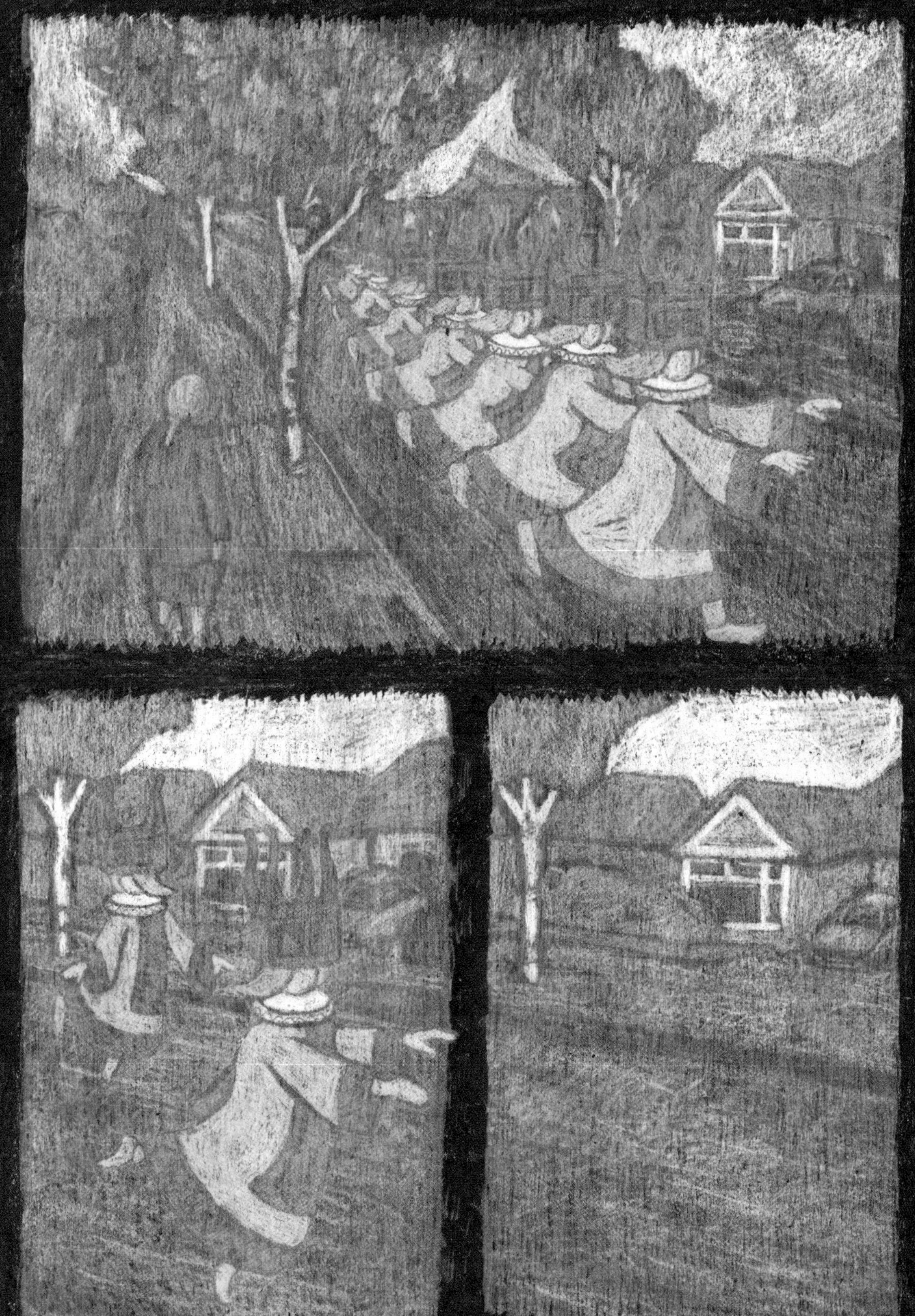

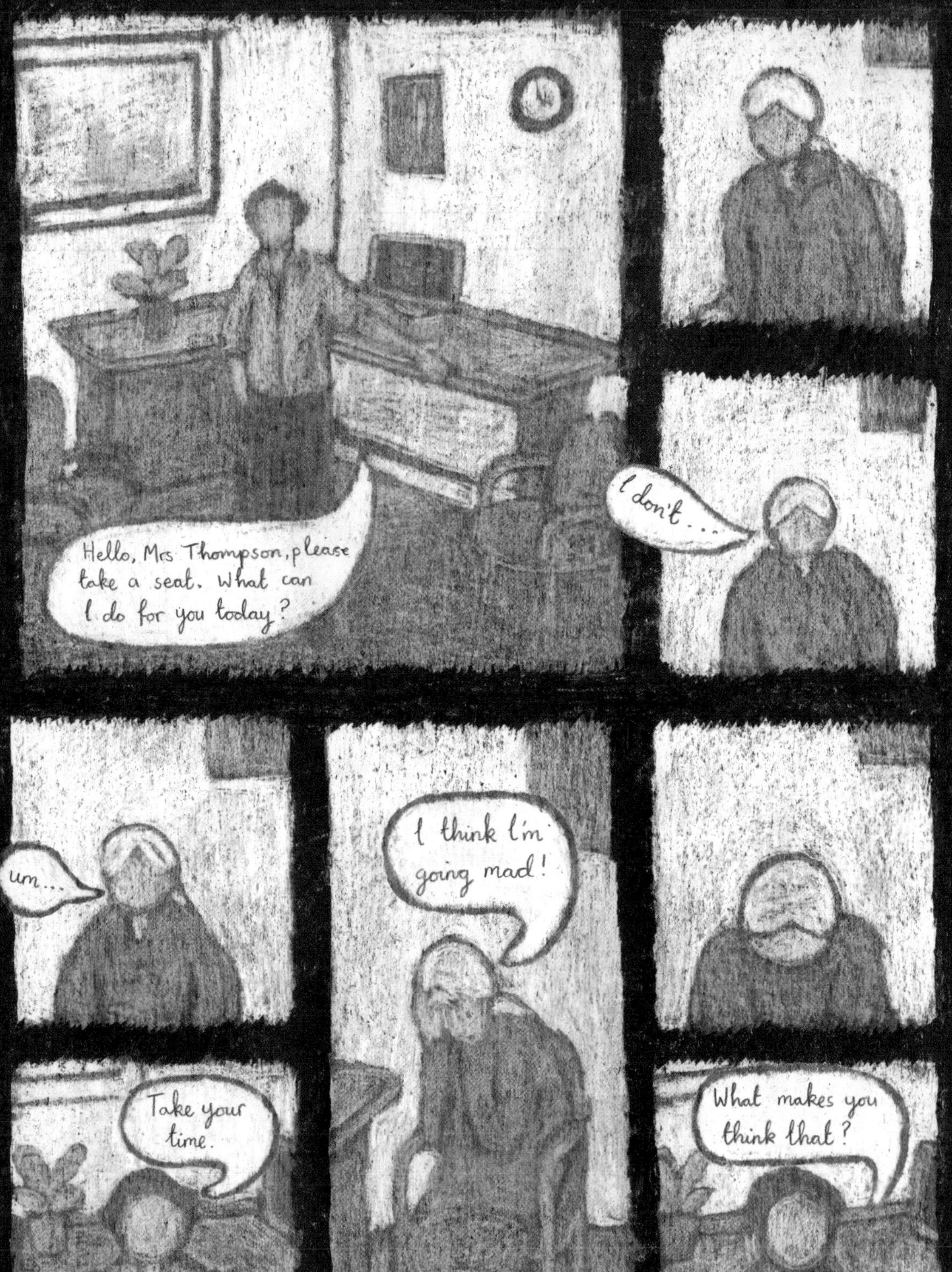
Hello, Mrs Thompson, please take a seat. What can I do for you today?
I don't...
um...
I think I'm going mad!
Take your time.
What makes you think that?

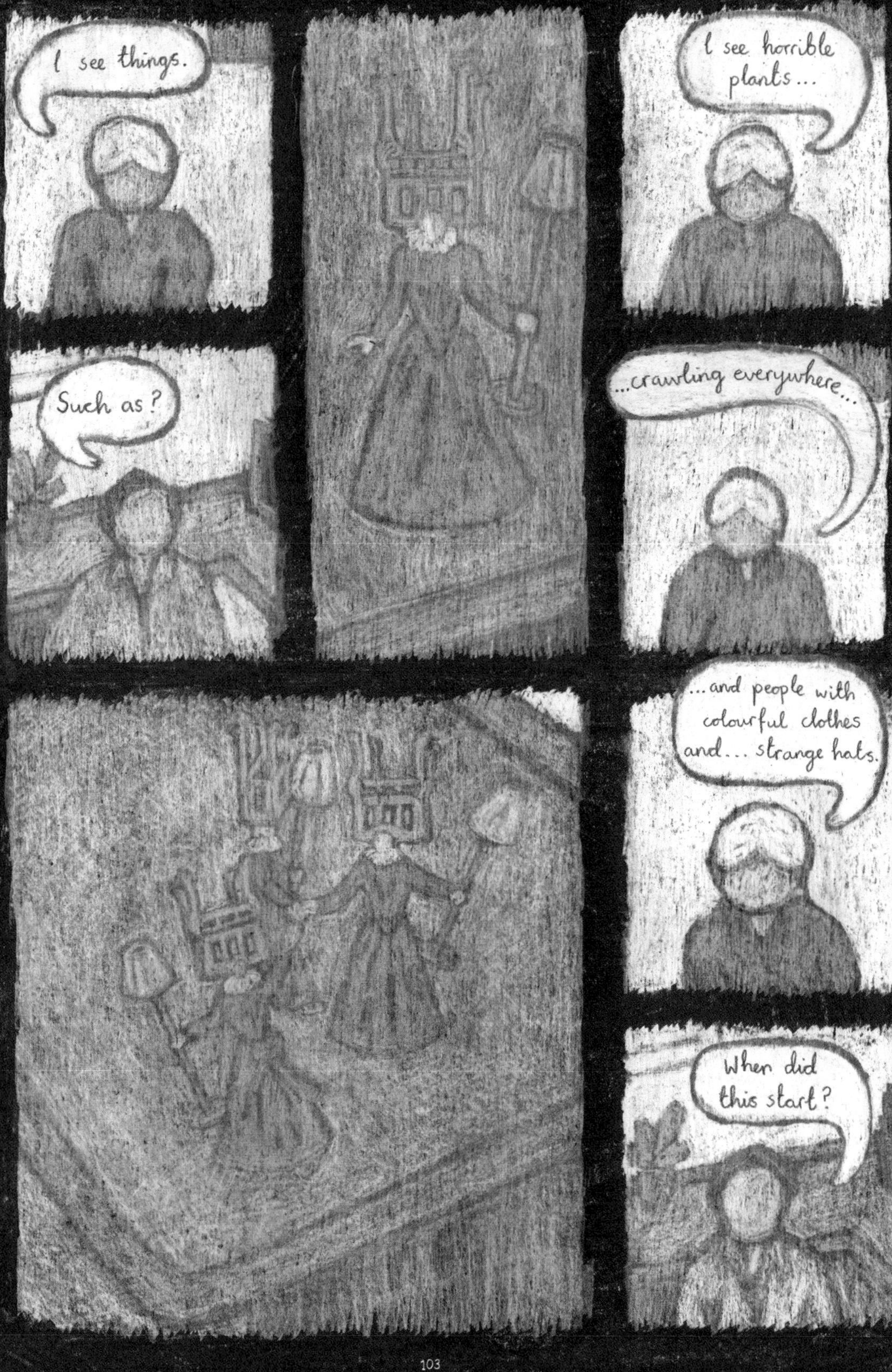
I see things.
Such as?
I see horrible plants...
...crawling everywhere...
...and people with colourful clothes and... strange hats.
When did this start?

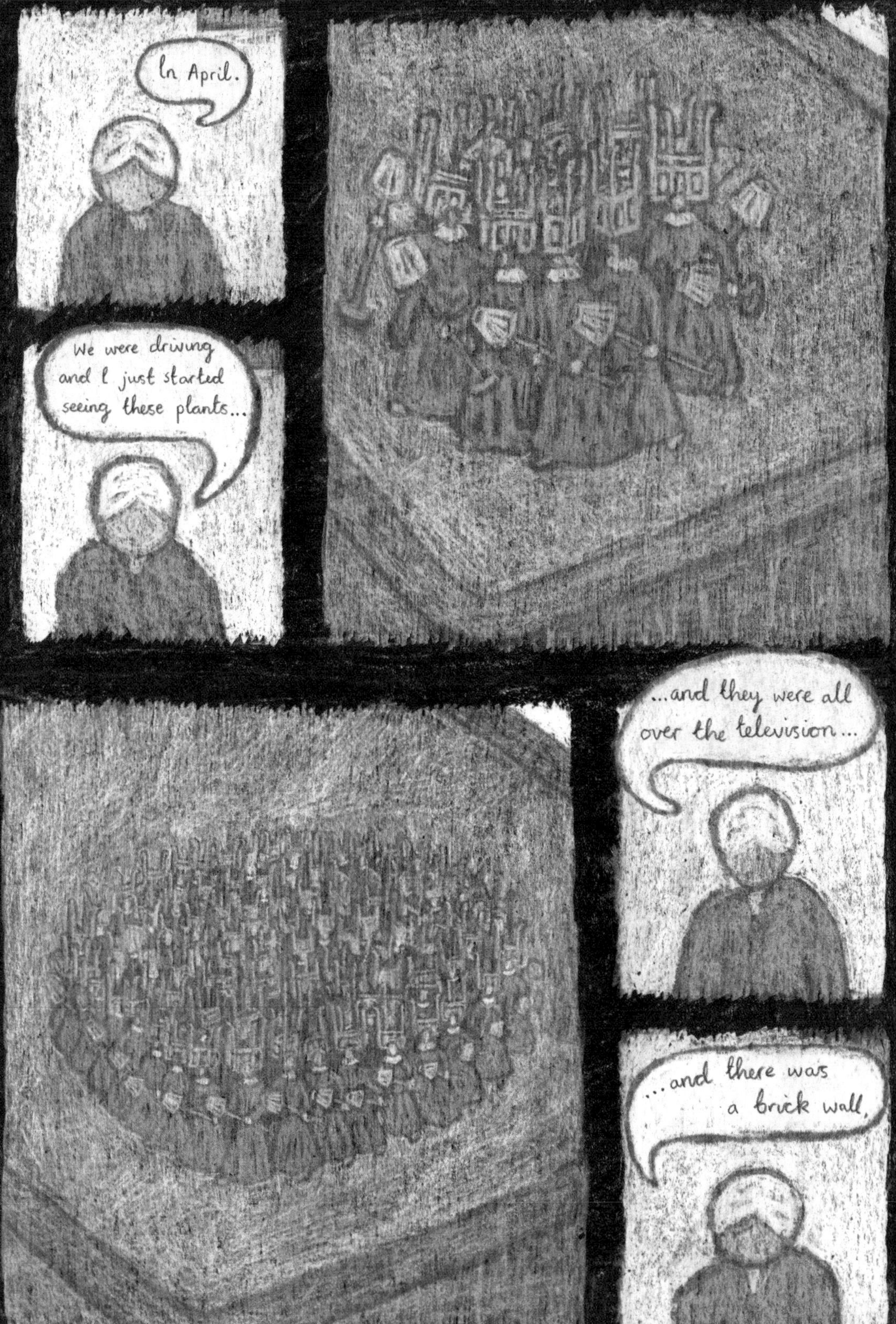
In April.
We were driving and I just started seeing these plants...
...and they were all over the television...
...and there was a brick wall,

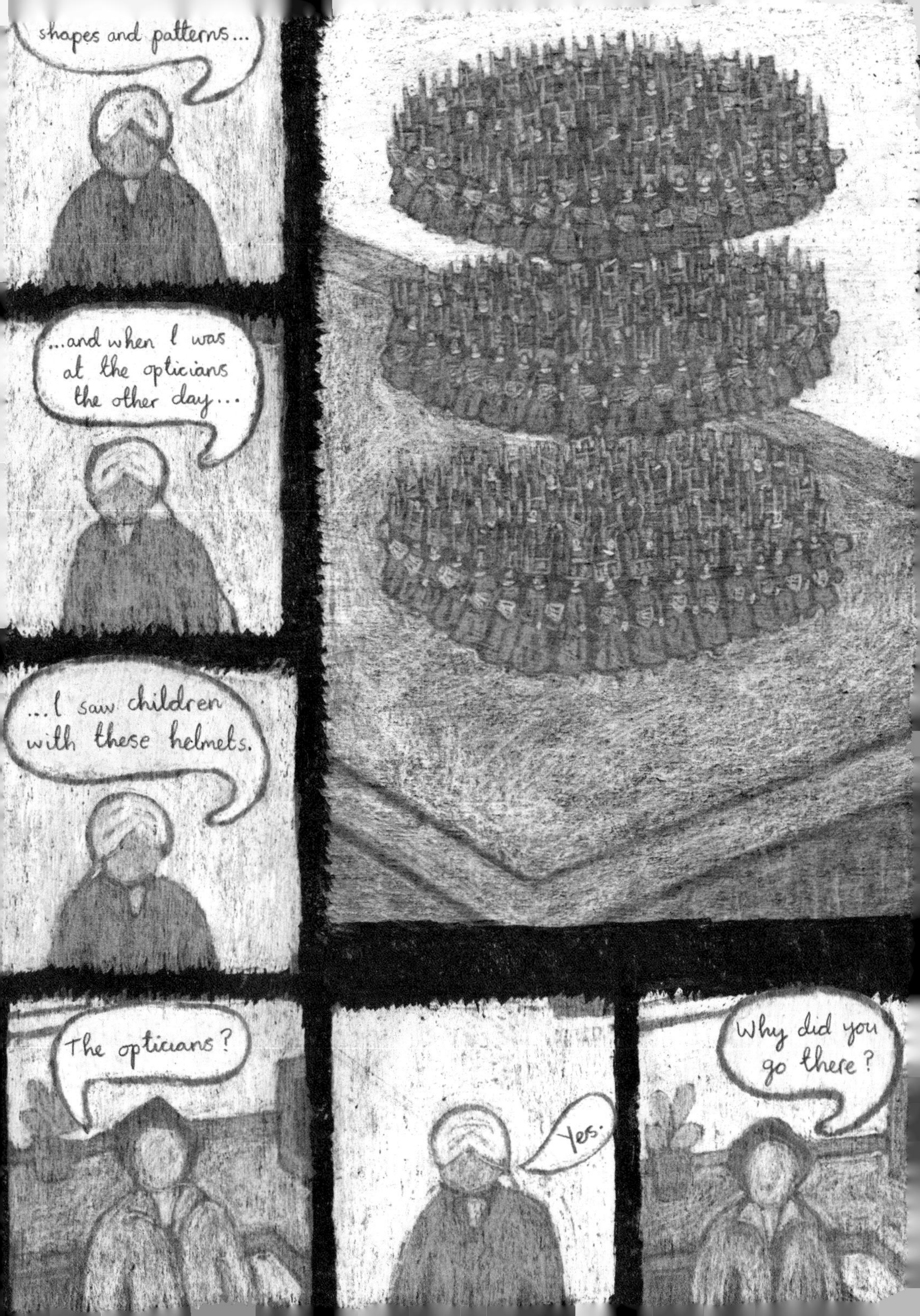

shapes and patterns...
...and when I was at the opticians the other day...
...I saw children with these helmets.
The opticians?
Yes.
Why did you go there?

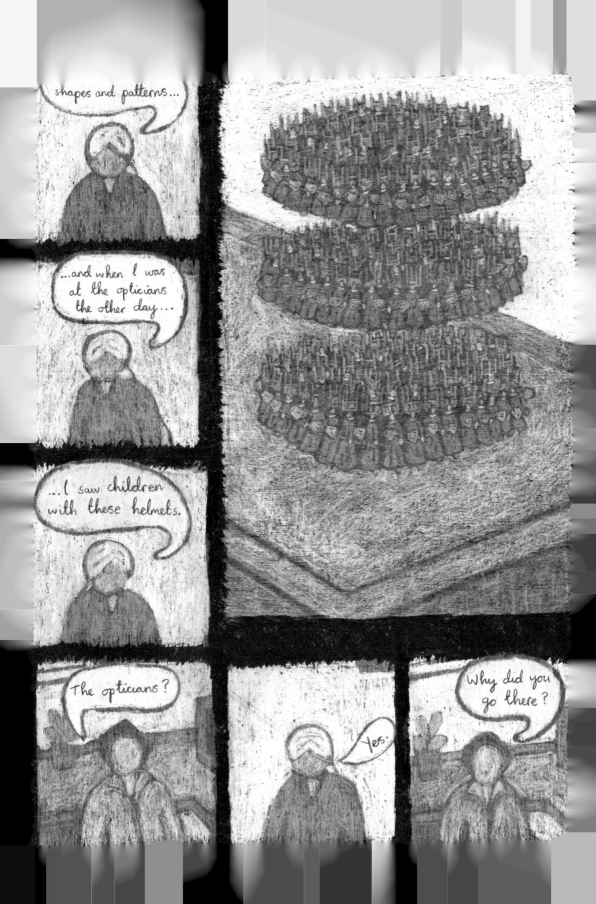

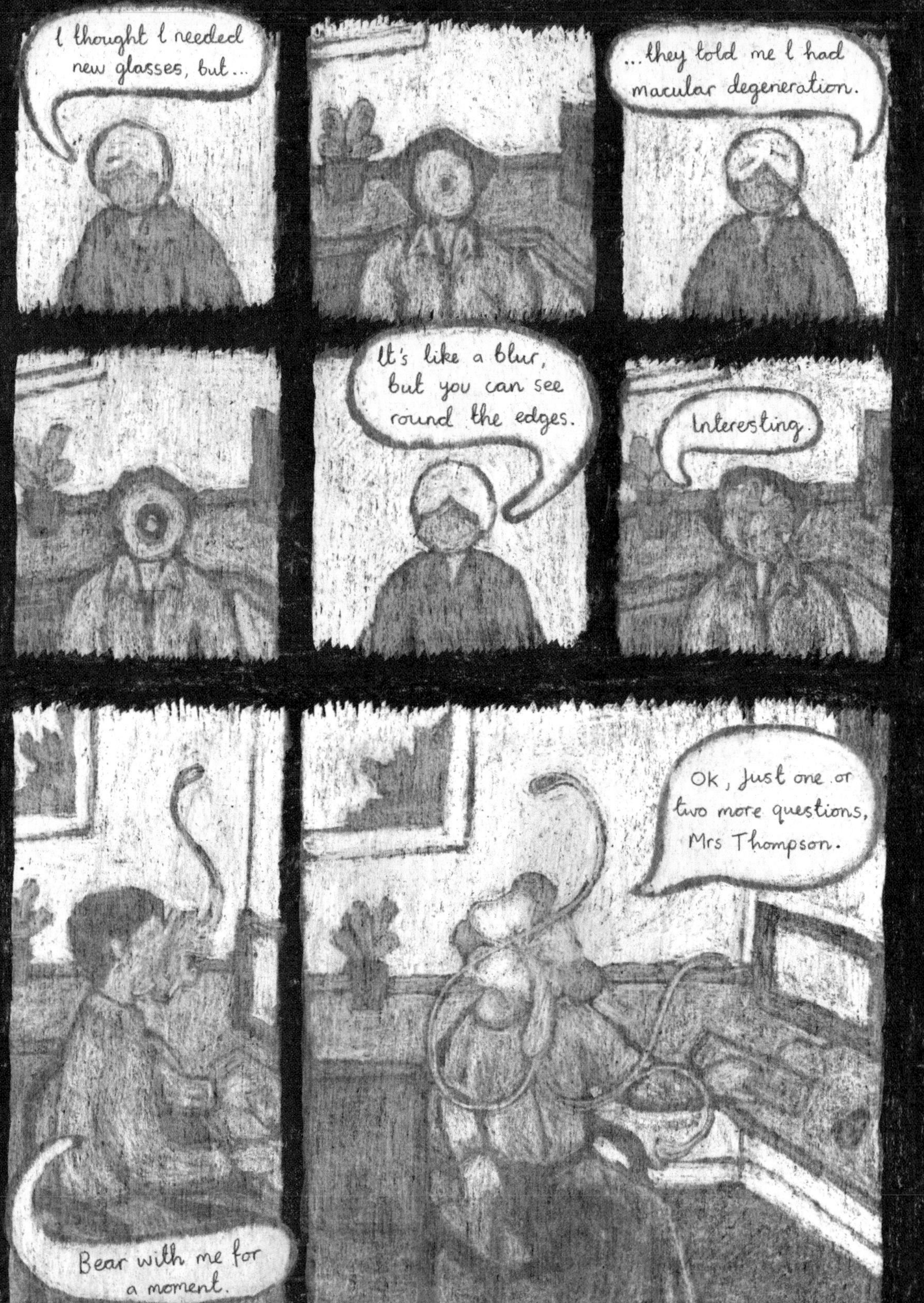
I thought I needed new glasses, but...
...they told me I had macular degeneration.
It's like a blur, but you can see round the edges.
Interesting.
Bear with me for a moment.
Ok, Just one or two more questions, Mrs Thompson.

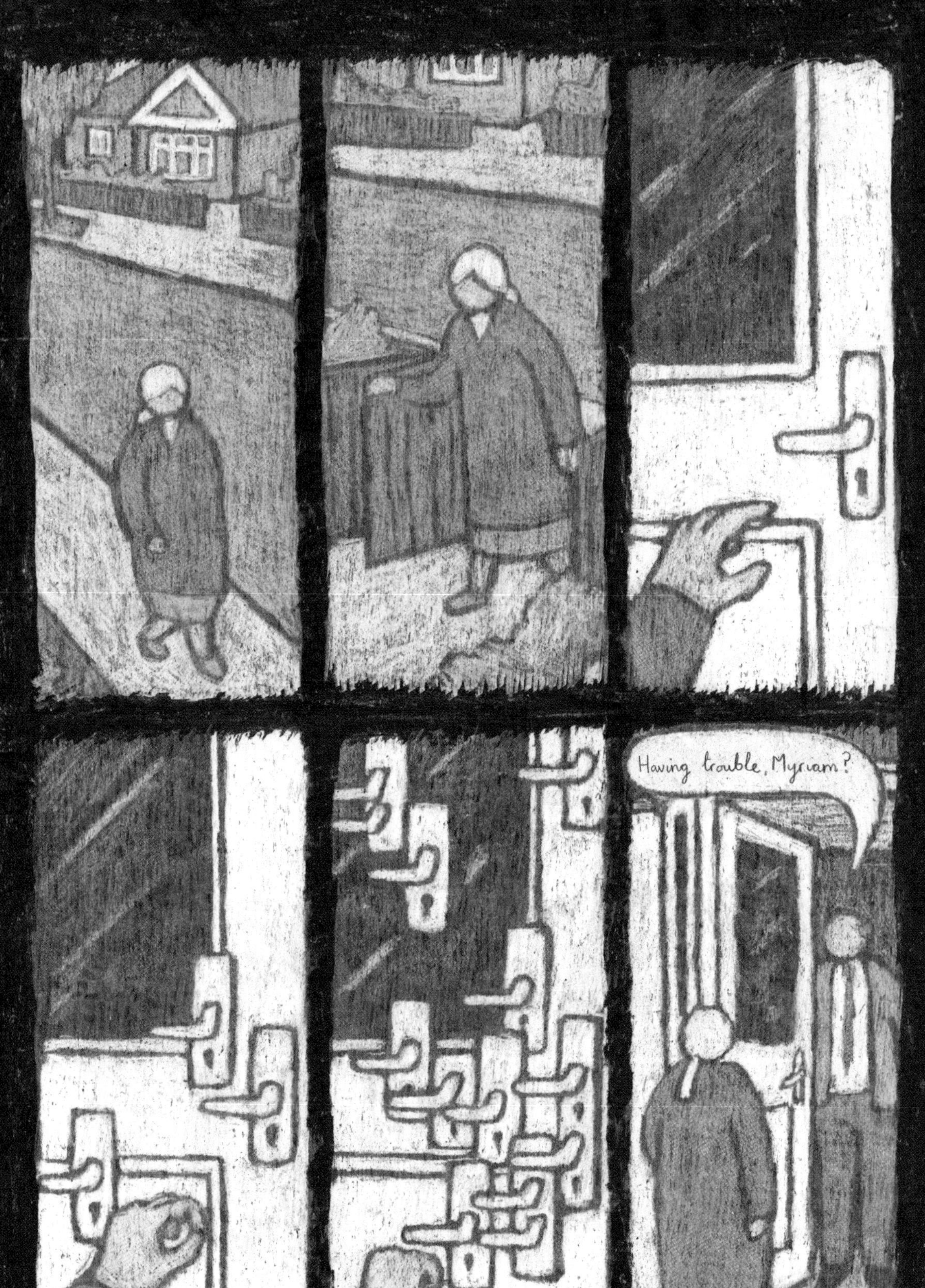
Having trouble, Myriam?

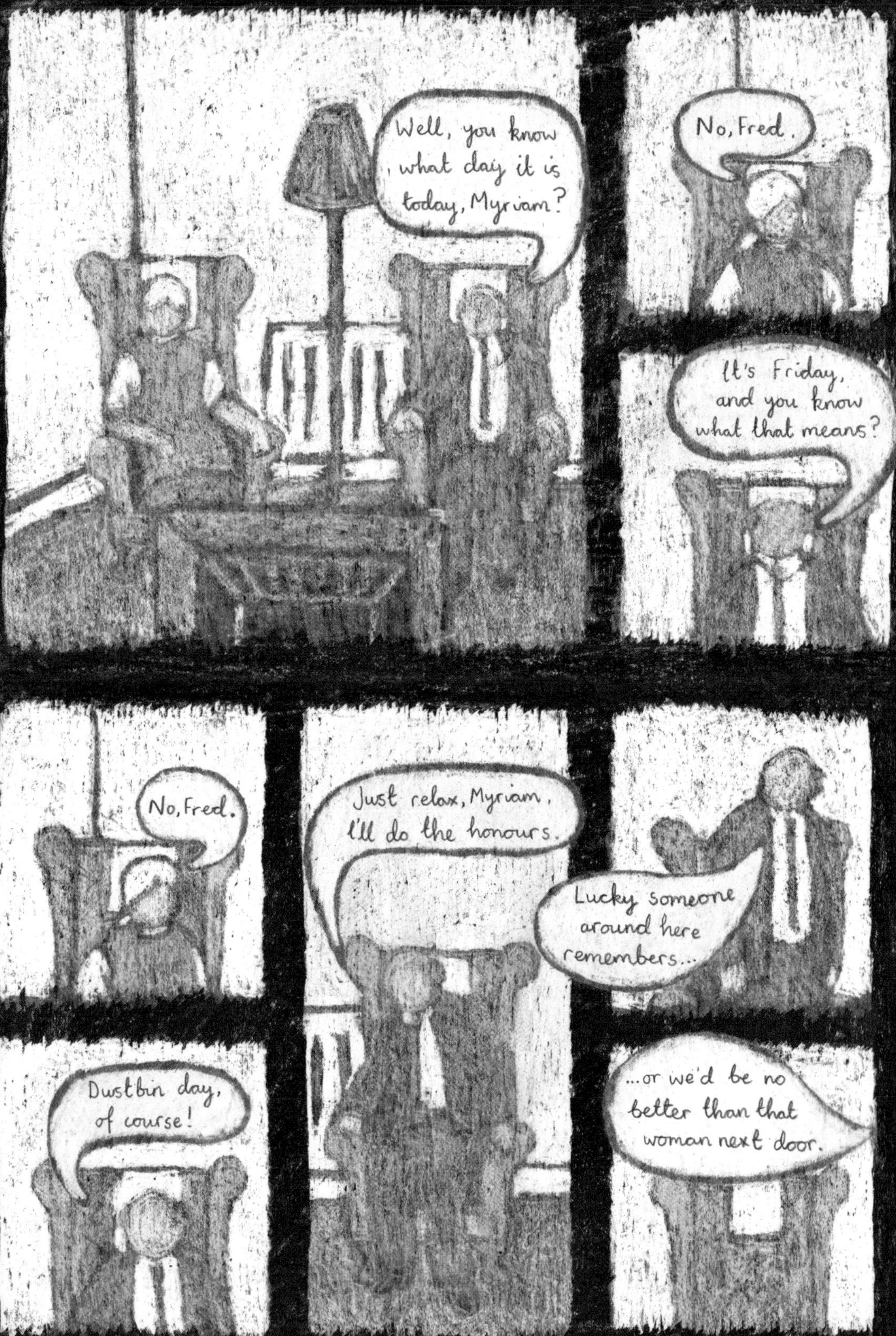
Well, you know what day it is today, Myriam?
No, Fred.
It's Friday, and you know what that means?
No, Fred.
Dustbin day, of course!
Just relax, Myriam, I'll do the honours.
Lucky someone around here remembers...
...or we'd be no better than that woman next door.

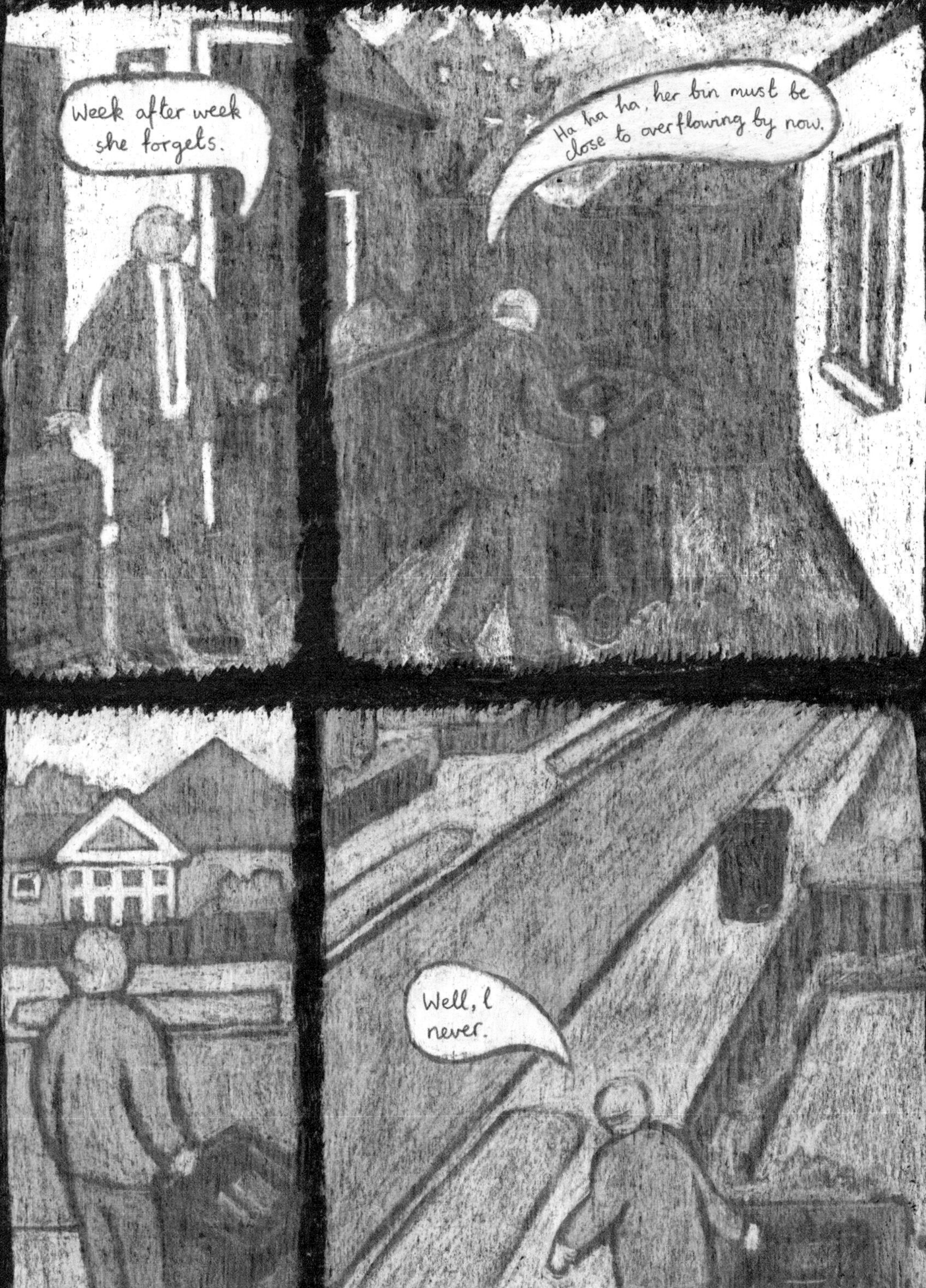
Week after week she forgets.
Ha ha ha, her bin must be close to overflowing by now.
Well, I never.

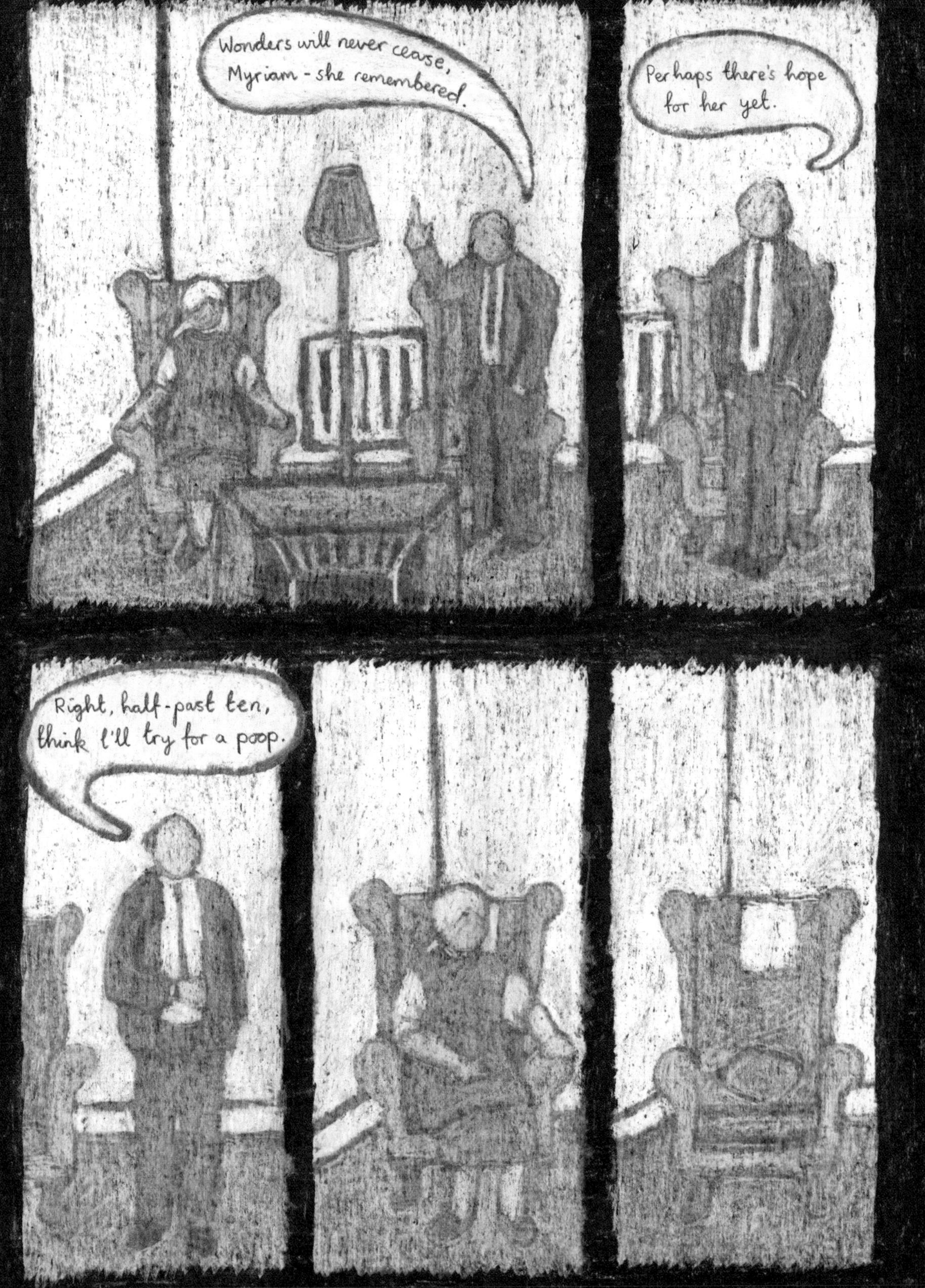
Wonders will never cease, Myriam - she remembered.
Perhaps there's hope for her yet.
Right, half-past ten, think I'll try for a poop.

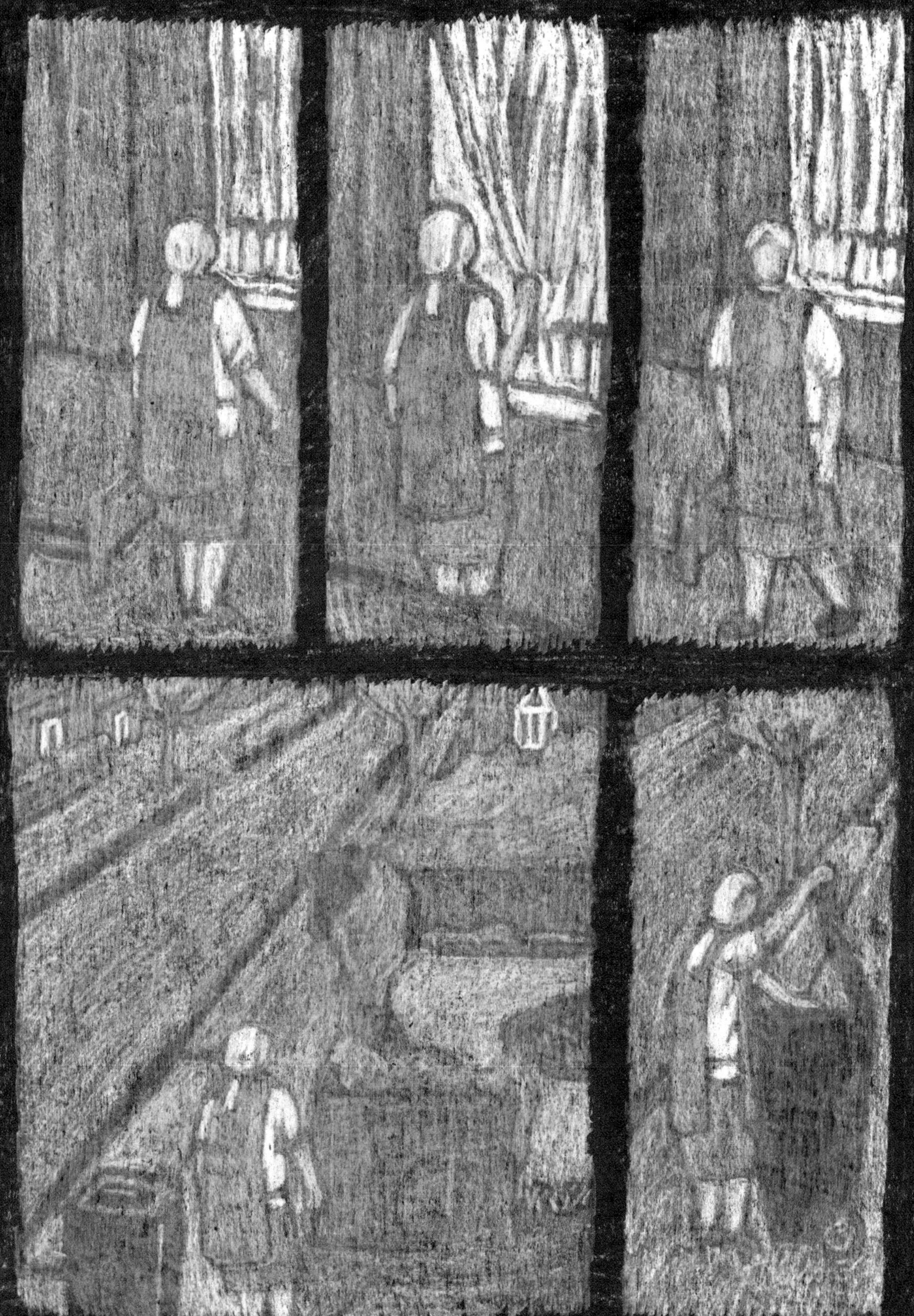

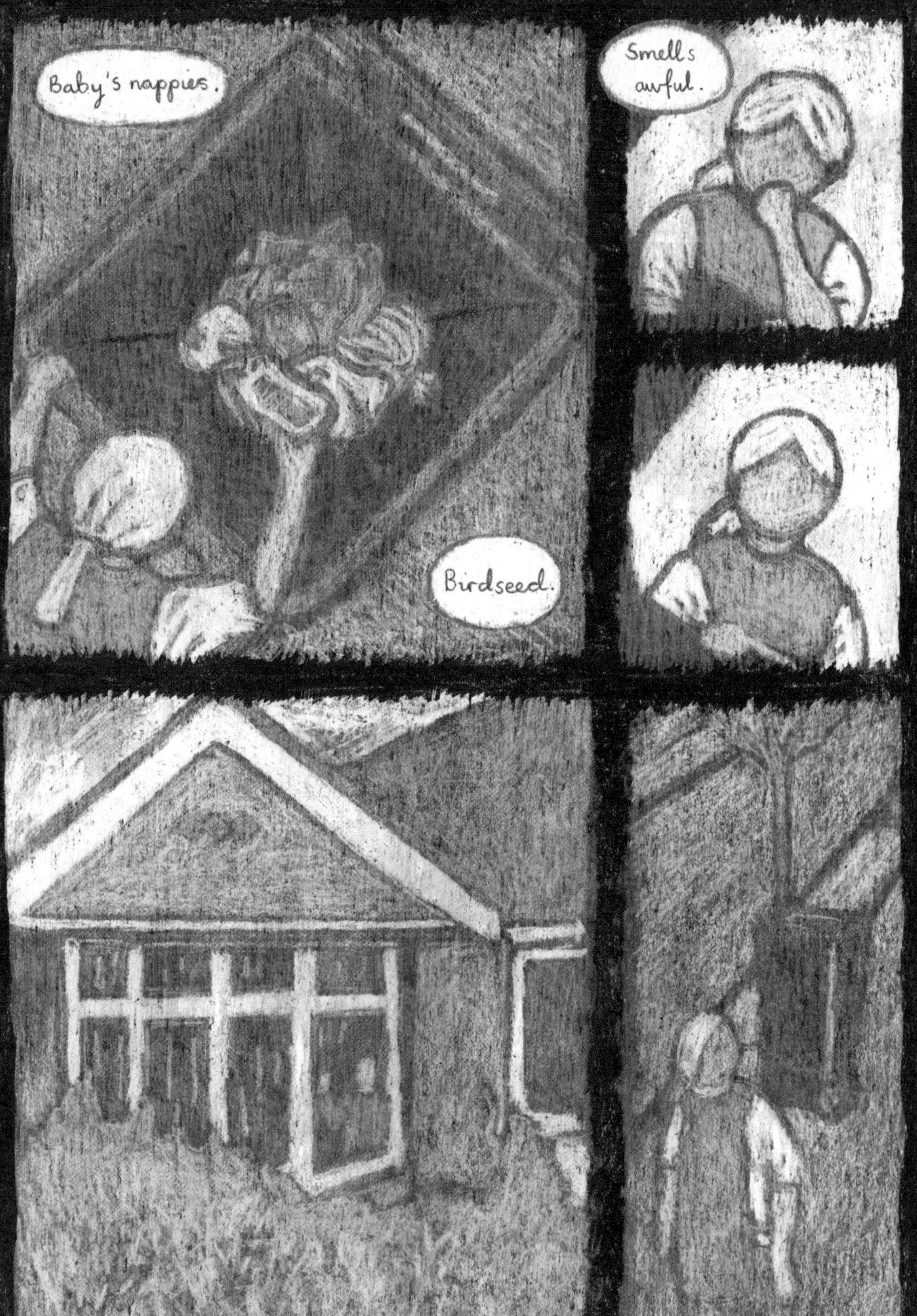
Baby's nappies.
Birdseed.
Smells awful.

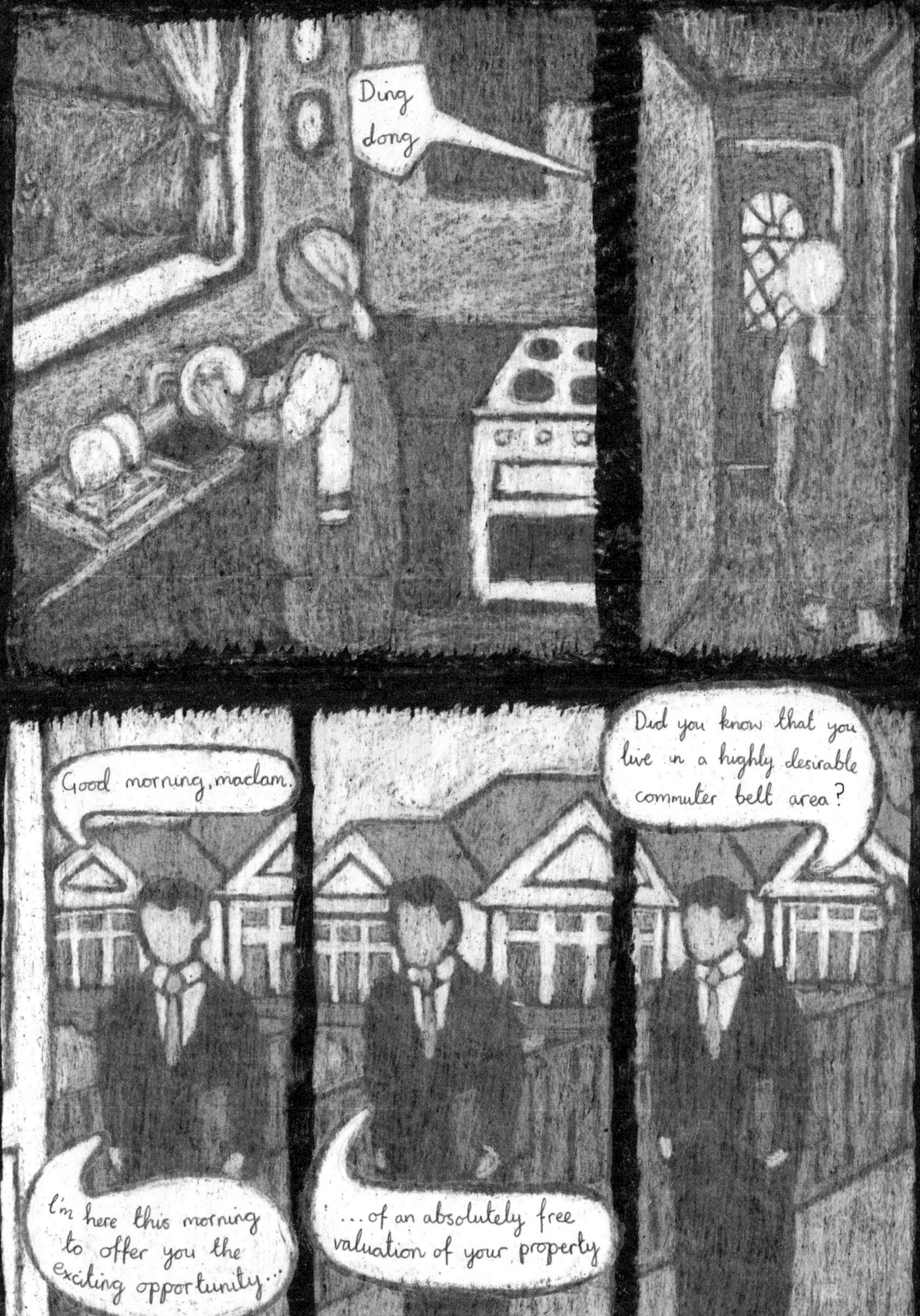
Ding dong
Good morning, madam.
I'm here this morning to offer you the exciting opportunity...
...of an absolutely free valuation of your property
Did you know that you live in a highly desirable commuter belt area?

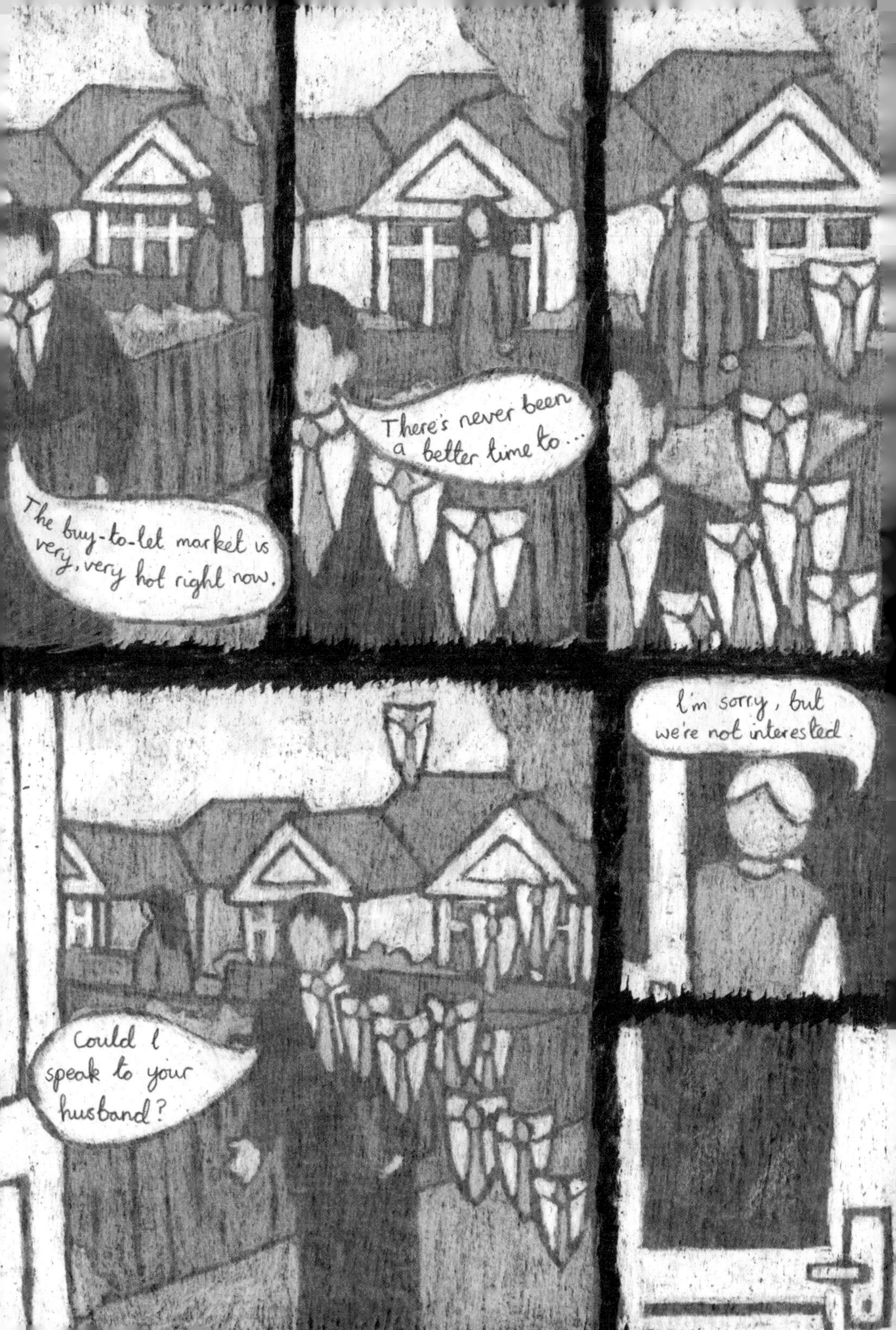
The buy-to-let market is very, very hot right now.
There's never been a better time to...
I'm sorry, but we're not interested
Could I speak to your husband?

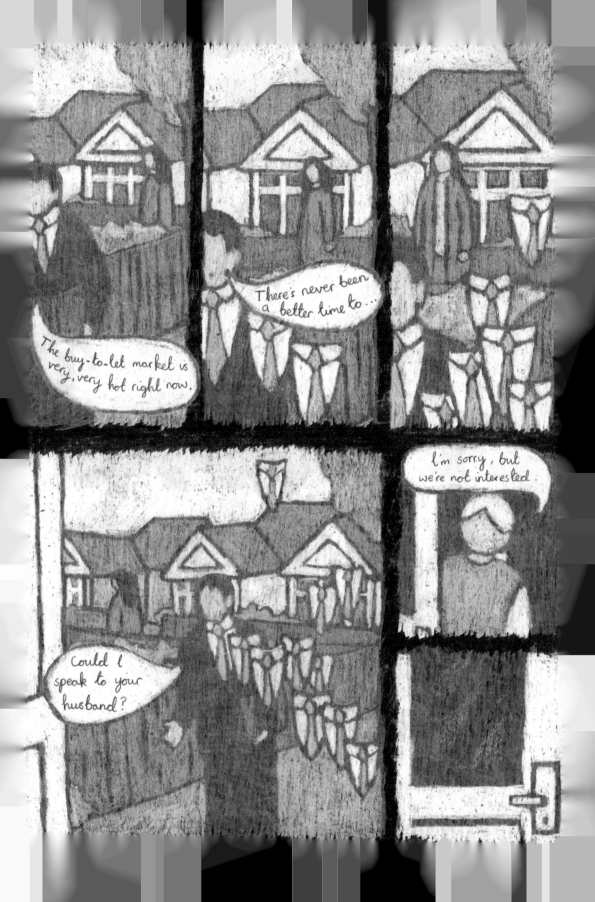

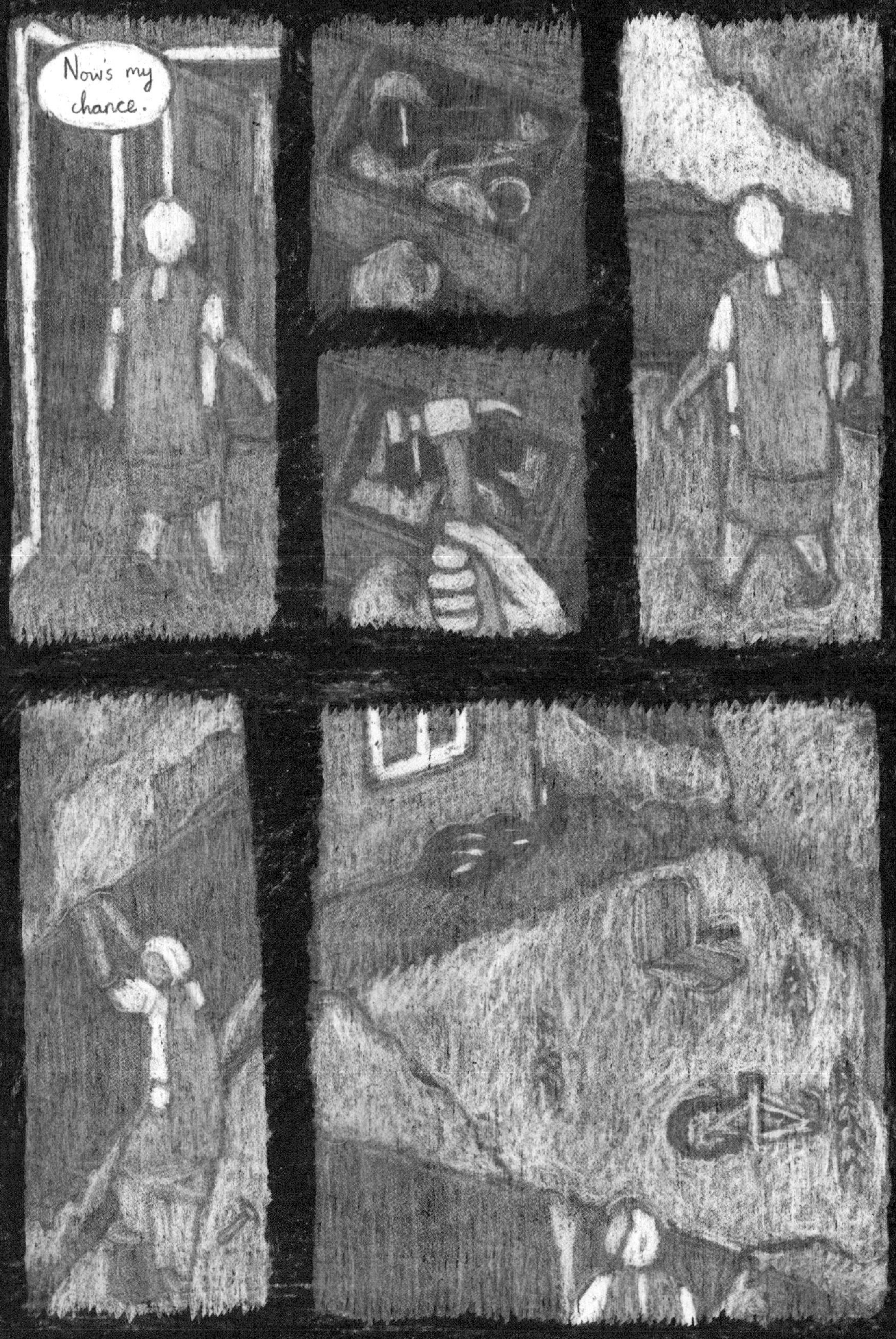
Now's my chance.

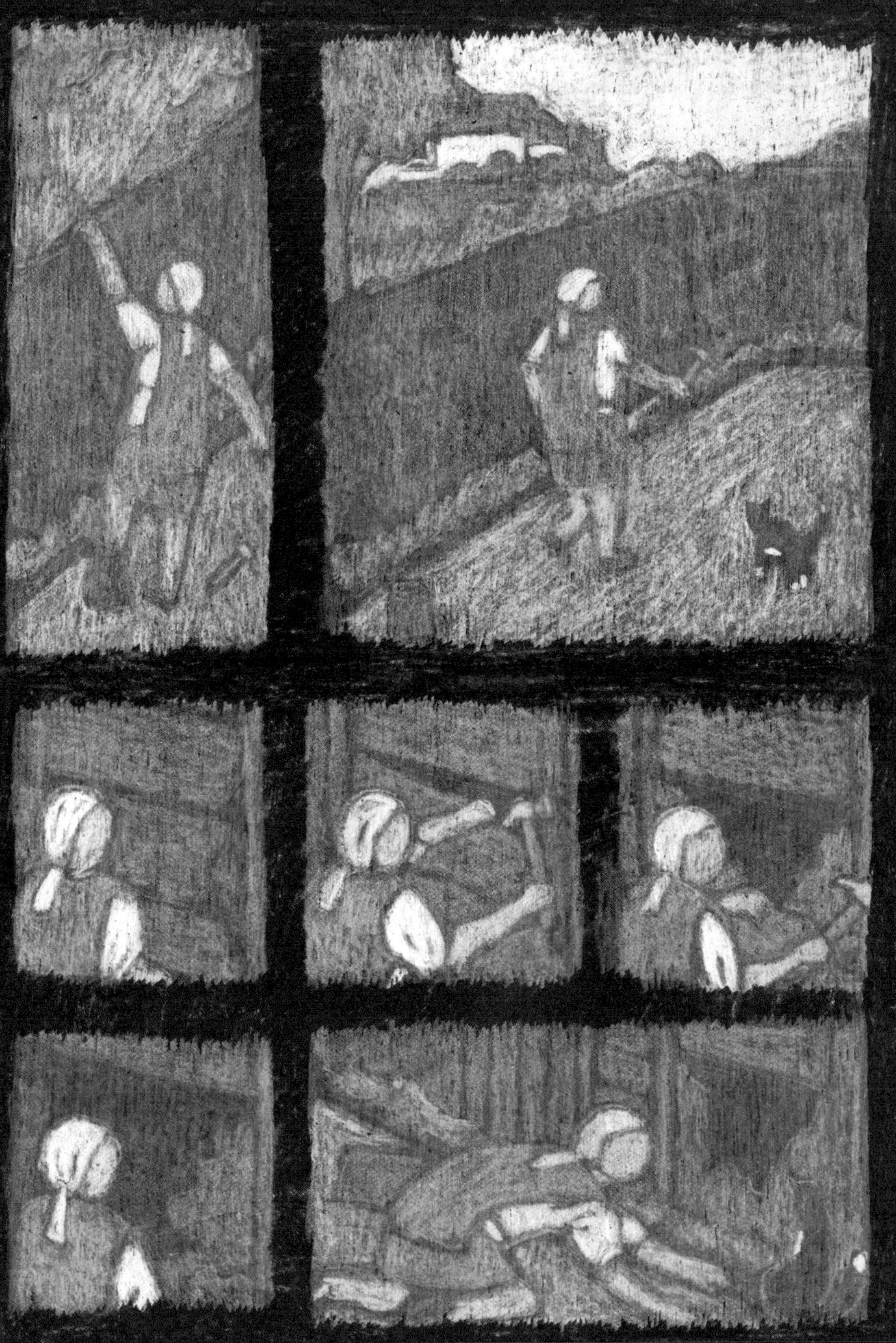

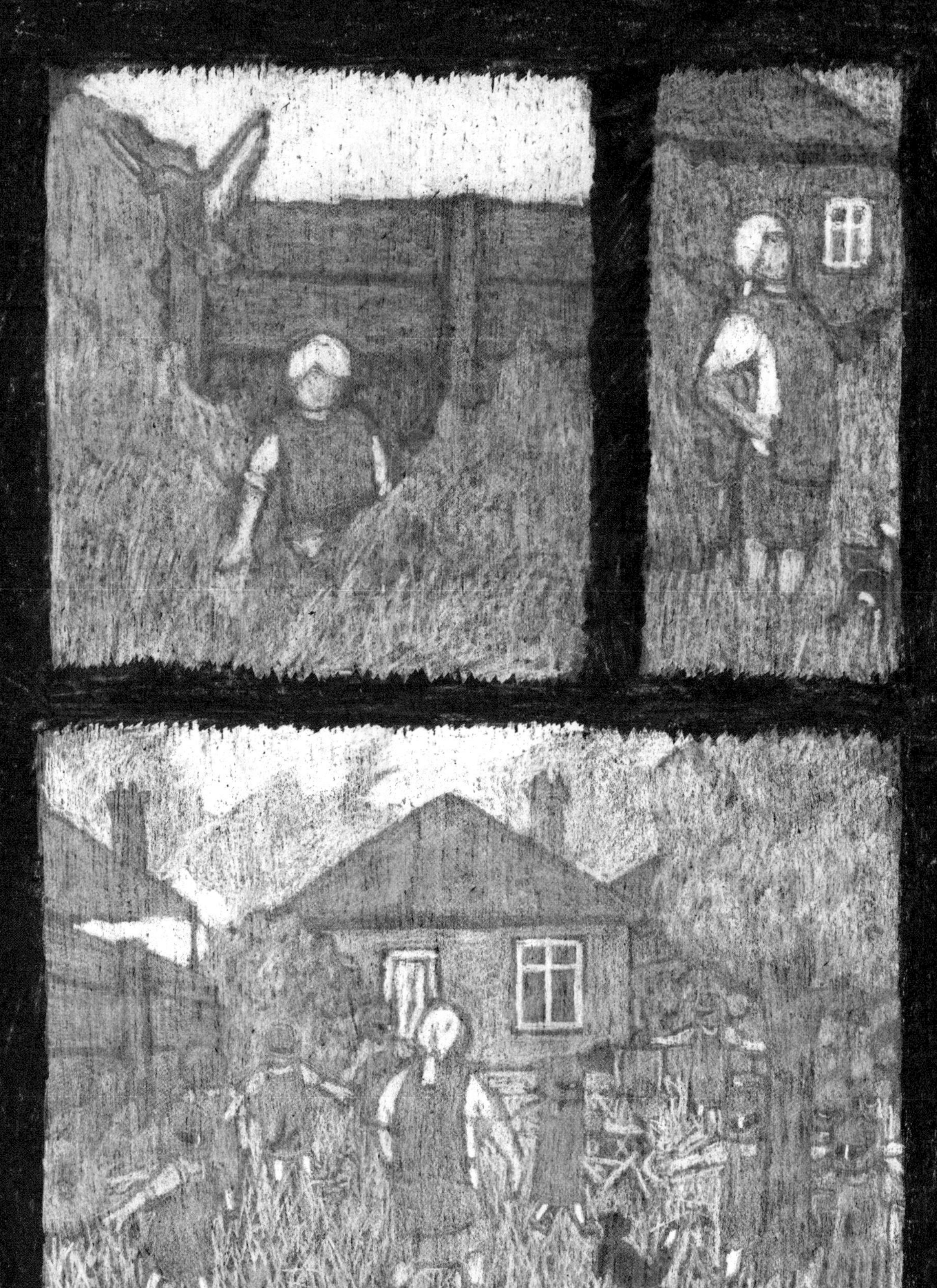

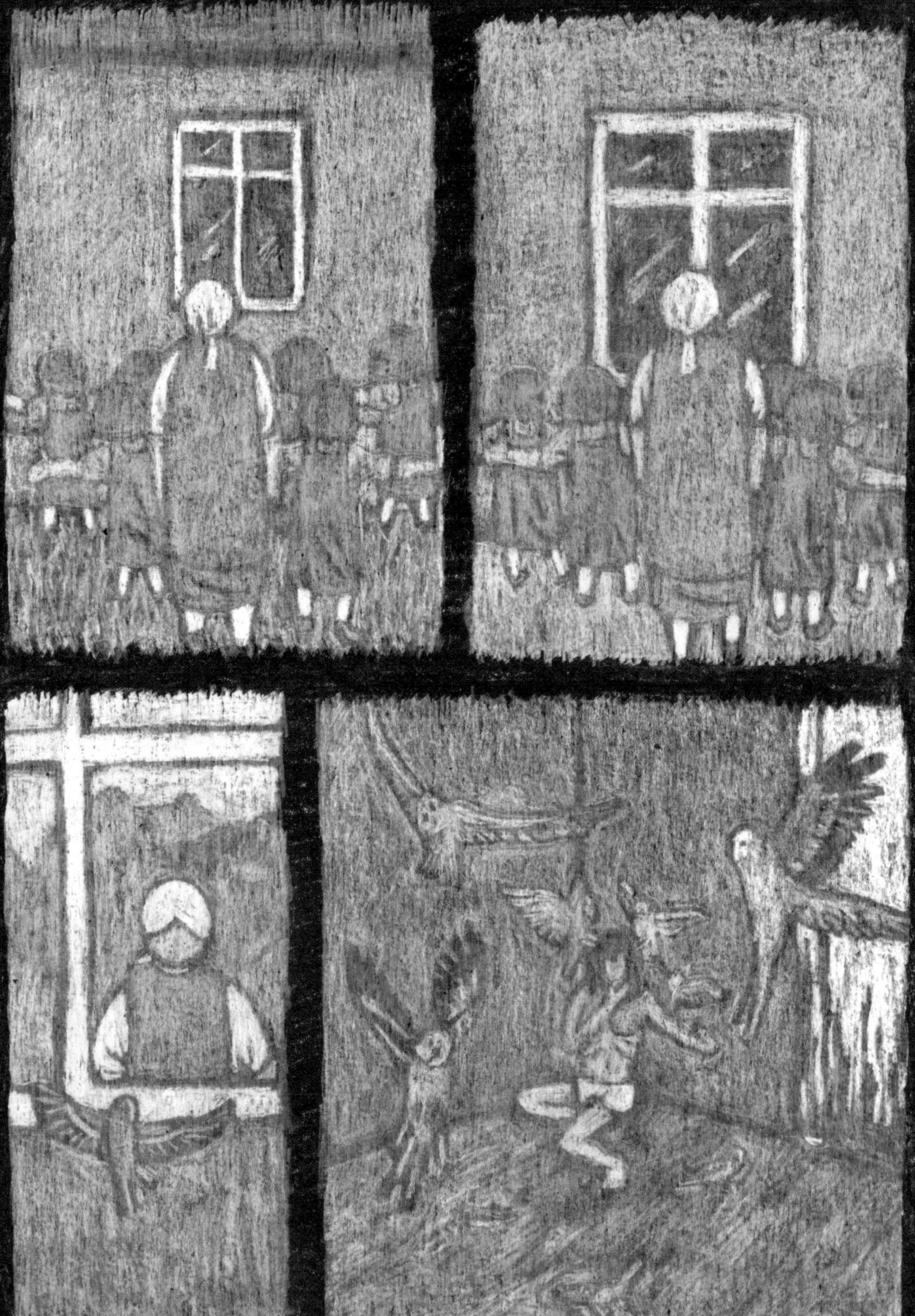

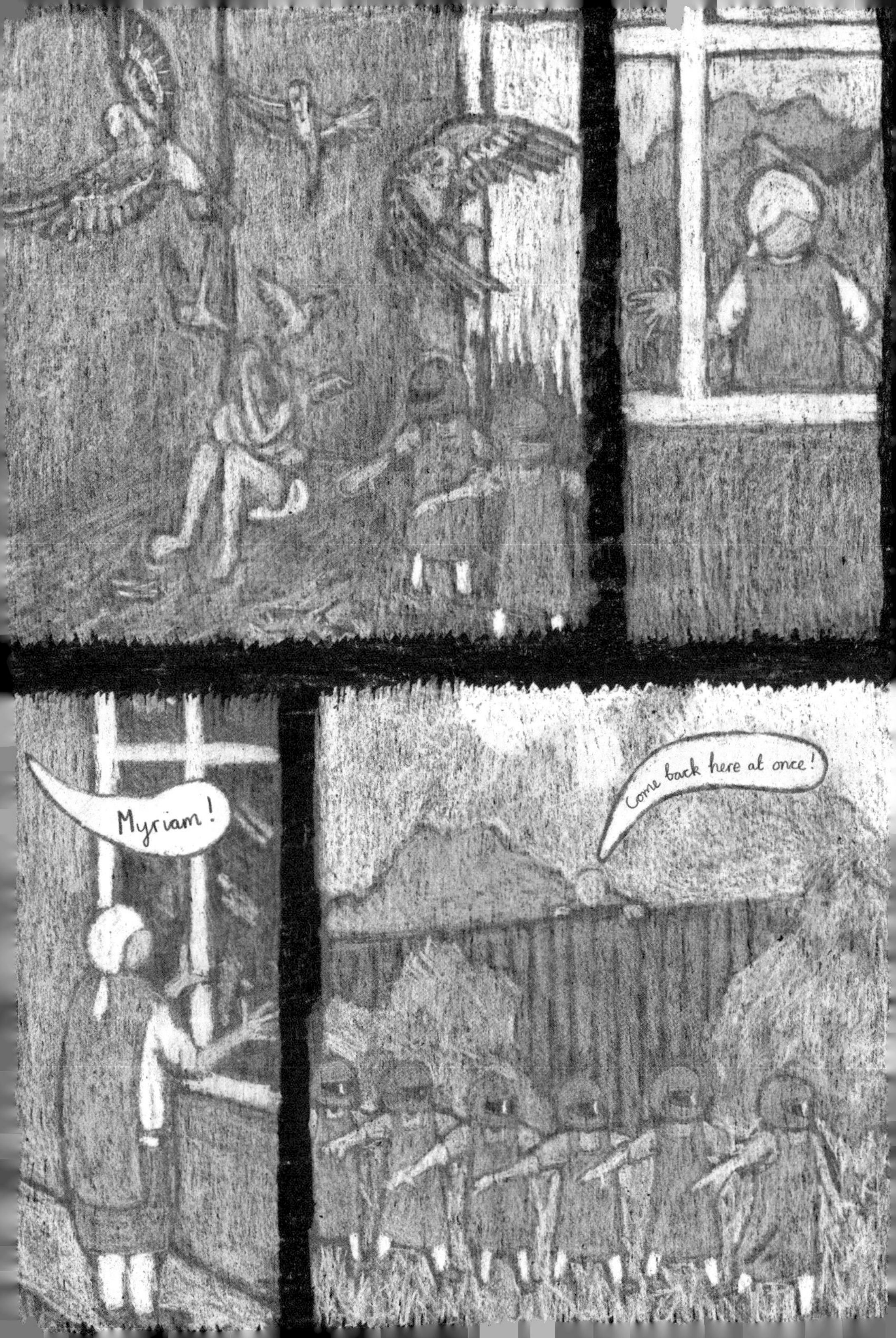
Myriam!
Come back here at once!

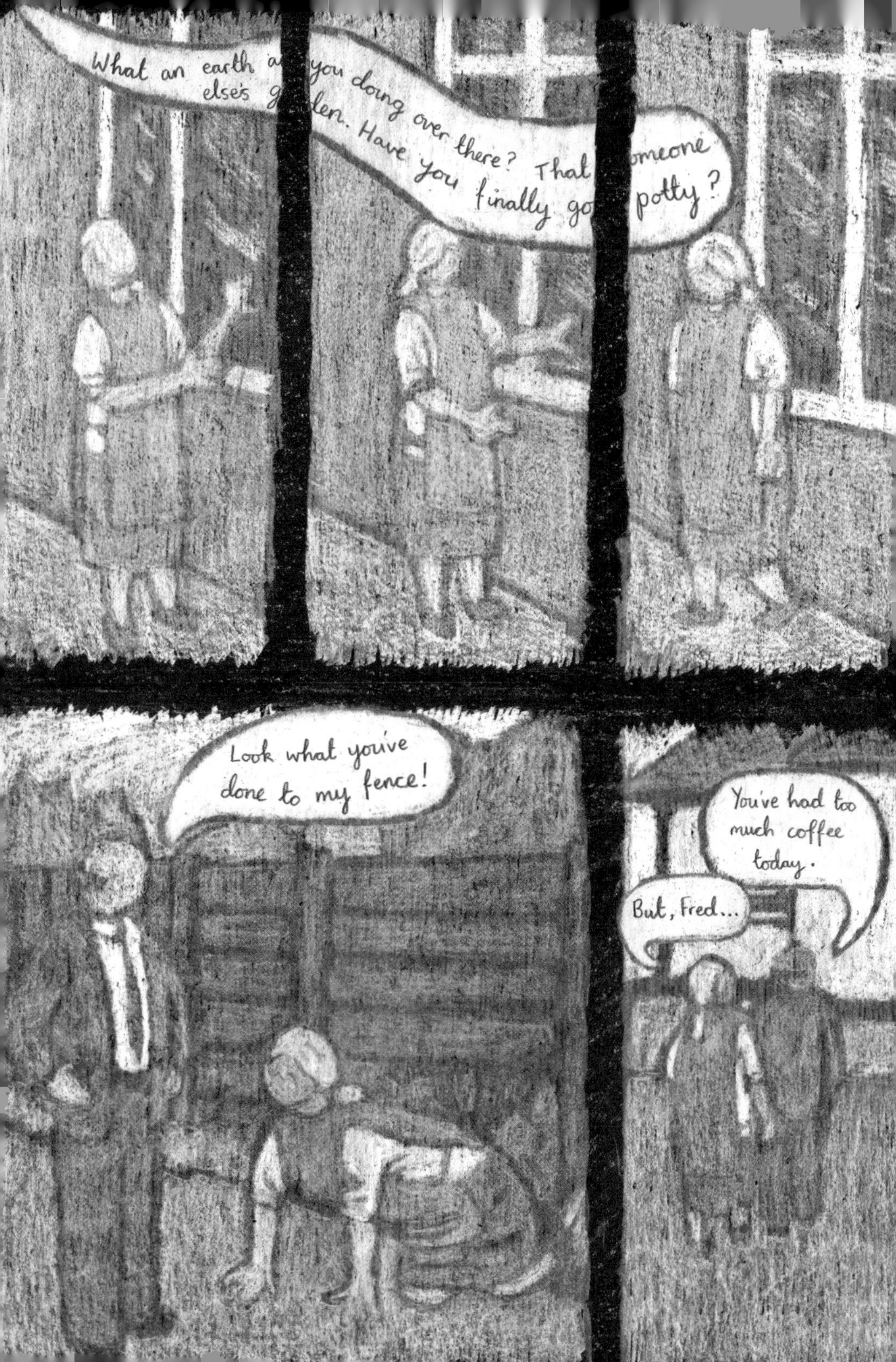
What an earth a you doing over there? That omeone else's g den. Have you finally go potty?
Look what you've done to my fence!
You've had too much coffee today.
But, Fred...

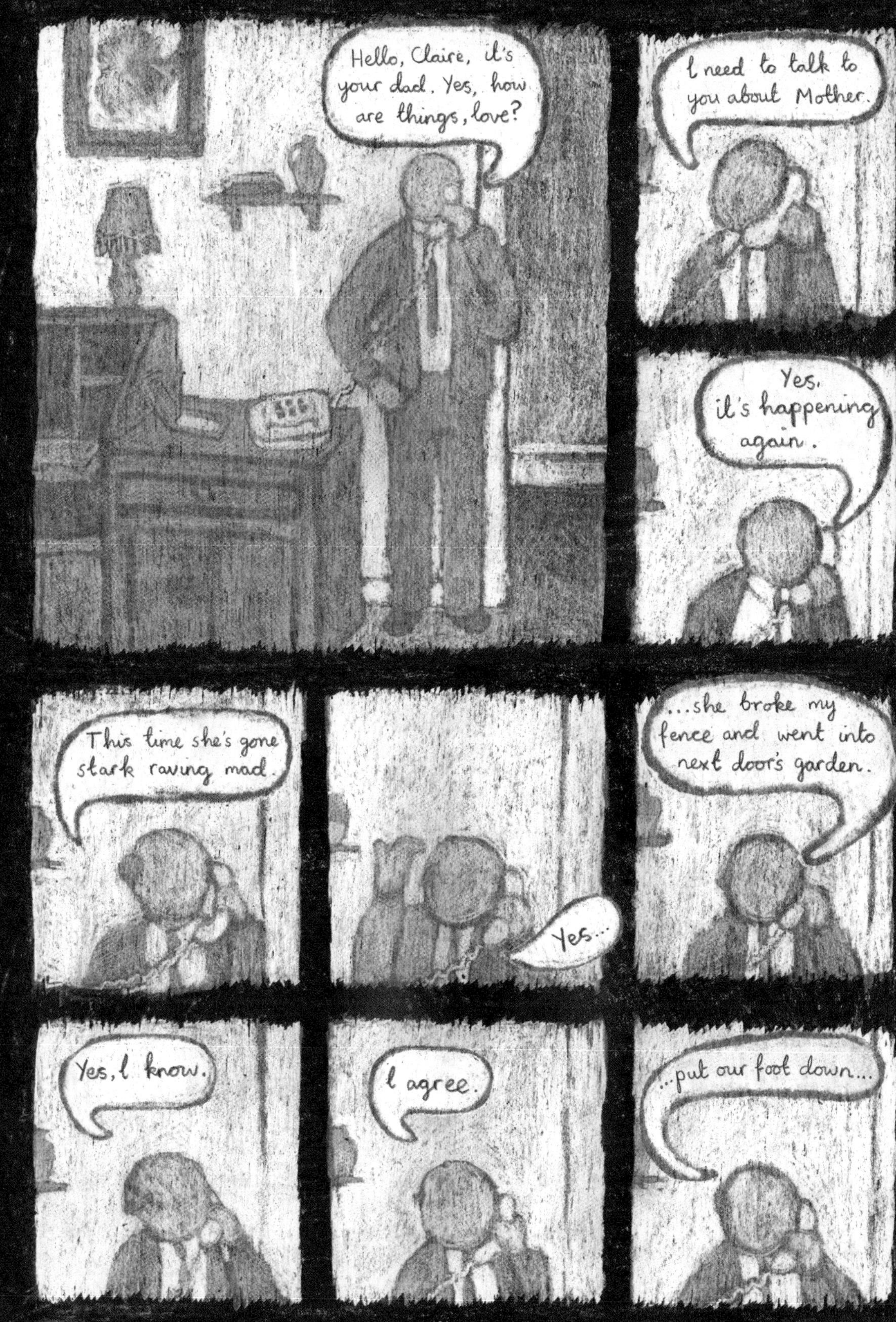
Hello, Claire, it's your dad. Yes, how are things, love?
I need to talk to you about Mother.
Yes, it's happening again.
This time she's gone stark raving mad.
Yes...
...she broke my fence and went into next door's garden.
Yes, I know.
I agree.
...put our foot down...

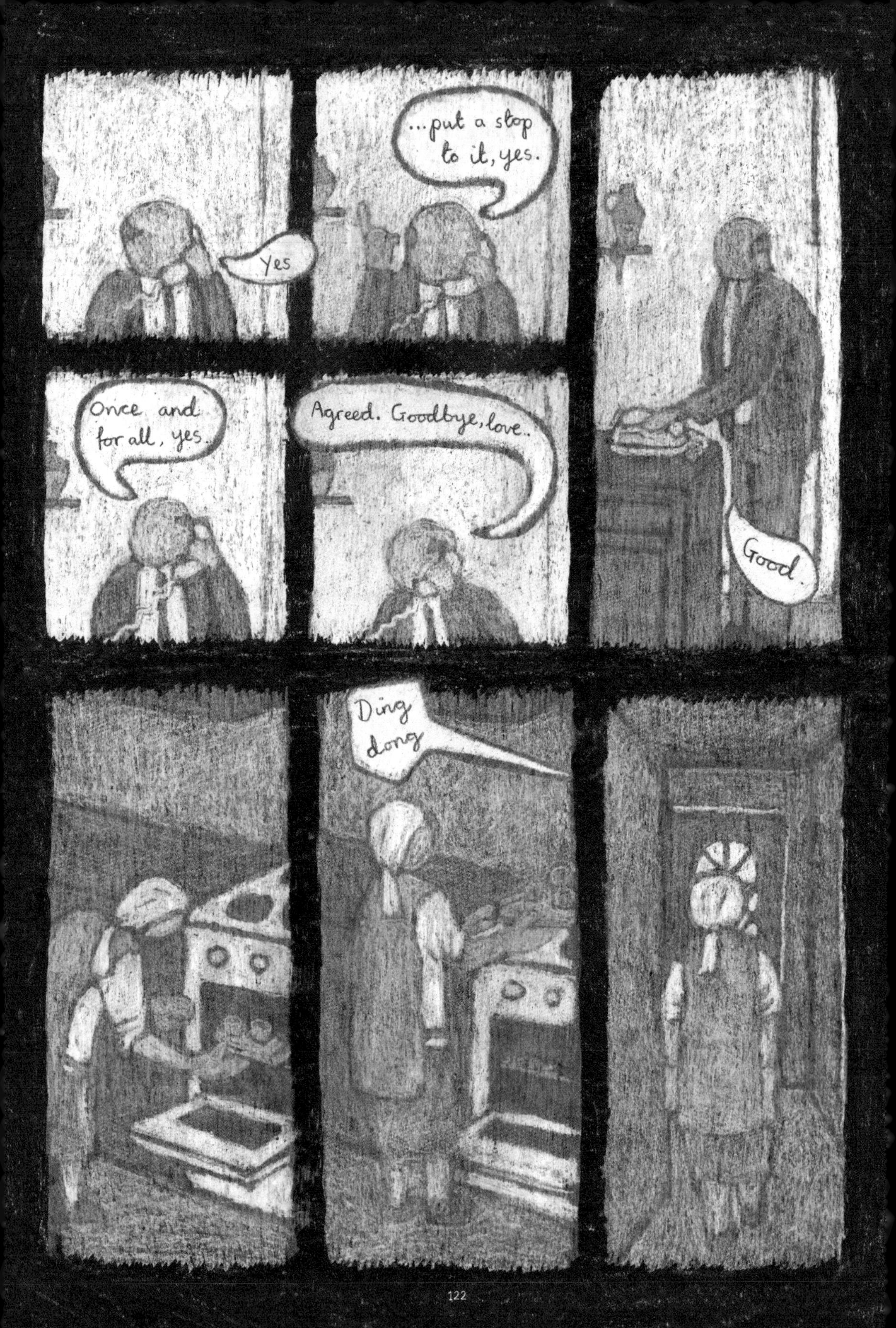
Yes
...put a stop to it, yes.
Once and for all, yes.
Agreed. Goodbye, love..
Good.
Ding dong

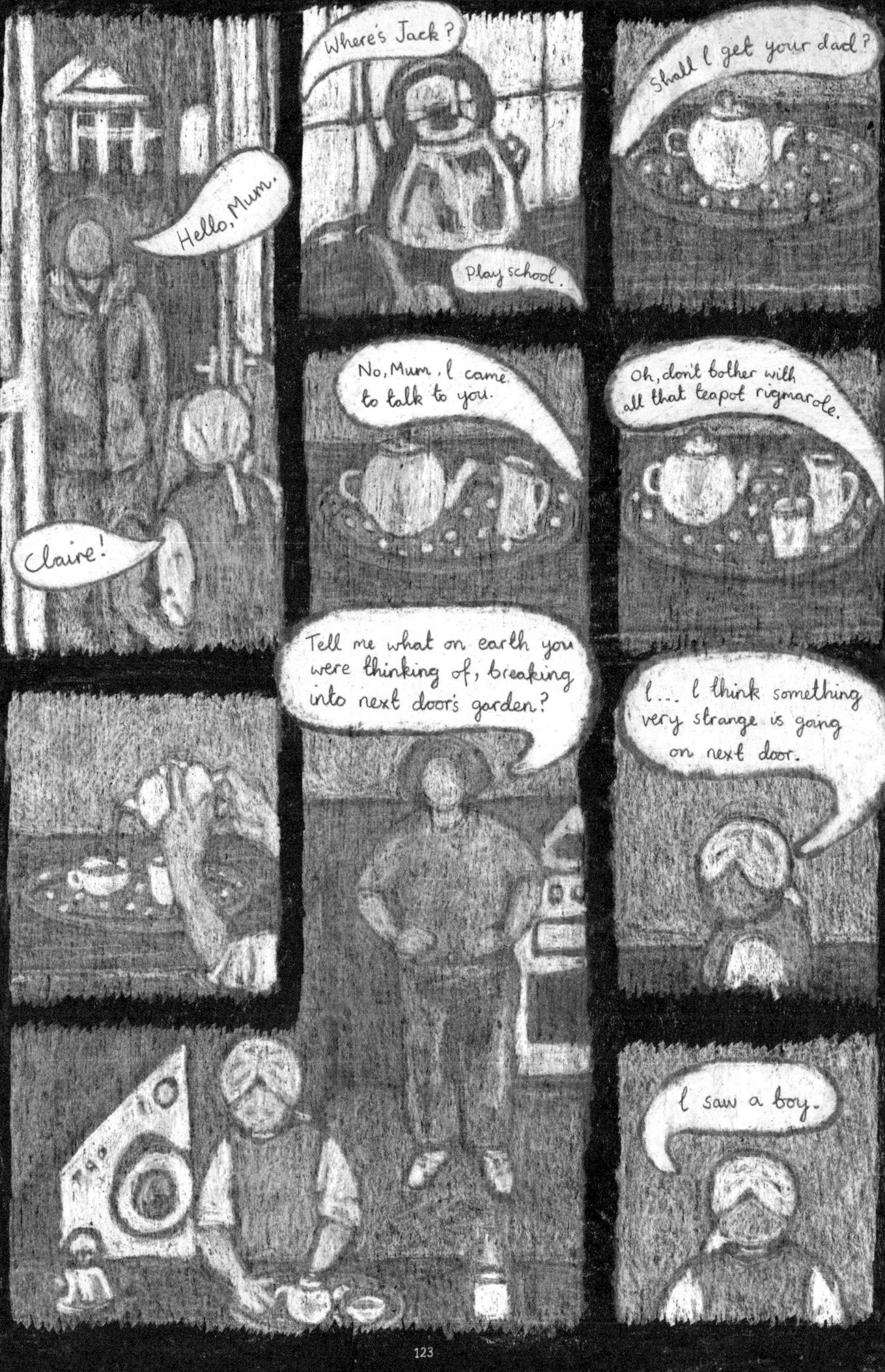
Hello, Mum.
Claire!
Where's Jack?
Play school.
Shall I get your dad?
No, Mum, I came to talk to you.
Oh, don't bother with all that teapot rigmarole.
Tell me what on earth you were thinking of, breaking into next door's garden?
I... I think something very strange is going on next door.
I saw a boy.

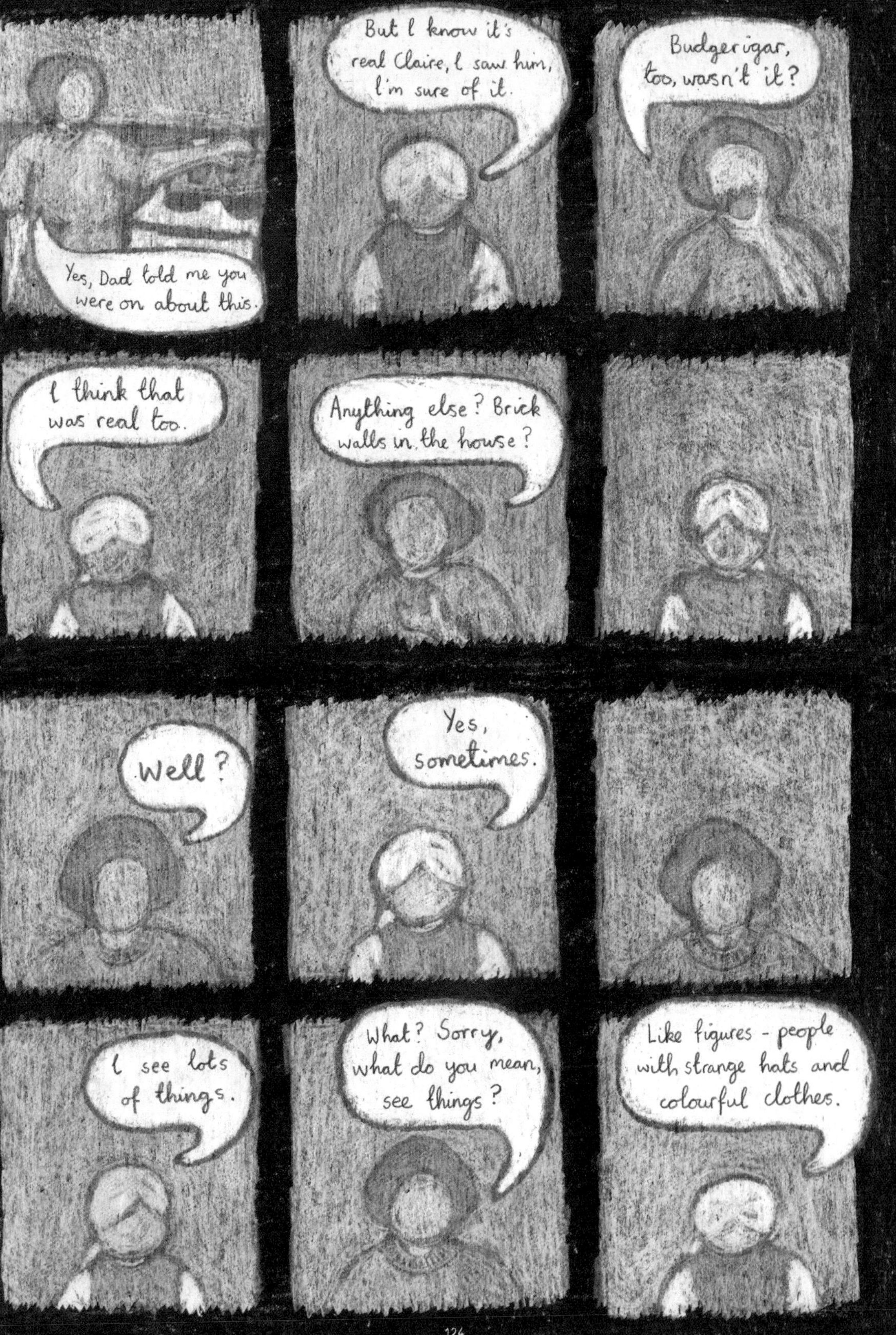
Yes, Dad told me you were on about this.
But I know it's real Claire, I saw him, I'm sure of it.
Budgerigar, too, wasn't it?
I think that was real too.
Anything else? Brick walls in the house?
Well?
Yes, sometimes.
I see lots of things.
What? Sorry, what do you mean, see things?
Like figures - people with strange hats and colourful clothes.

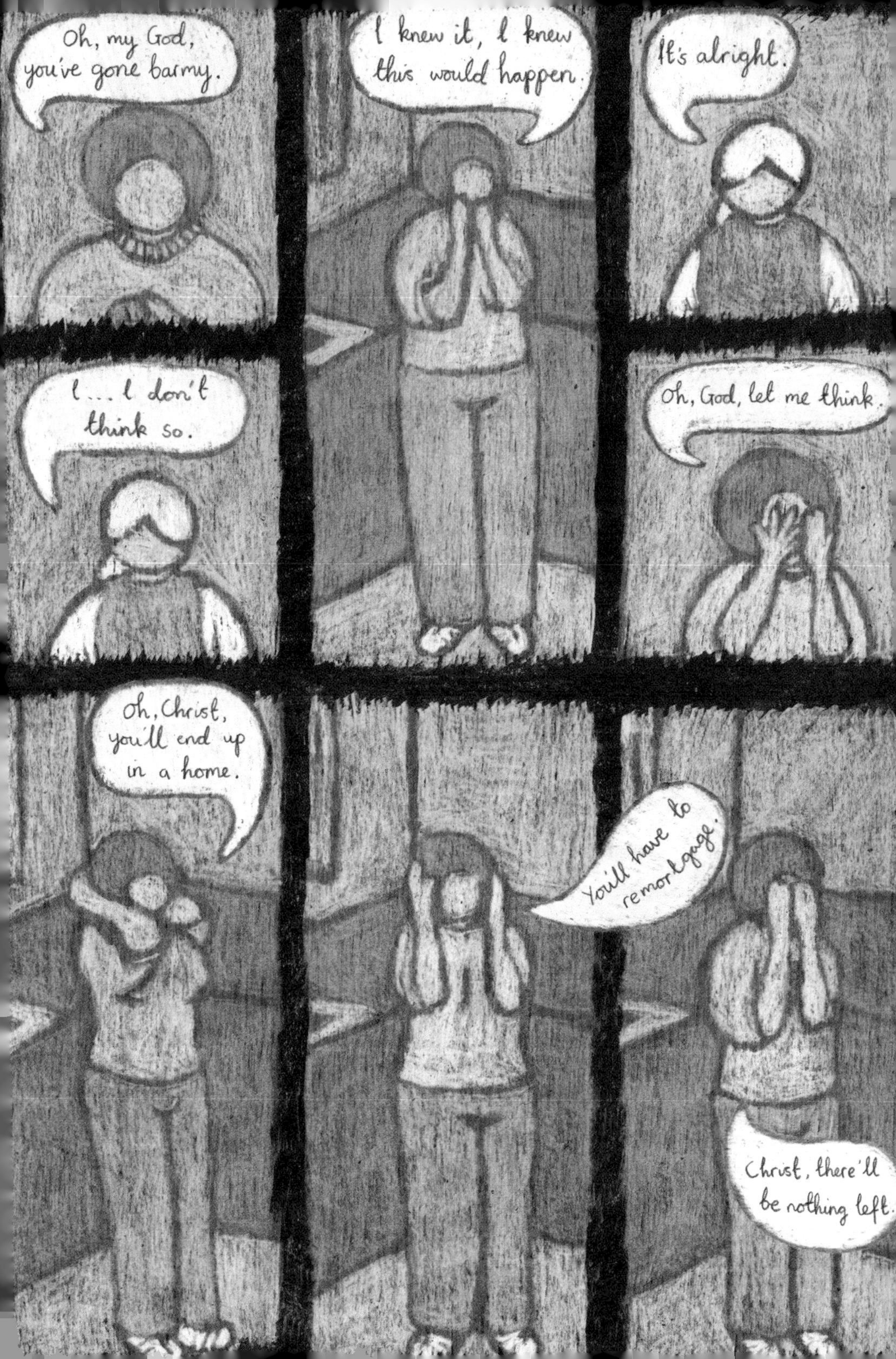
Oh, my God, you've gone barmy.
I knew it, I knew this would happen.
It's alright.
I... I don't think so.
Oh, God, let me think.
Oh, Christ, you'll end up in a home.
You'll have to remortgage.
Christ, there'll be nothing left.

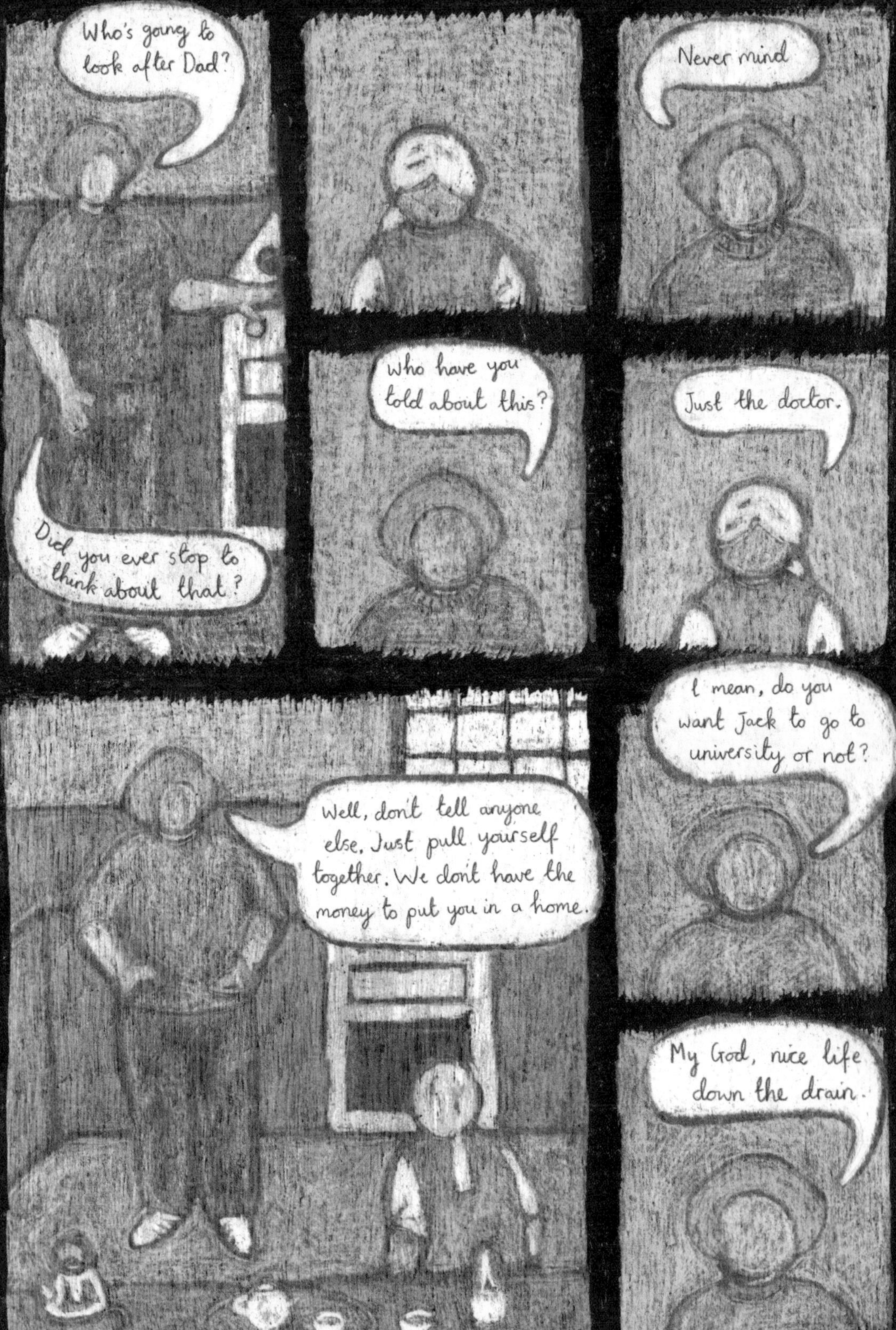
Who's going to look after Dad?
Did you ever stop to think about that?
Never mind
Who have you told about this?
Just the doctor.
Well, don't tell anyone else. Just pull yourself together. We don't have the money to put you in a home.
I mean, do you want Jack to go to university or not?
My God, nice life down the drain.

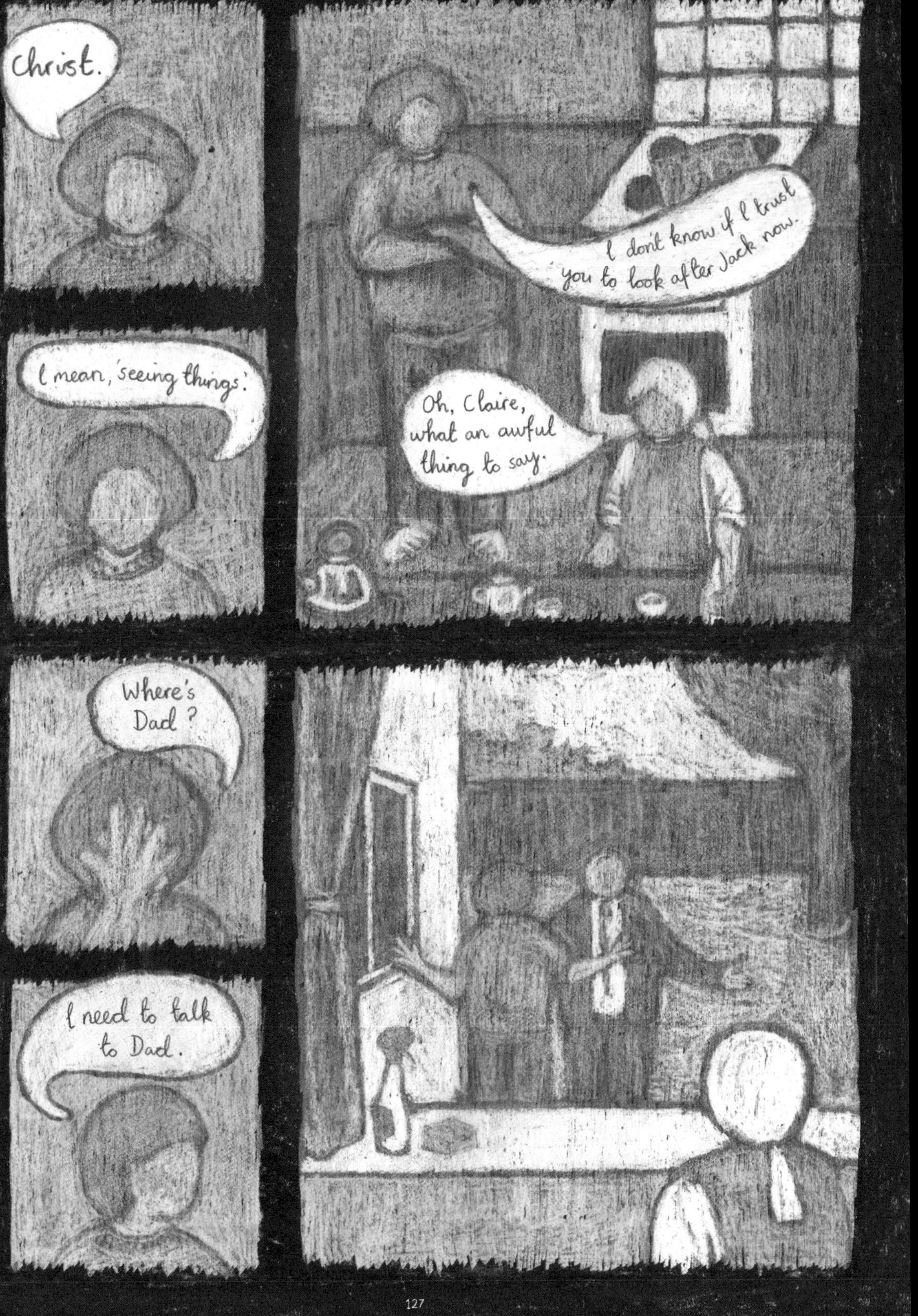
Christ.
I don't know if I trust you to look after Jack now.
I mean, 'seeing things'.
Oh, Claire, what an awful thing to say.
Where's Dad?
I need to talk to Dad.

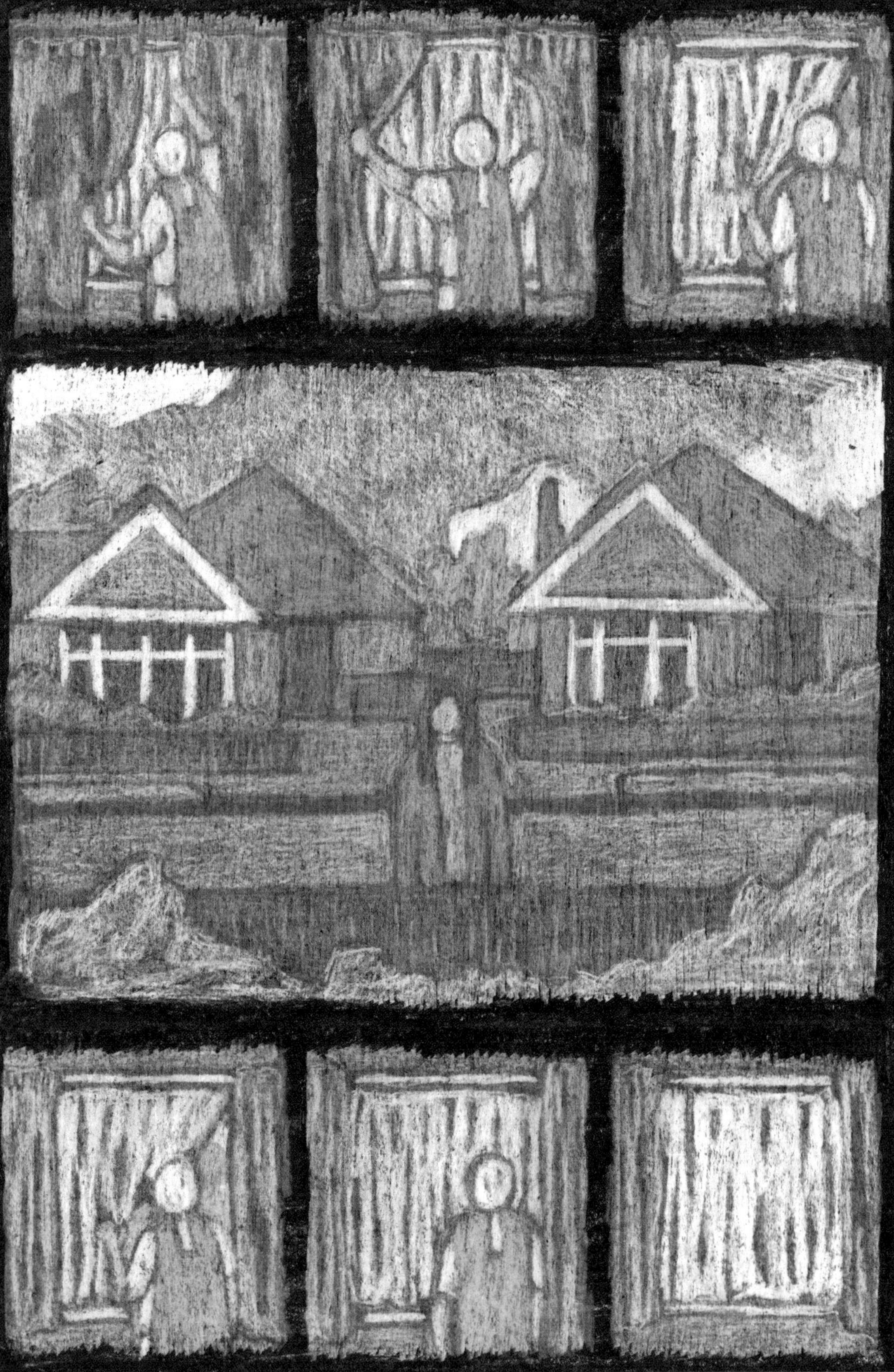

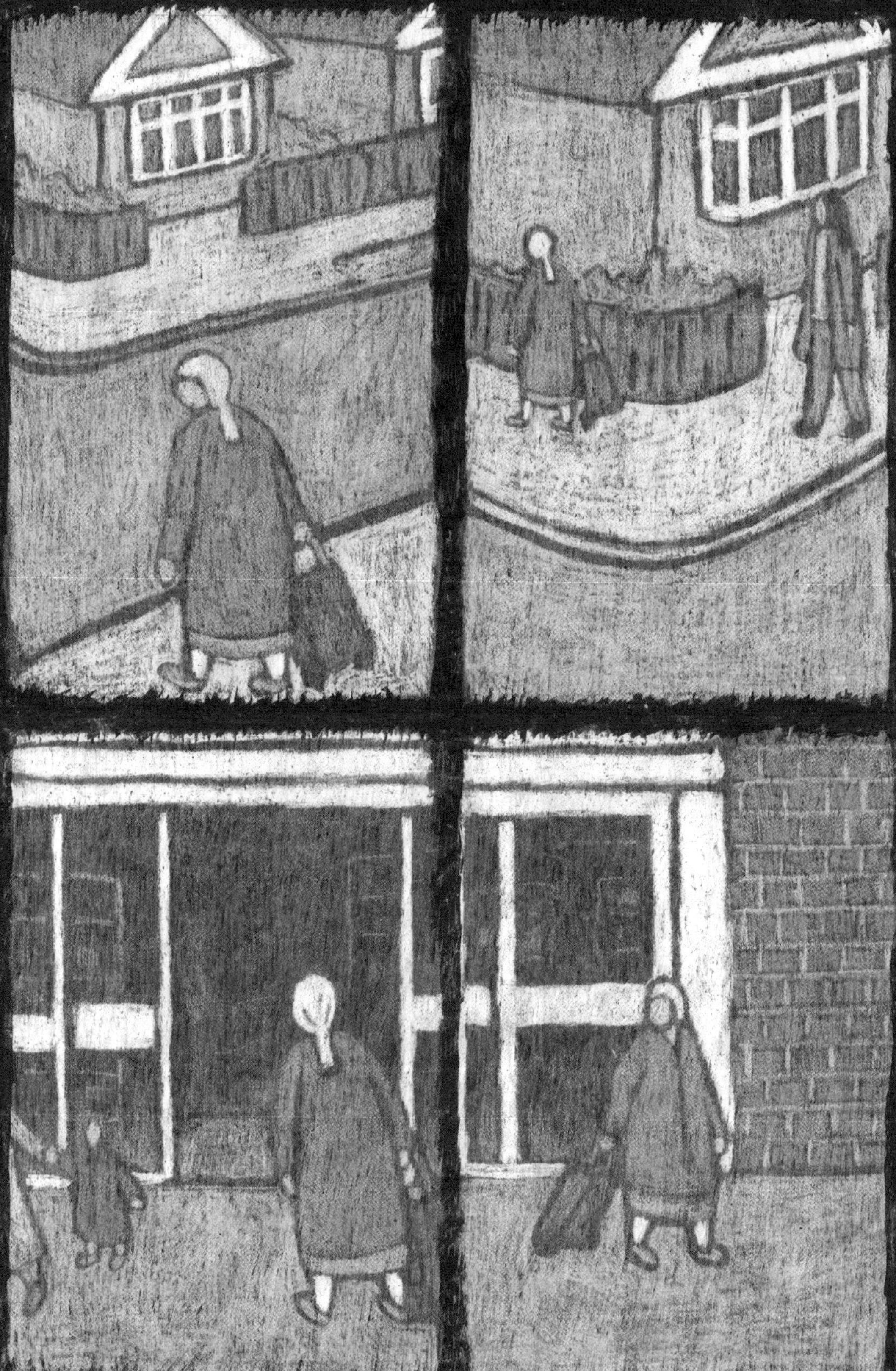

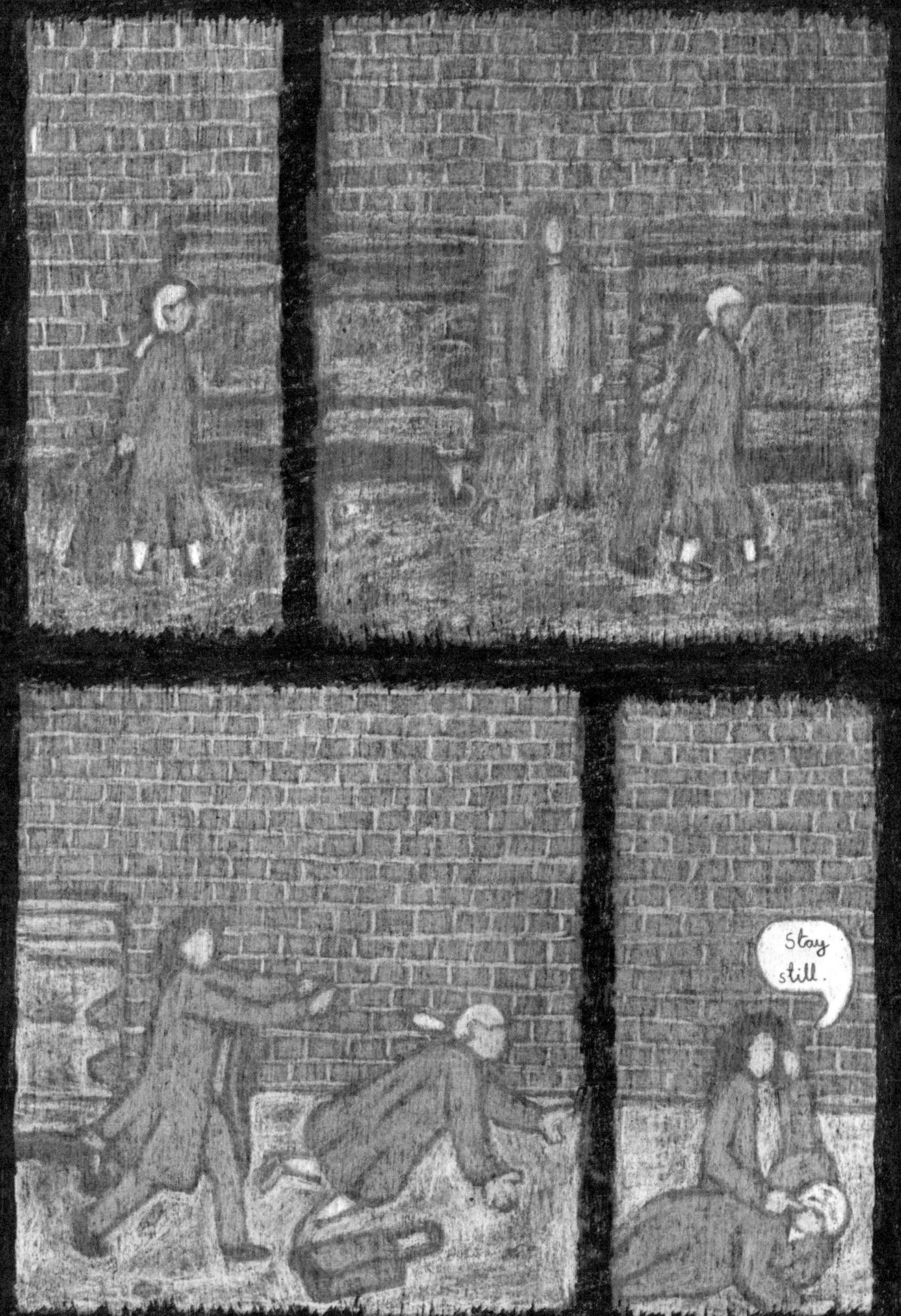
Stay still.

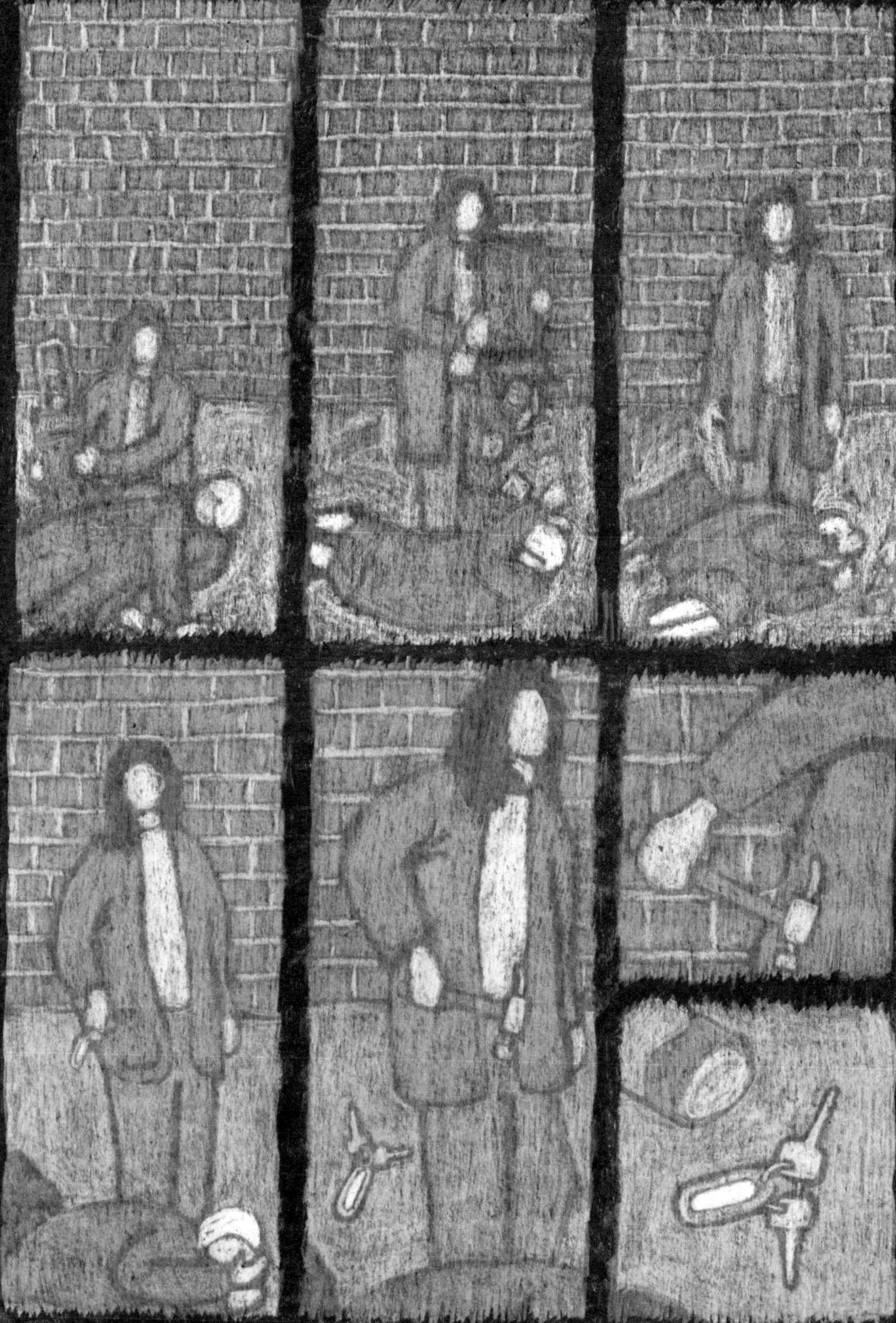

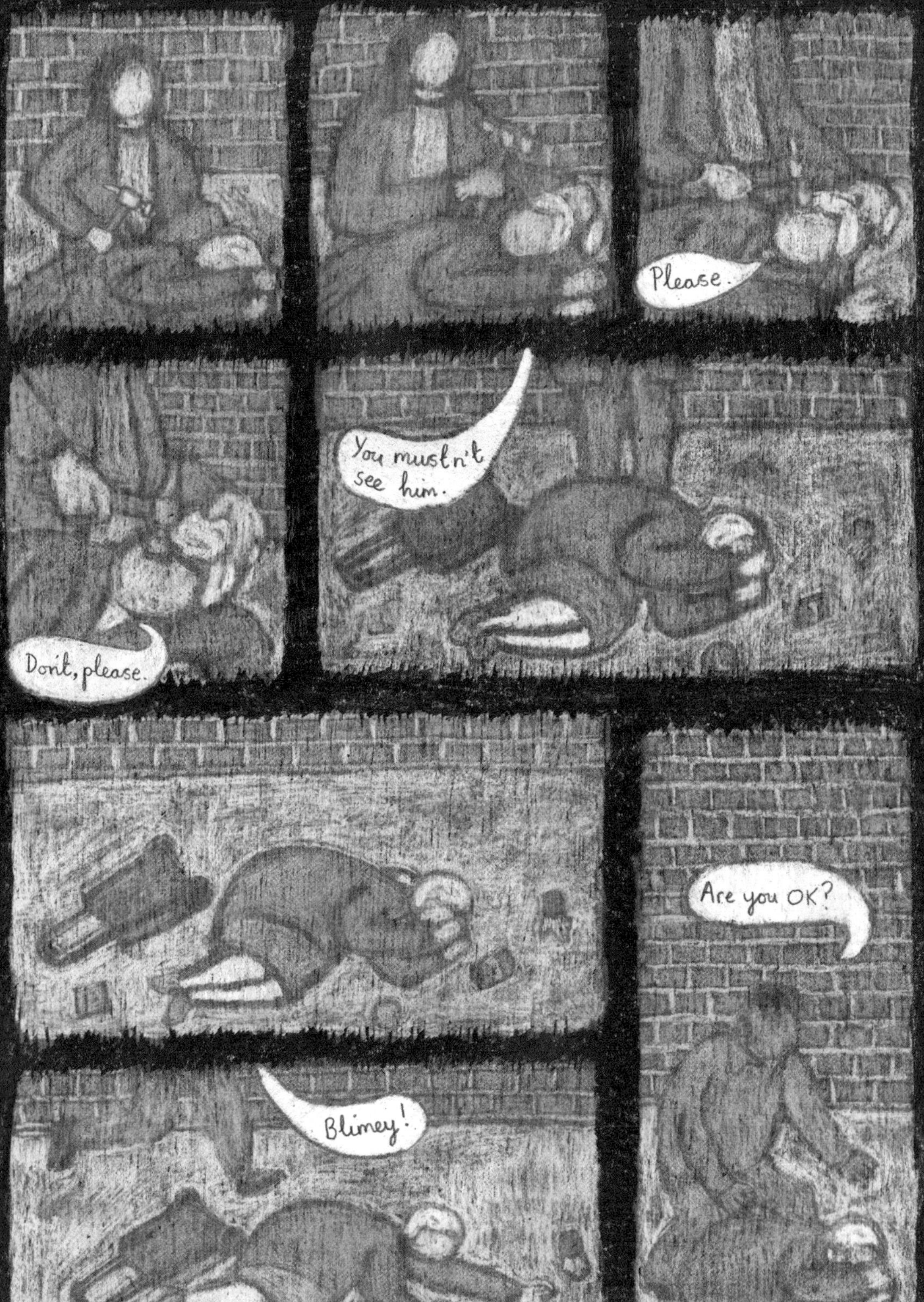
Please.
Don't, please.
You mustn't see him.
Are you OK?
Blimey!

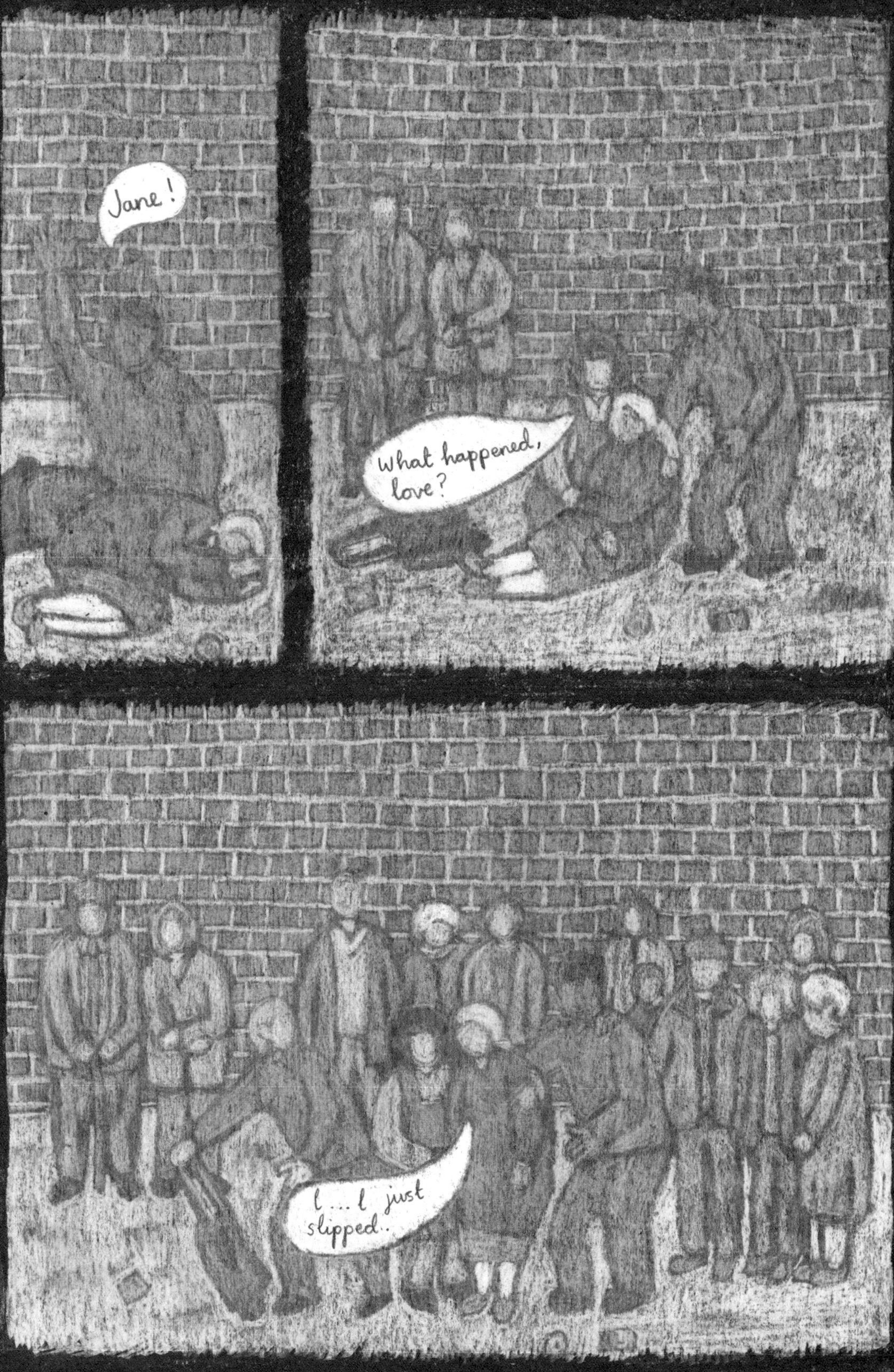
Jane!
What happened, love?
I... I just slipped...

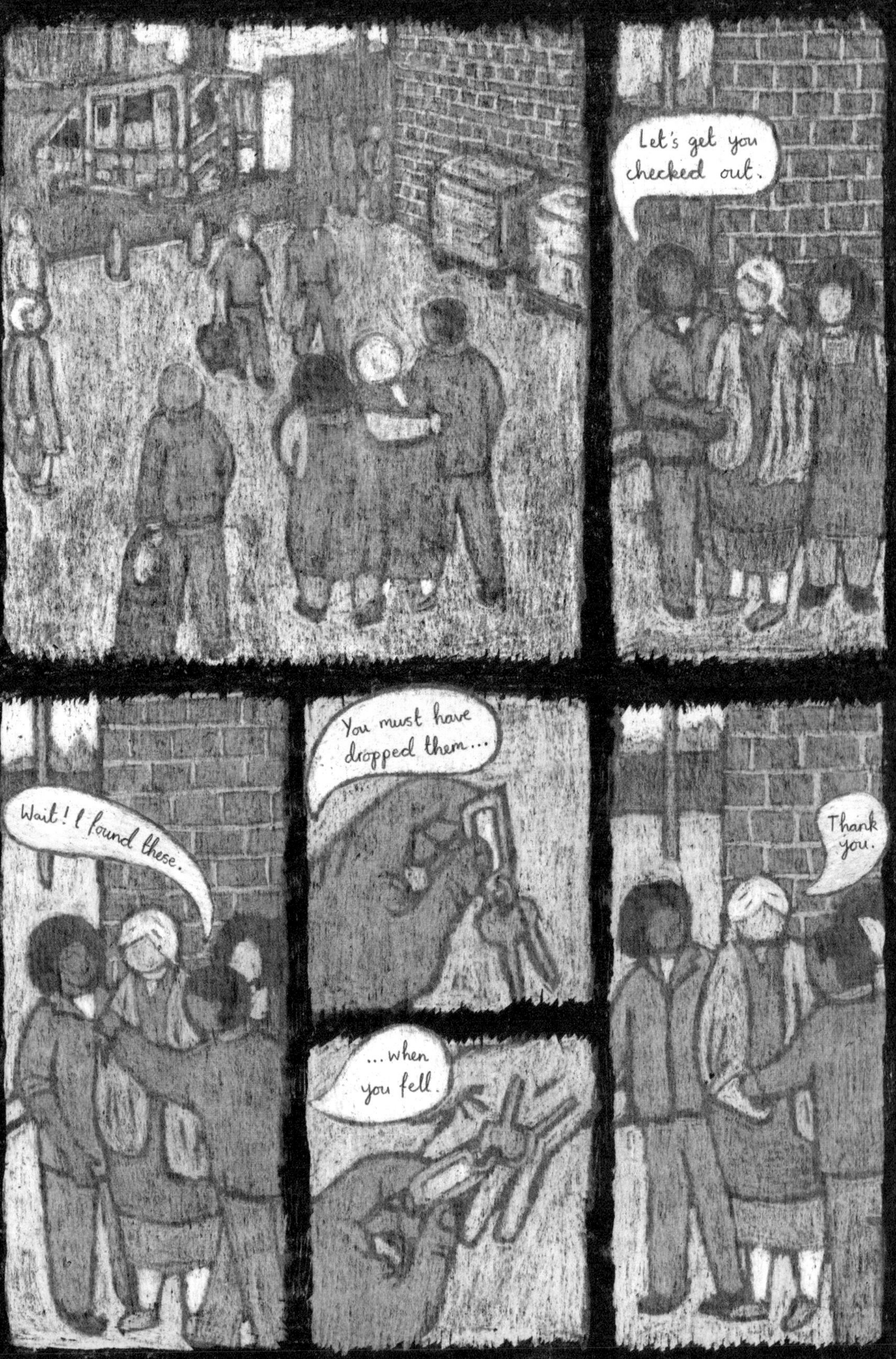
Let's get you checked out.
Wait! I found these.
You must have dropped them...
...when you fell.
Thank you.

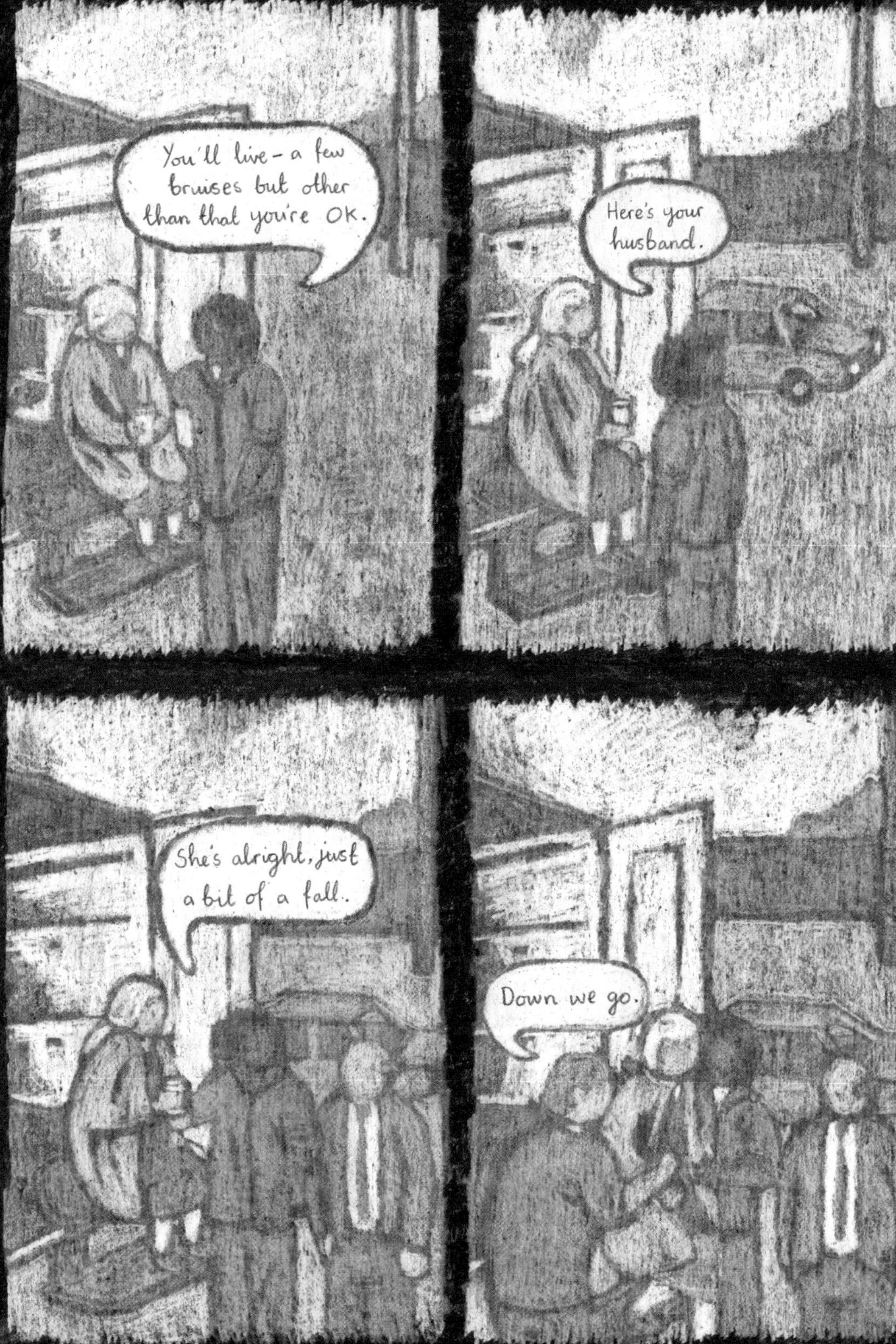
You'll live – a few bruises but other than that you're OK.
Here's your husband.
She's alright, just a bit of a fall.
Down we go.

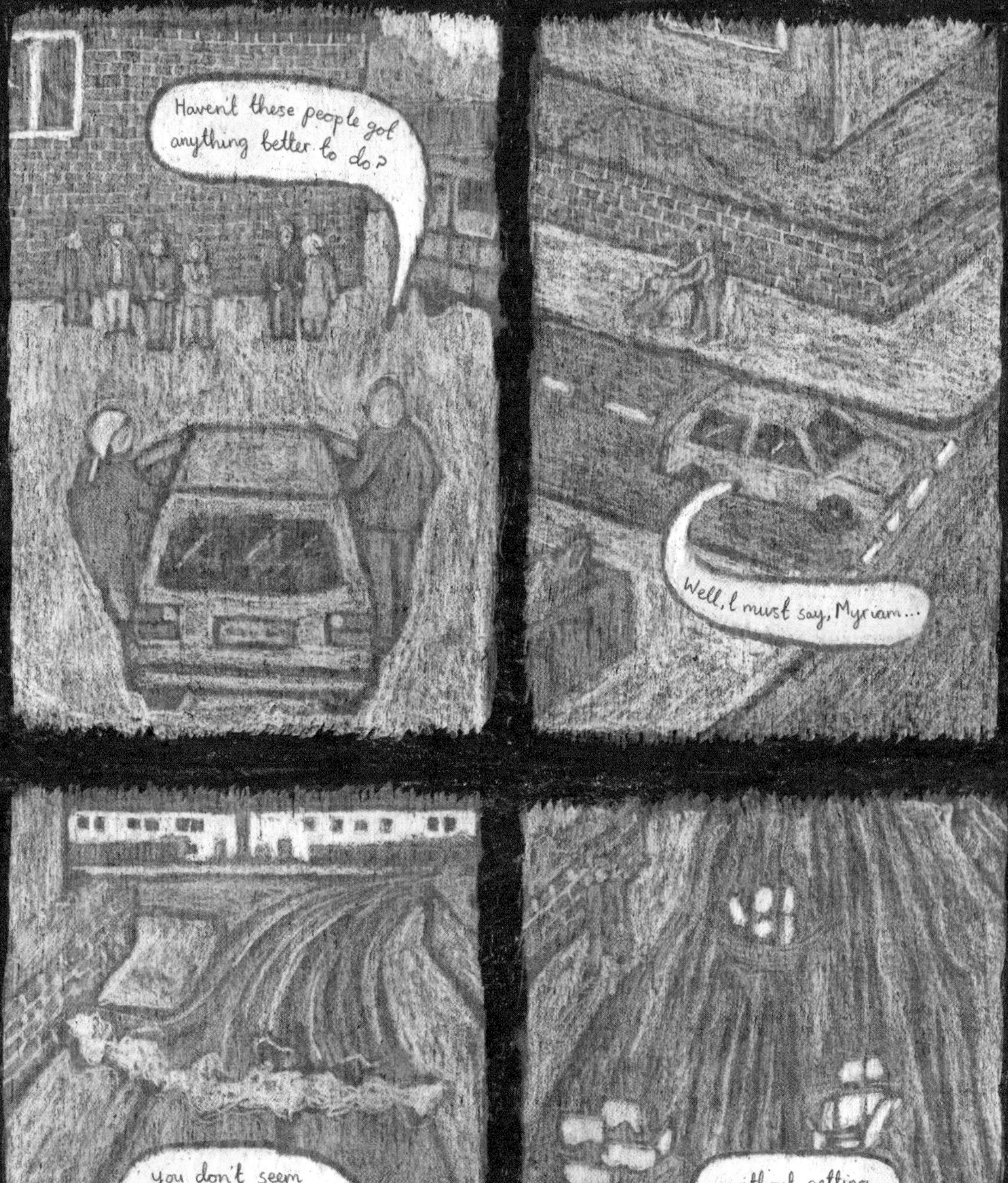
Haven't these people got anything better to do?
Well, I must say, Myriam...
you don't seem to be able to do anything these days...
...without getting yourself into some sort of trouble.

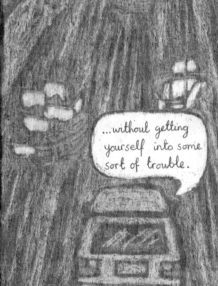

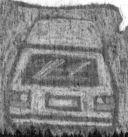

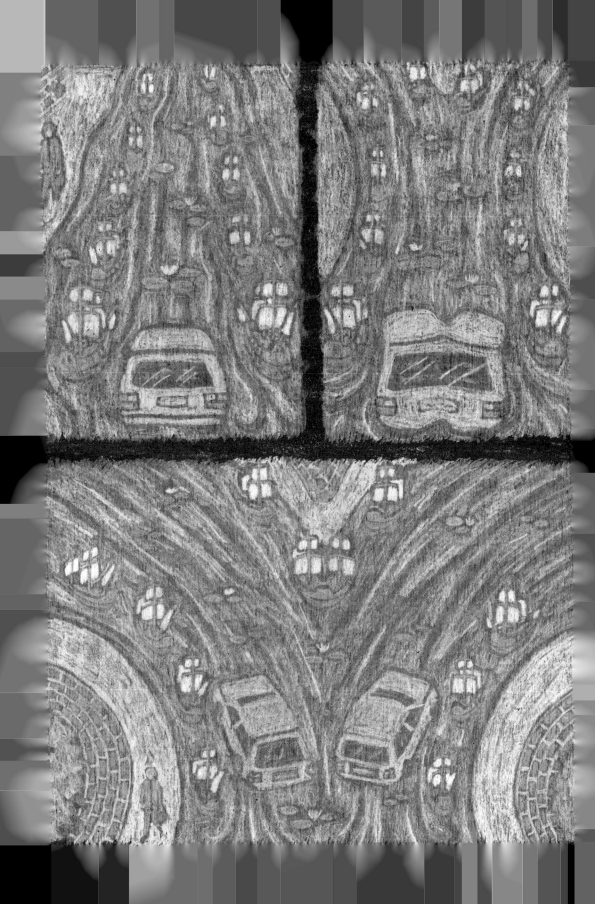

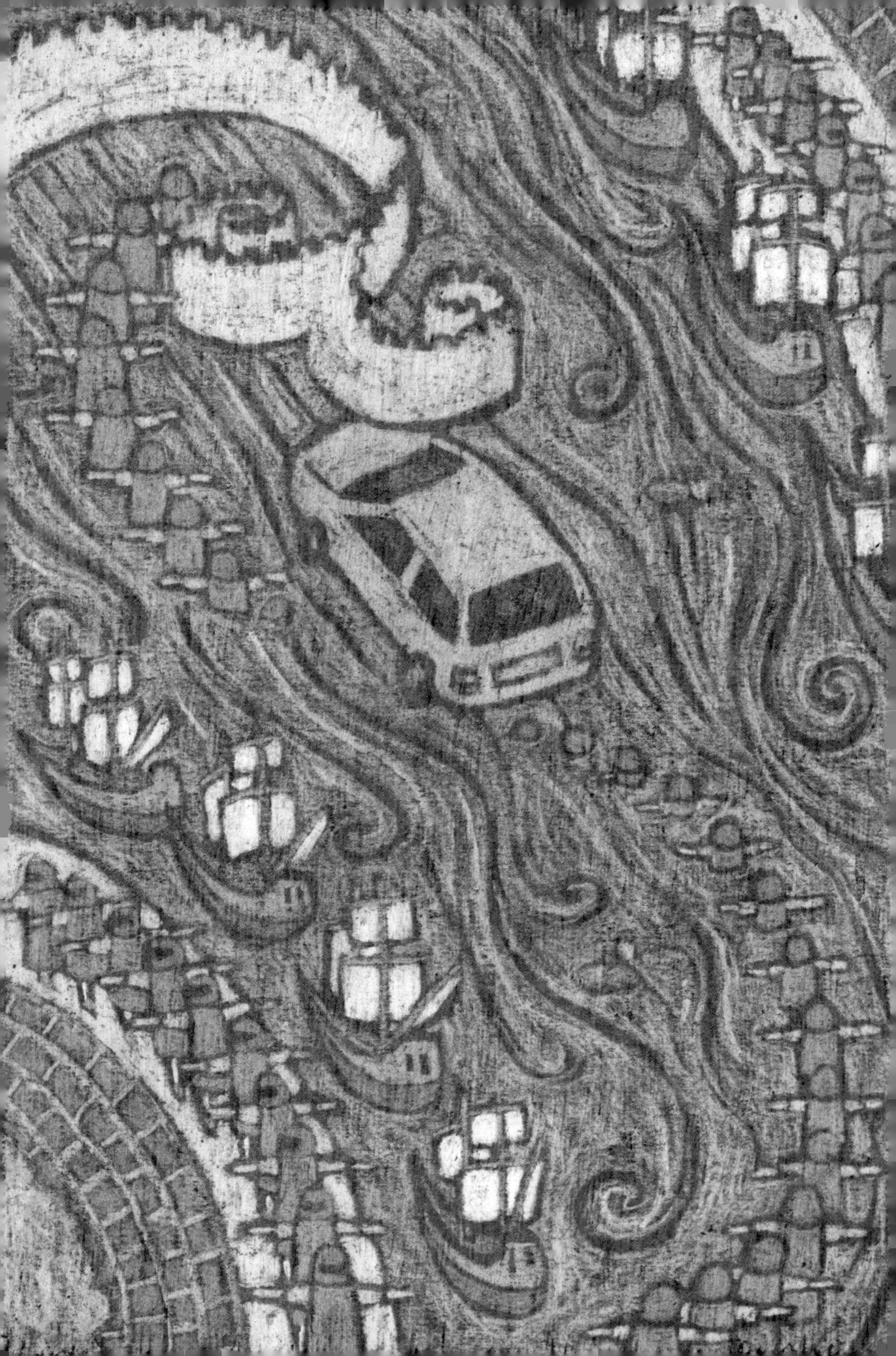

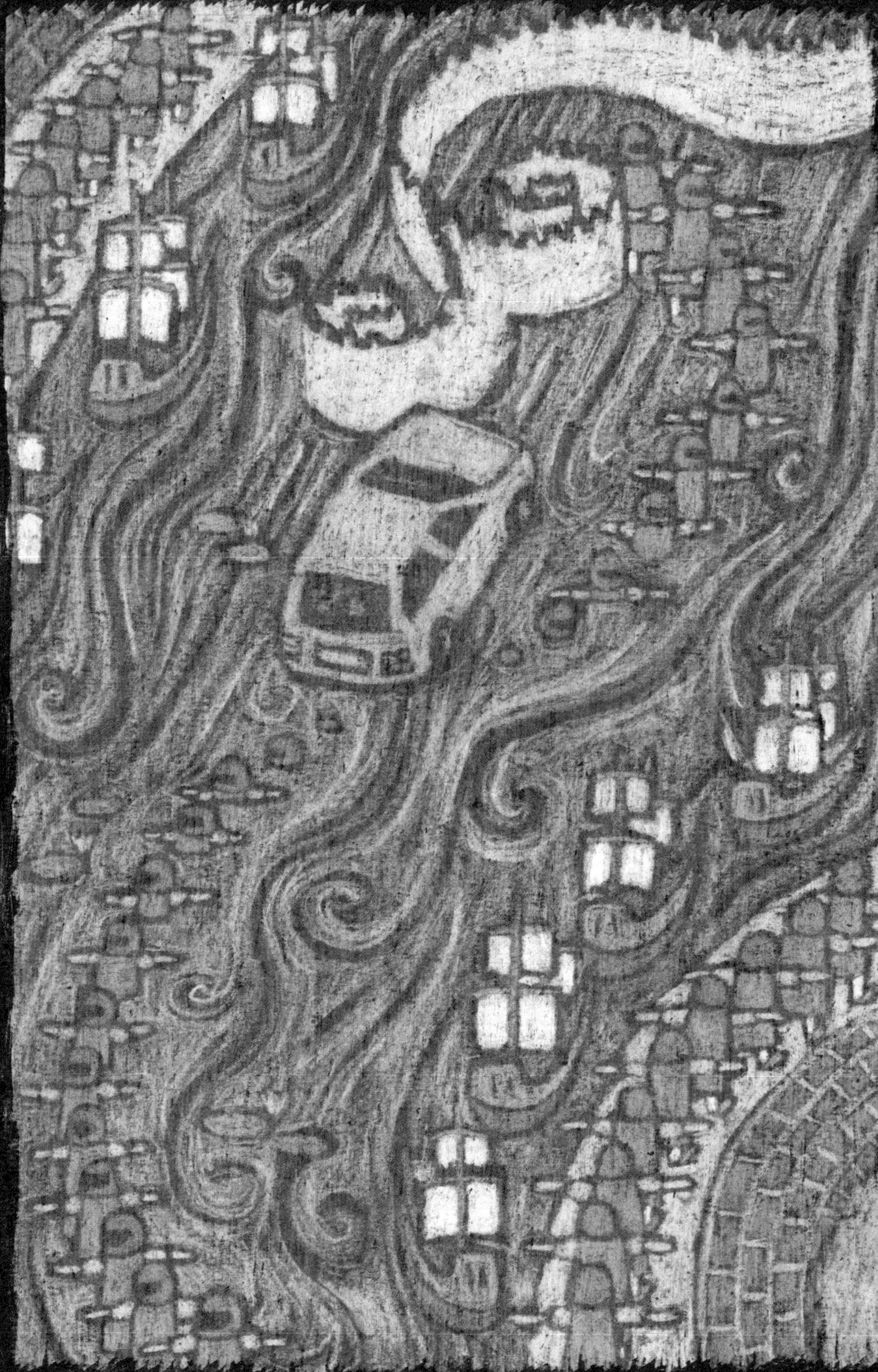

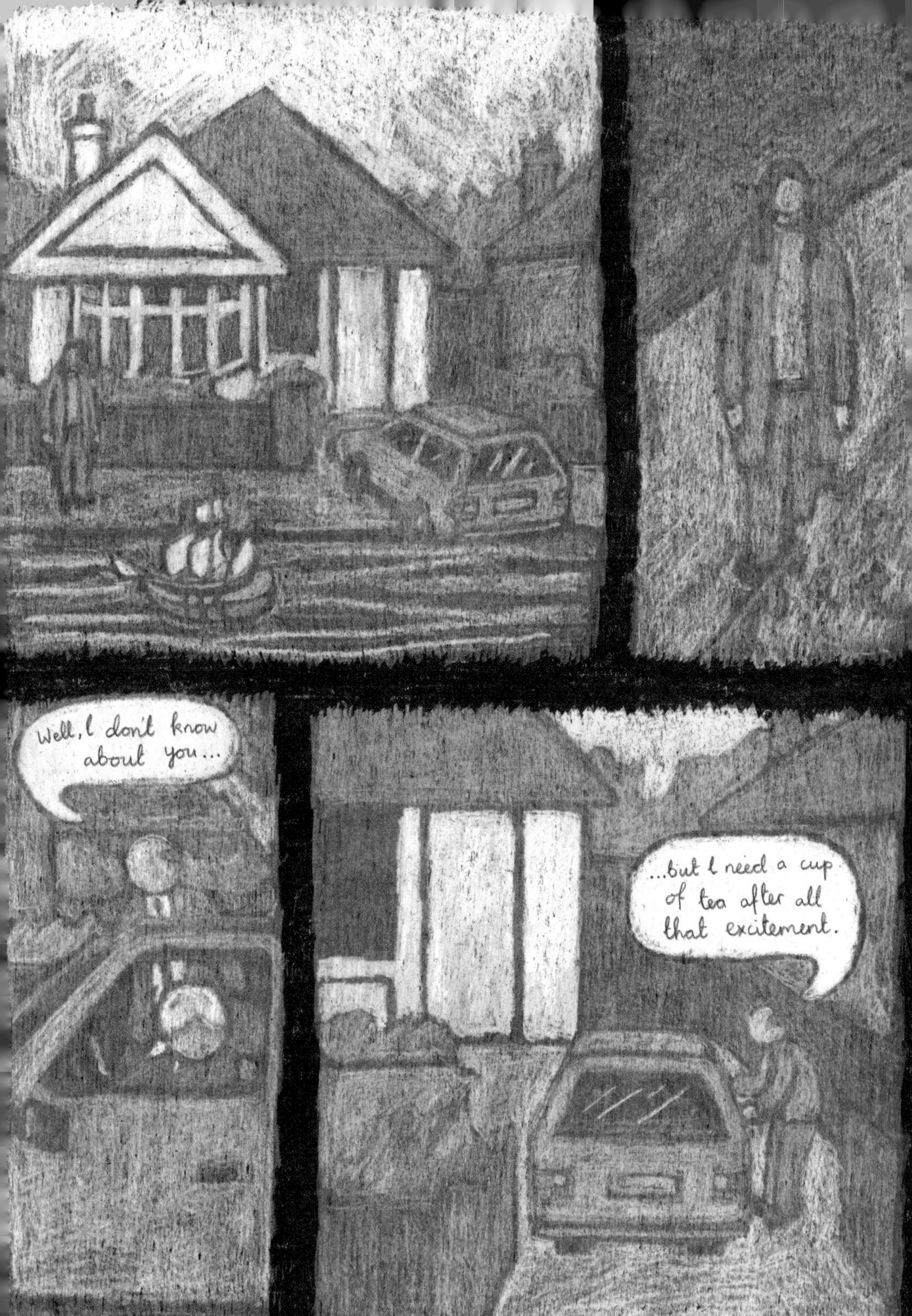
Well, I don't know about you...
...but I need a cup of tea after all that excitement.

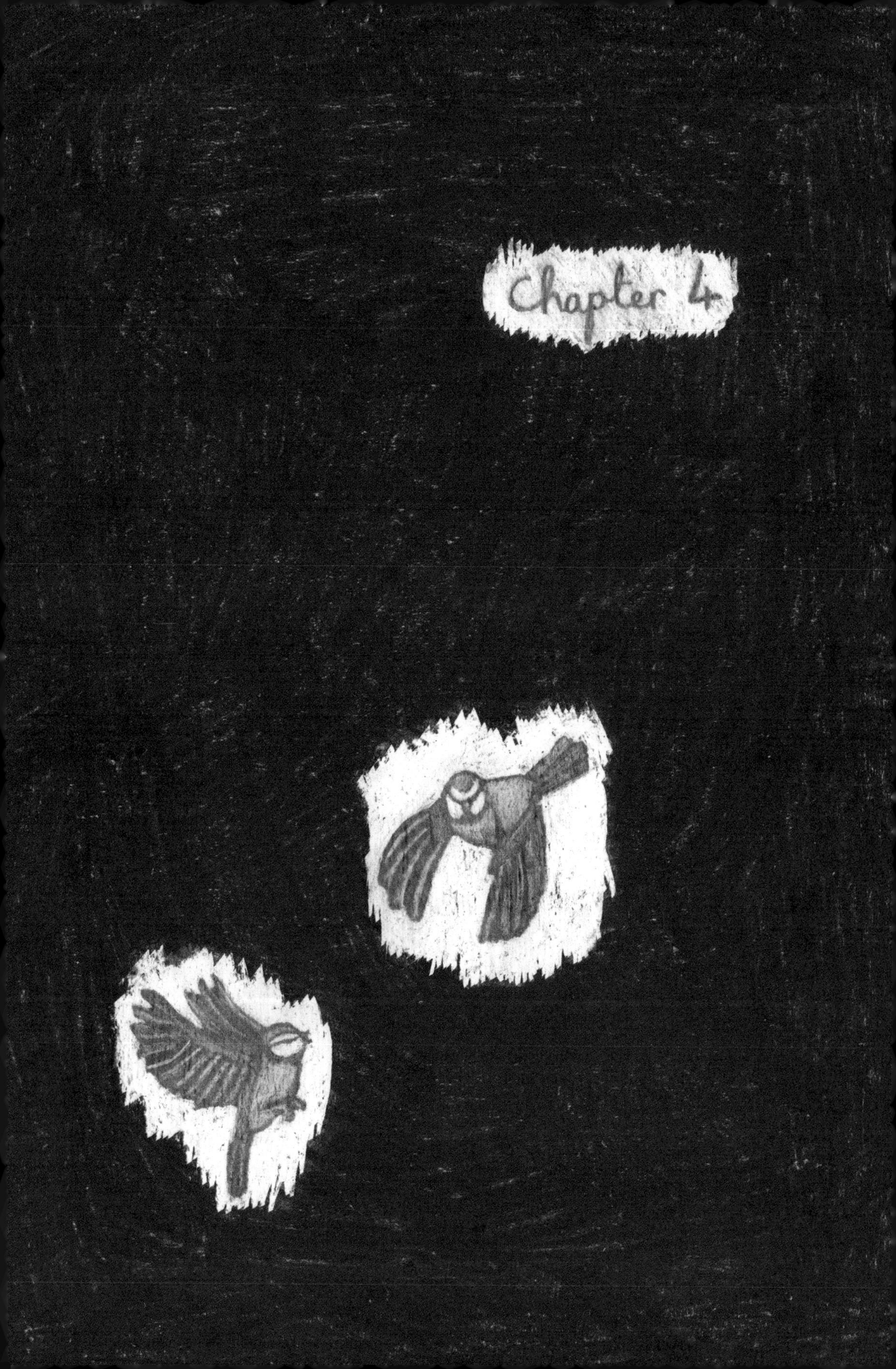
Chapter 4

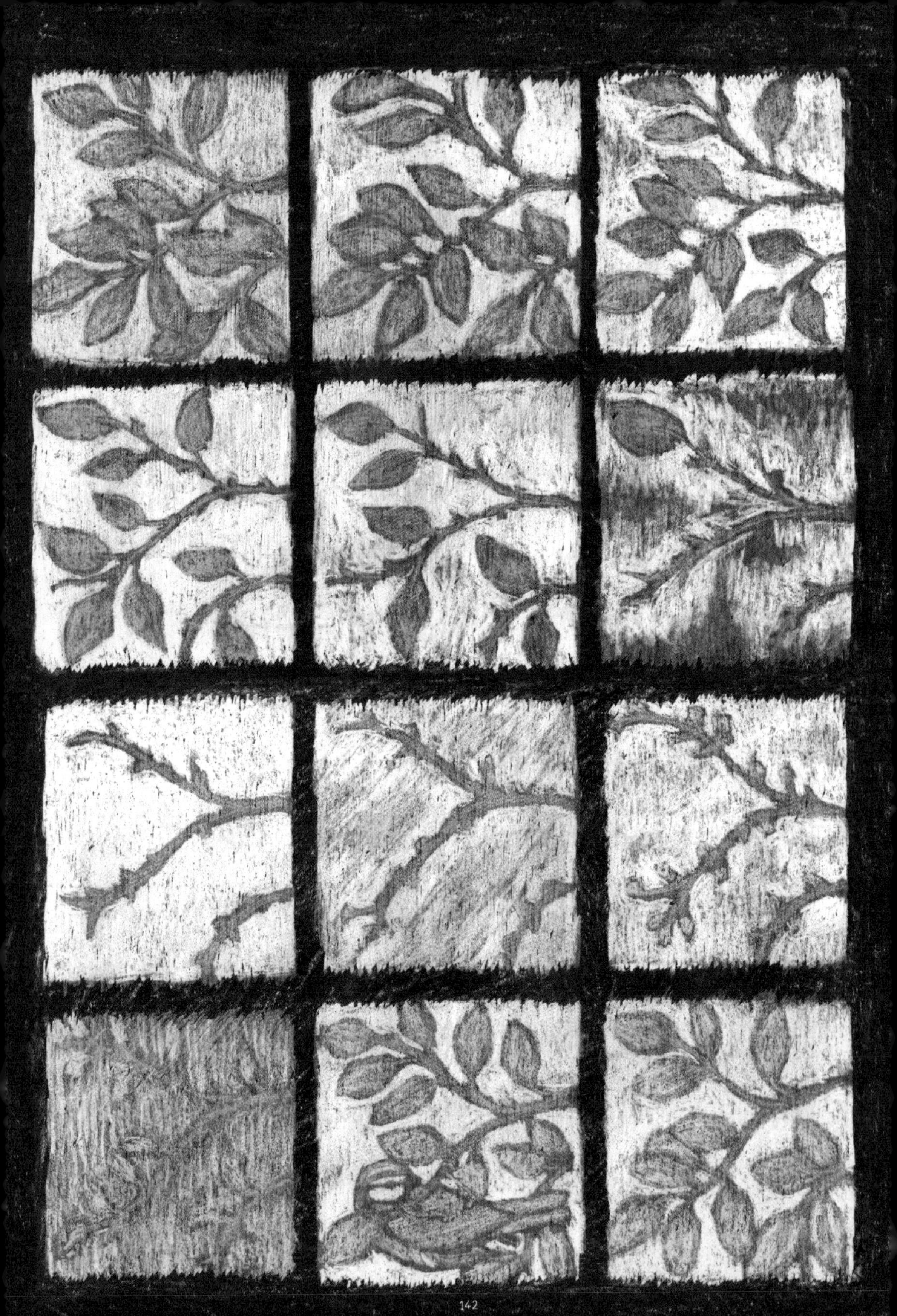

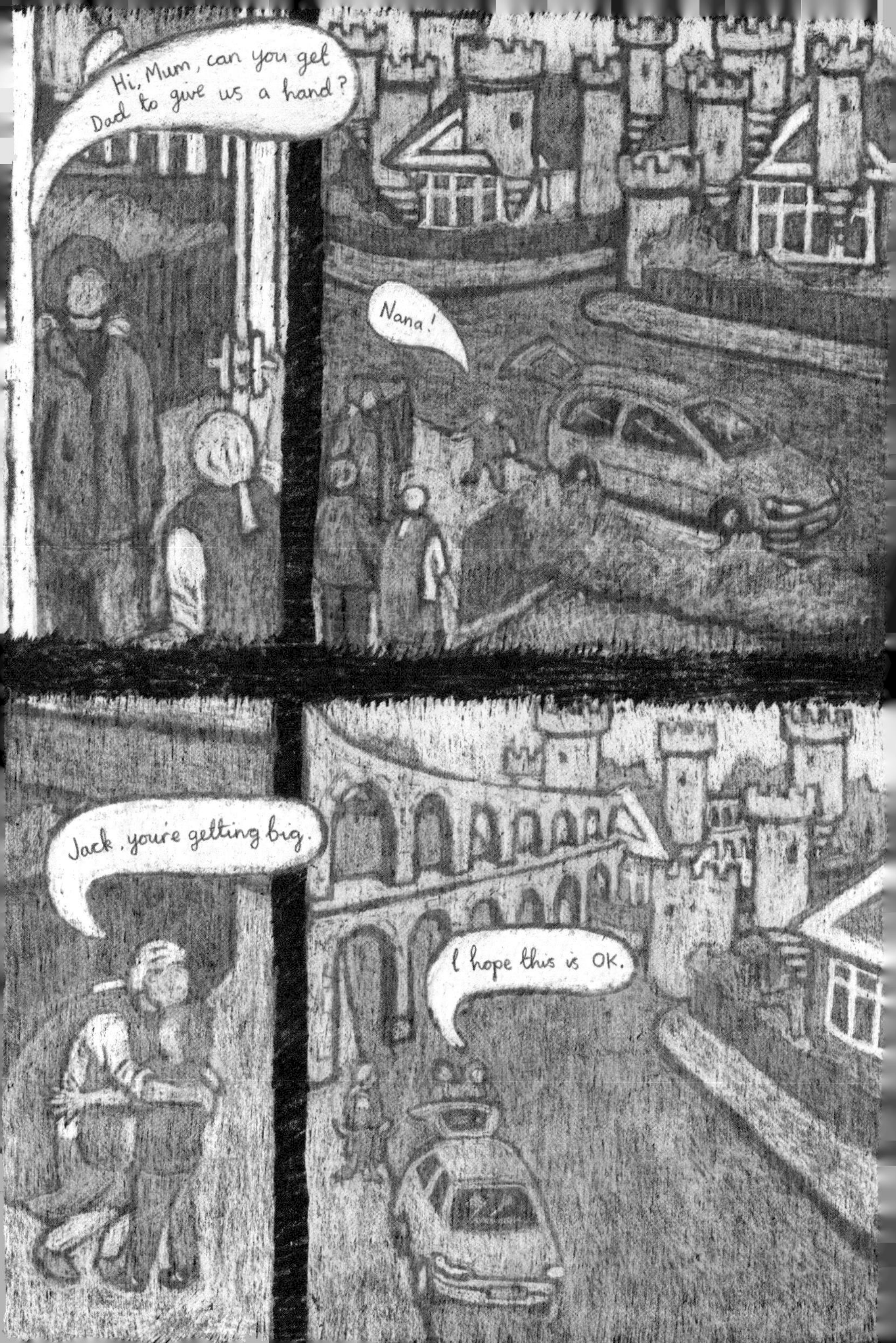
Hi, Mum, can you get Dad to give us a hand?
Nana!
Jack, you're getting big.
I hope this is OK.

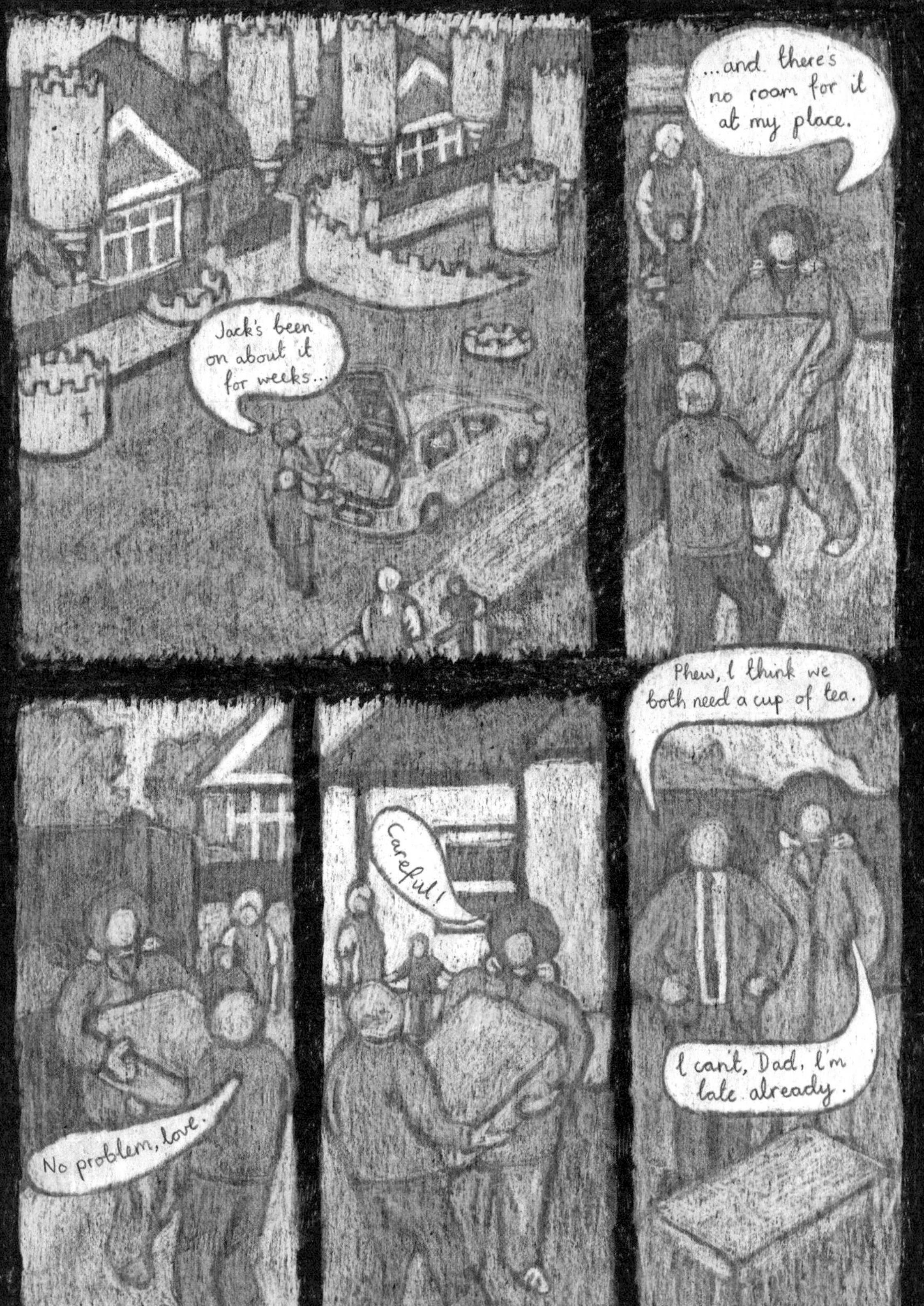
Jack's been on about it for weeks...
...and there's no room for it at my place.
No problem, love.
Careful!
Phew, I think we both need a cup of tea.
I can't, Dad, I'm late already.

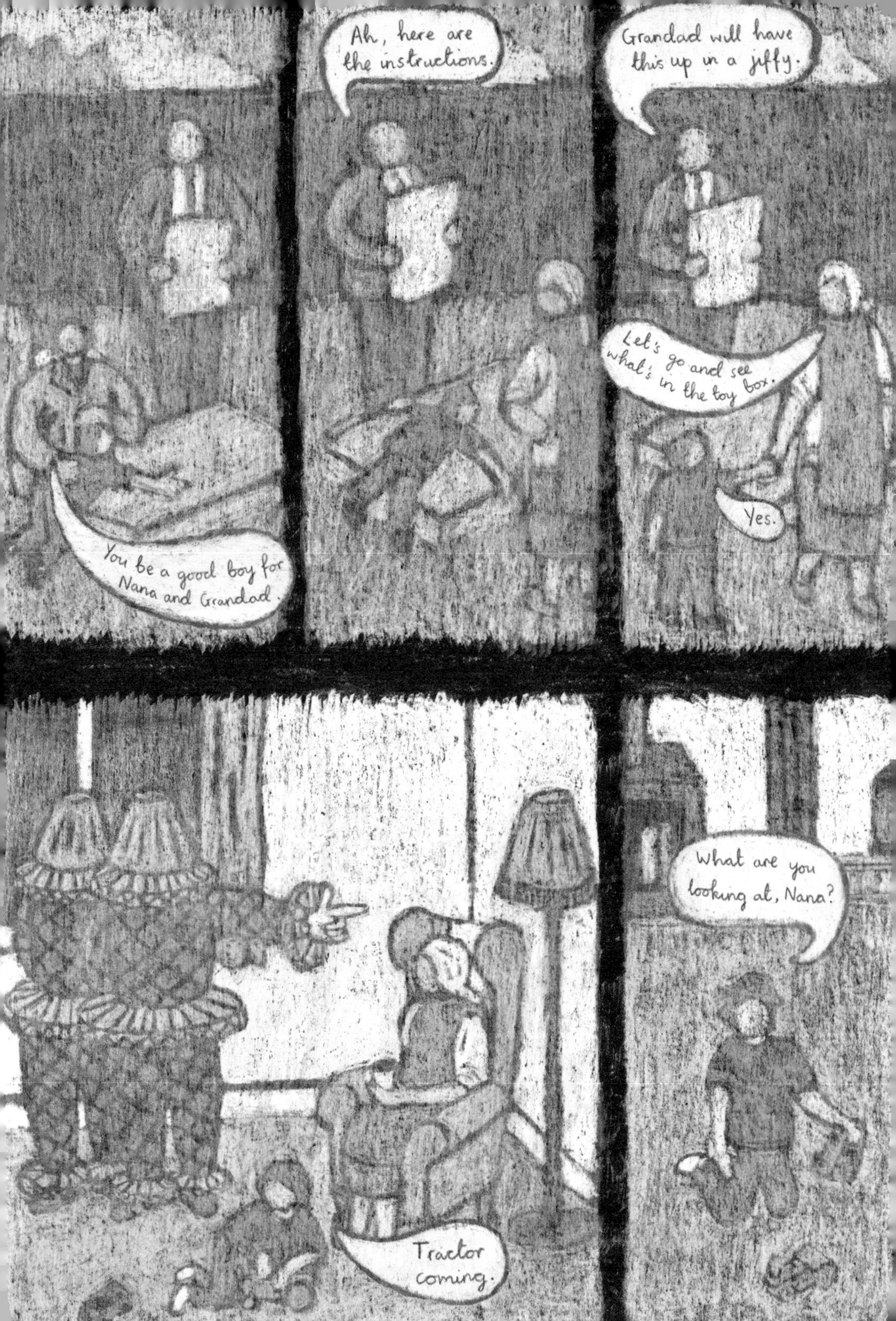
You be a good boy for Nana and Grandad.
Ah, here are the instructions.
Grandad will have this up in a jiffy.
Let's go and see what's in the toy box.
Yes.
Tractor coming.
What are you looking at, Nana?

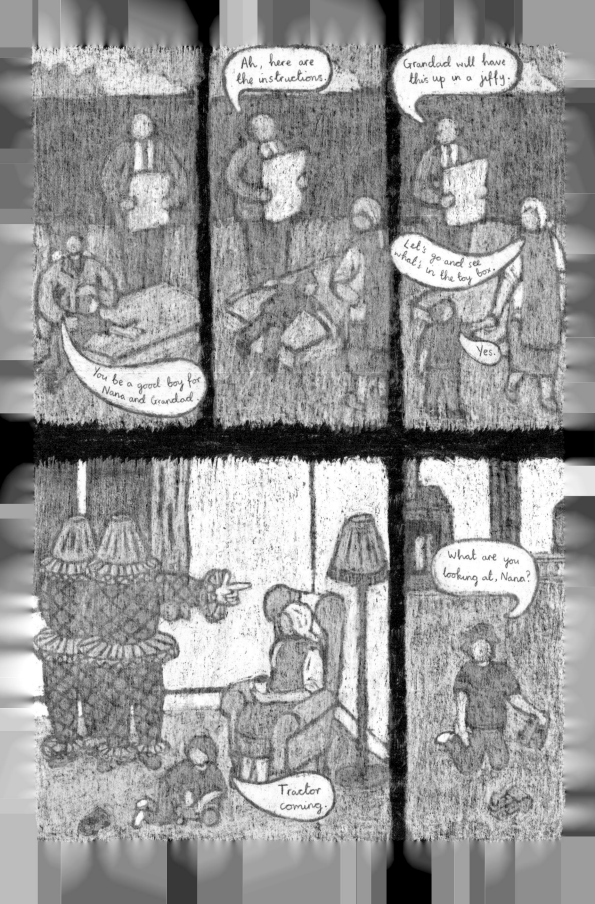

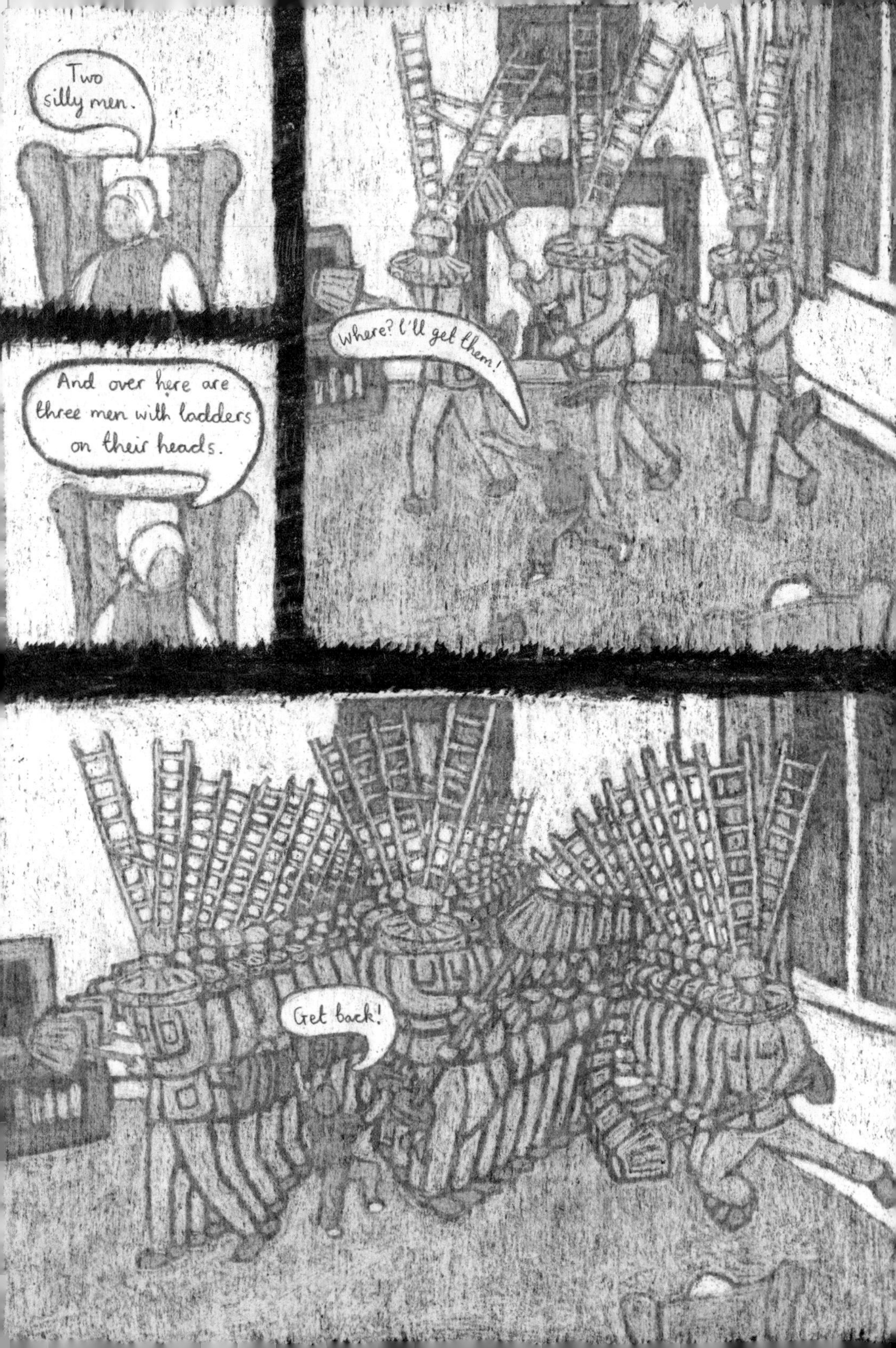
Two silly men.
And over here are three men with ladders on their heads.
Where? I'll get them!
Get back!

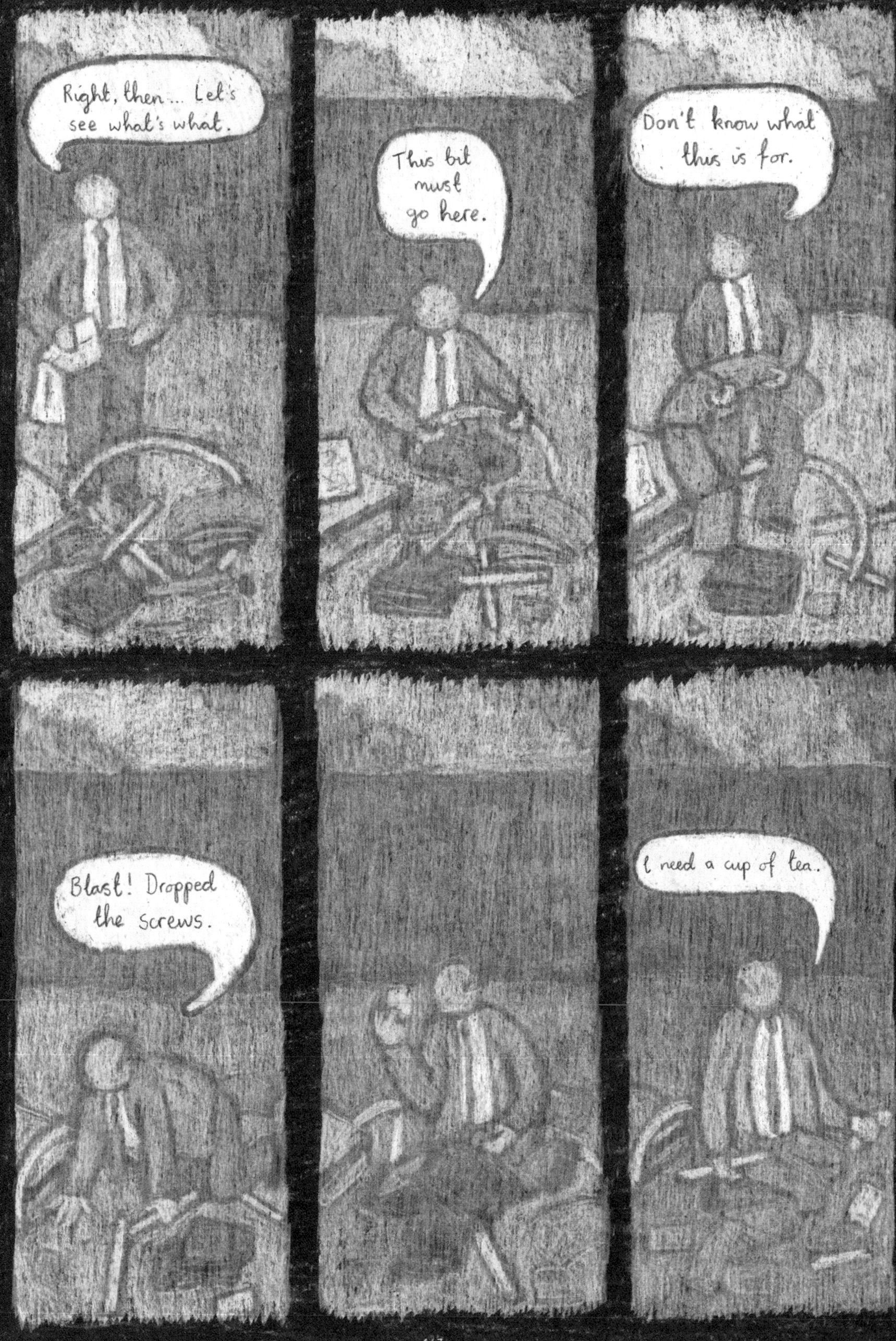
Right, then... Let's see what's what.
This bit must go here.
Don't know what this is for.
Blast! Dropped the screws.
I need a cup of tea.

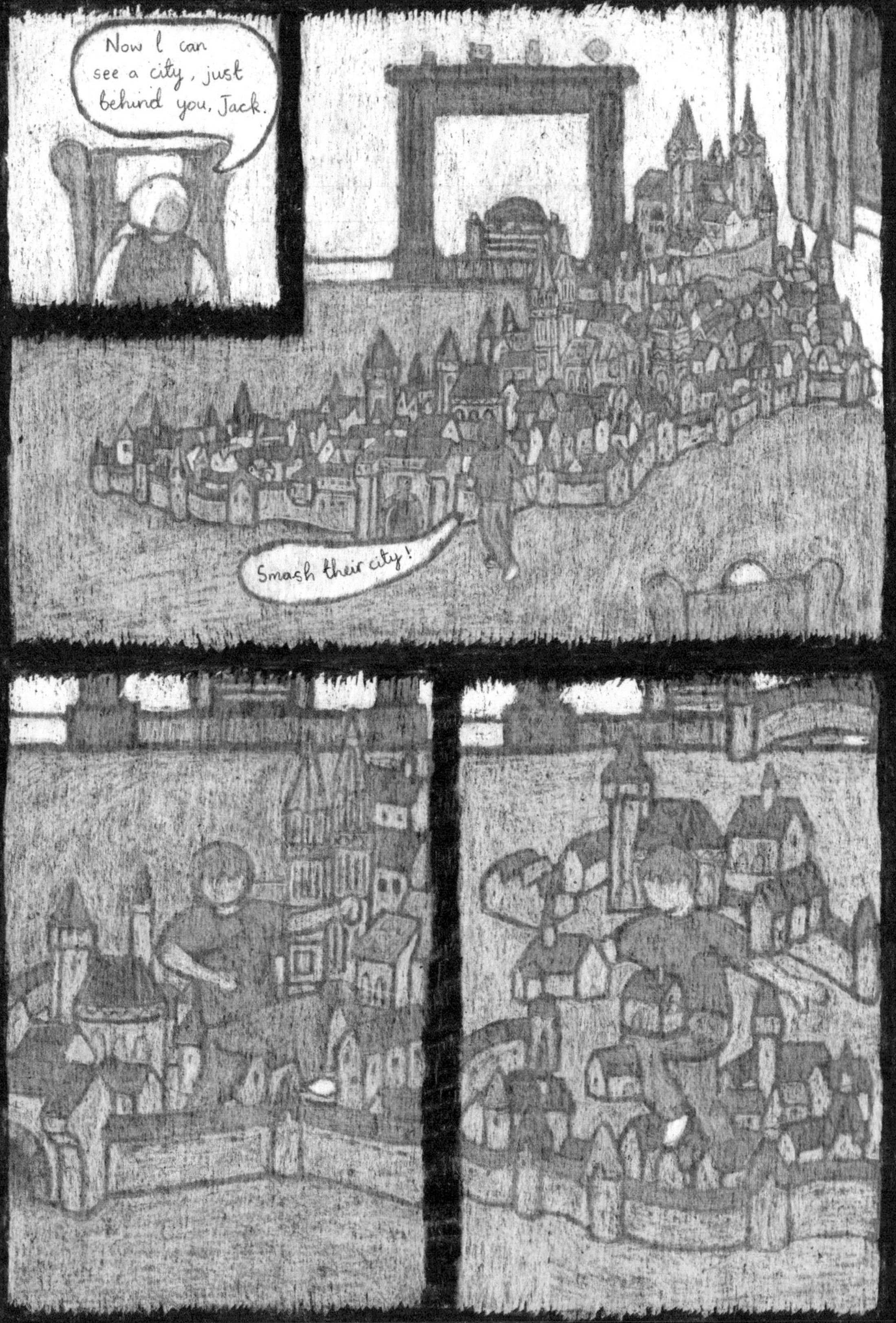
Now I can see a city, just behind you, Jack.
Smash their city!

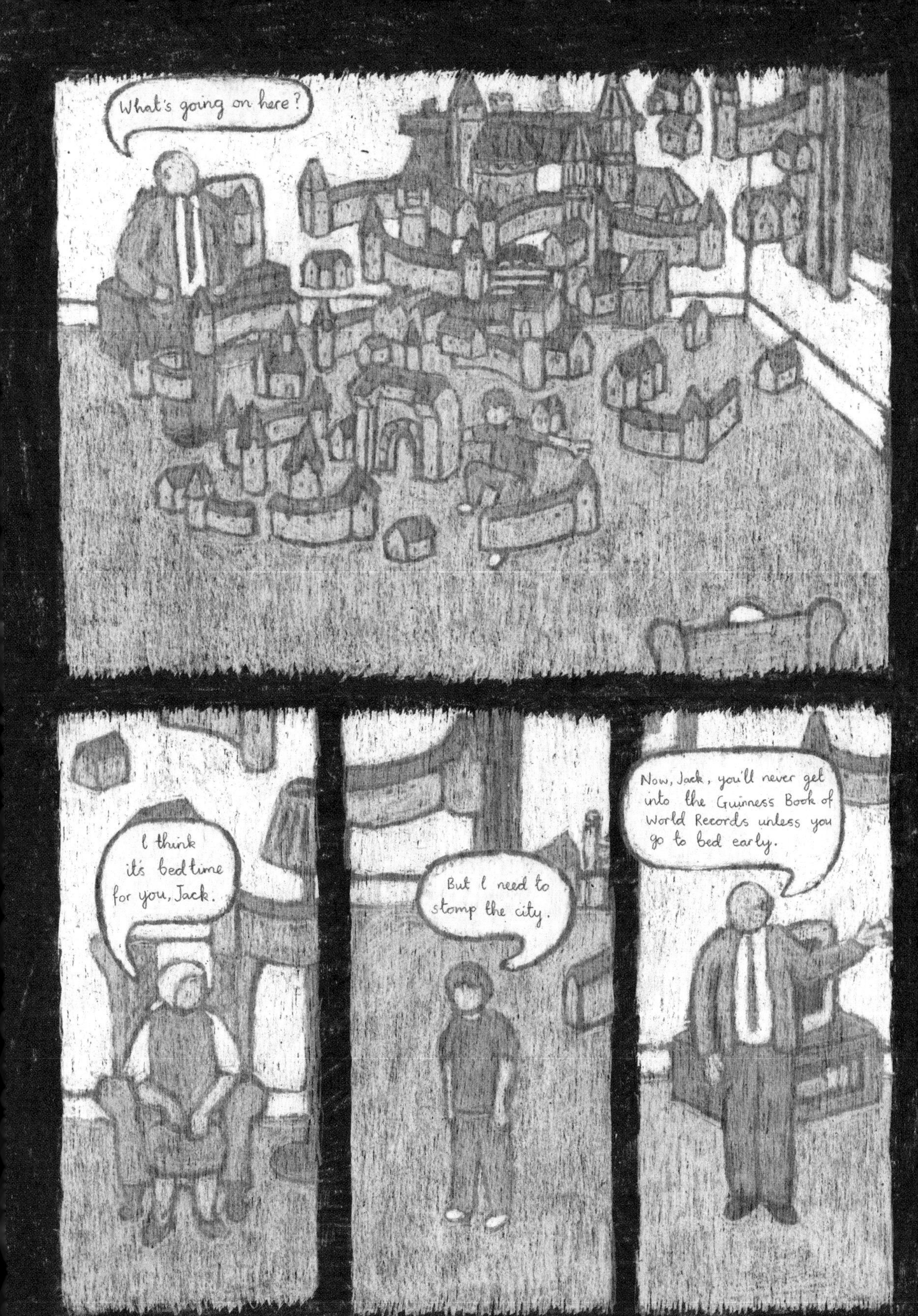
What's going on here?
I think it's bedtime for you, Jack.
But I need to stomp the city.
Now, Jack, you'll never get into the Guinness Book of World Records unless you go to bed early.

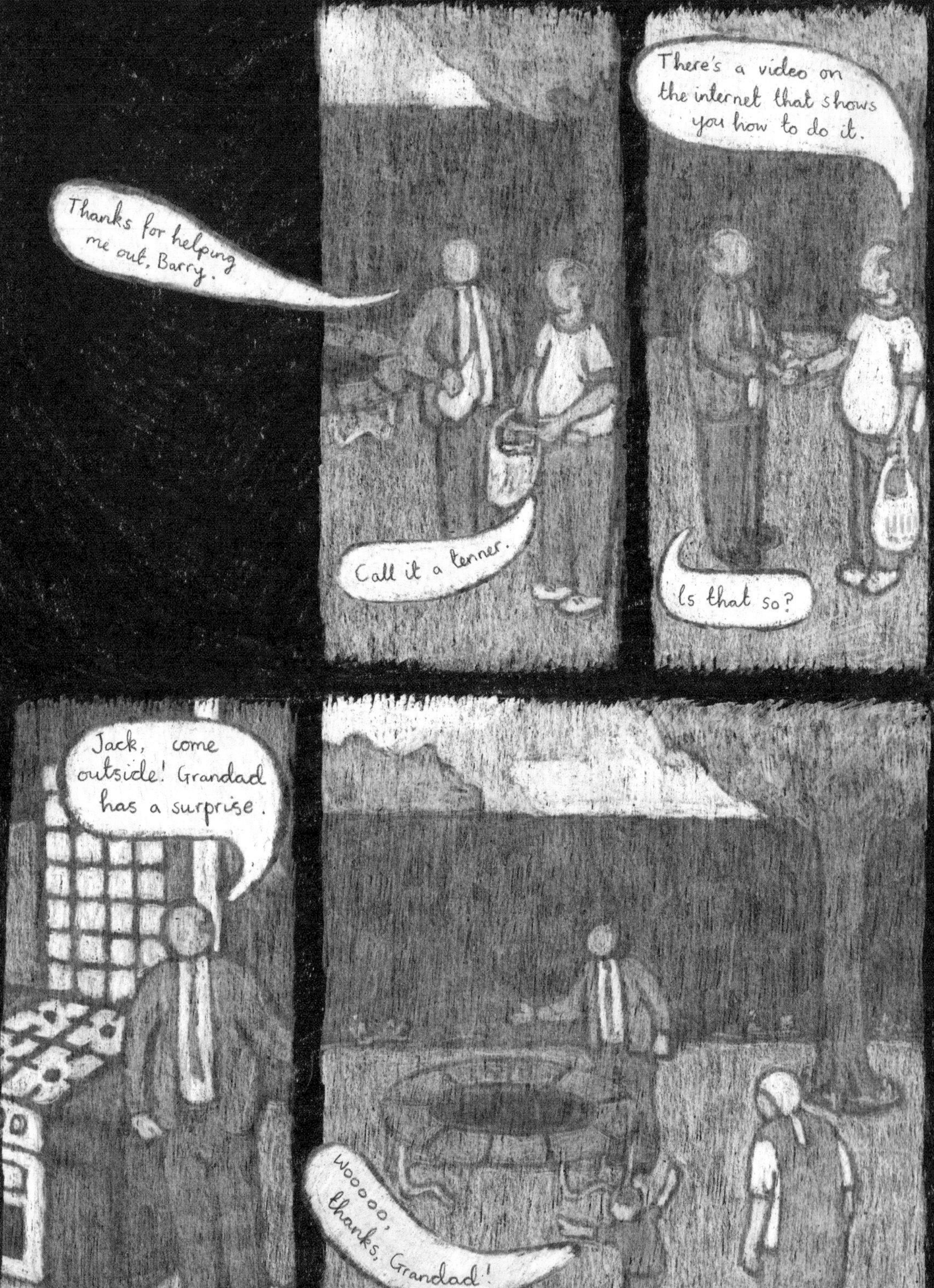
Thanks for helping me out, Barry.
Call it a tenner.
There's a video on the internet that shows you how to do it.
Is that so?
Jack, come outside! Grandad has a surprise.
Wooooo, thanks, Grandad!

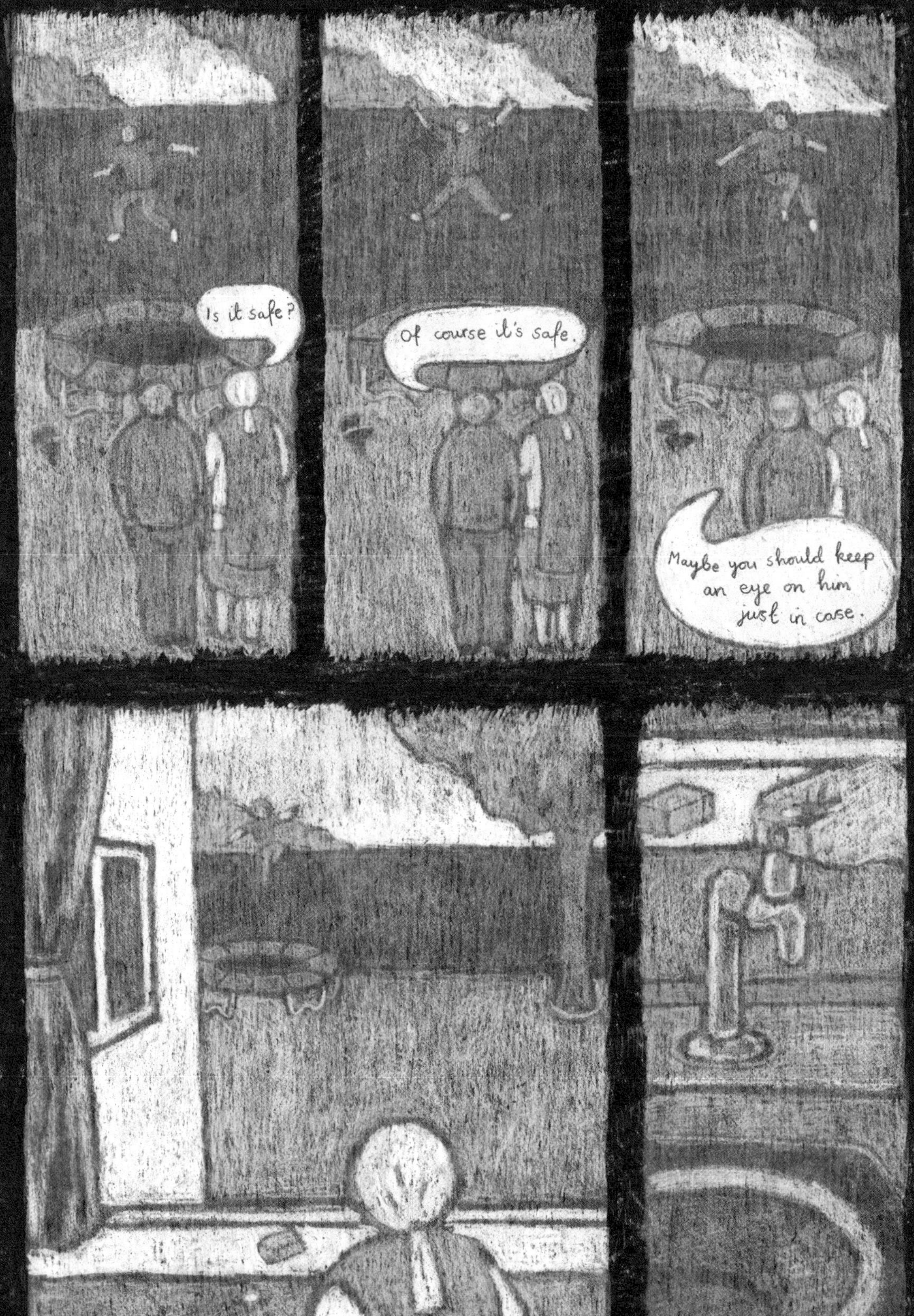
Is it safe?
Of course it's safe.
Maybe you should keep an eye on him just in case.

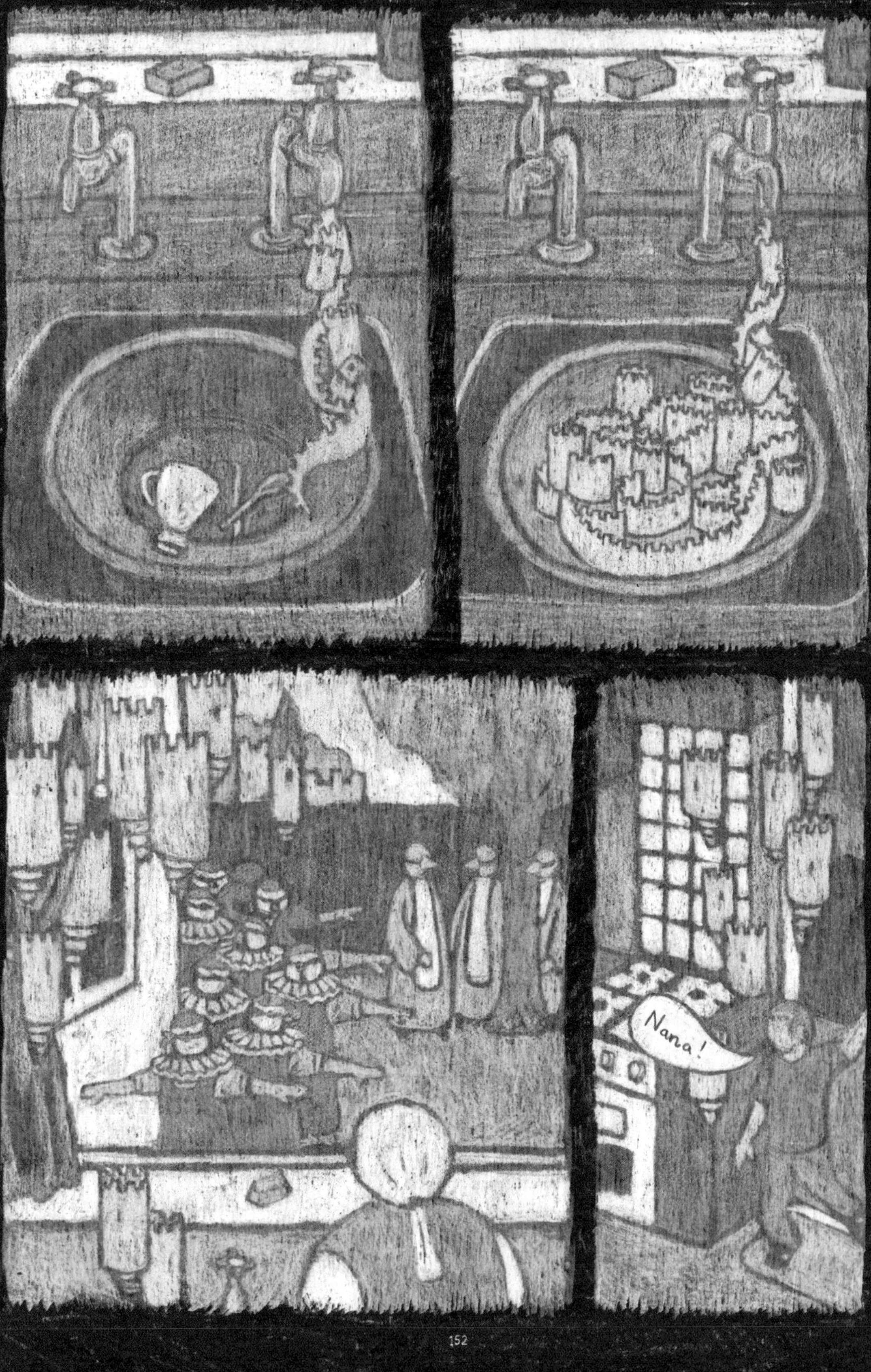
Nana!

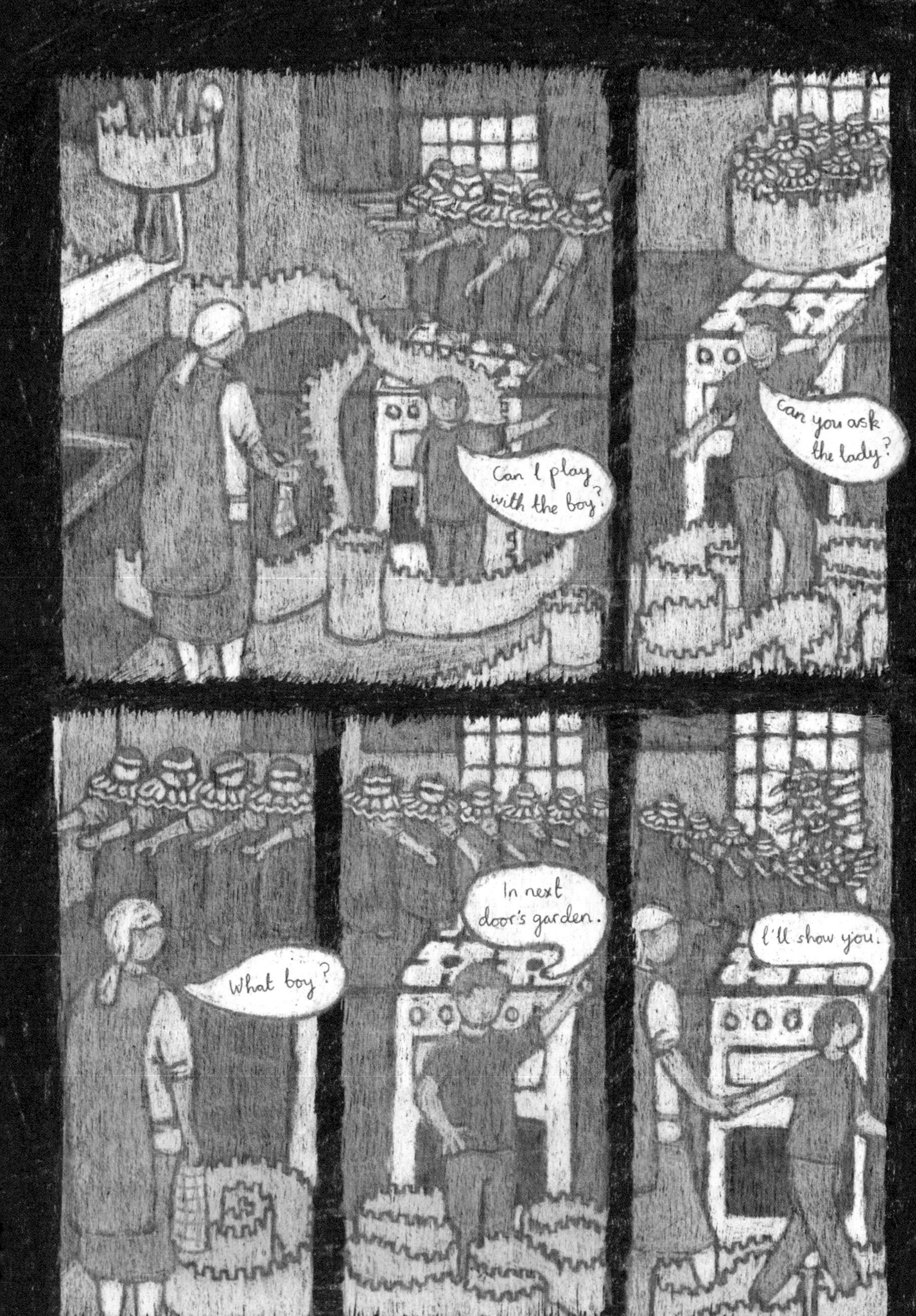
Can I play with the boy?
Can you ask the lady?
What boy?
In next door's garden.
I'll show you.

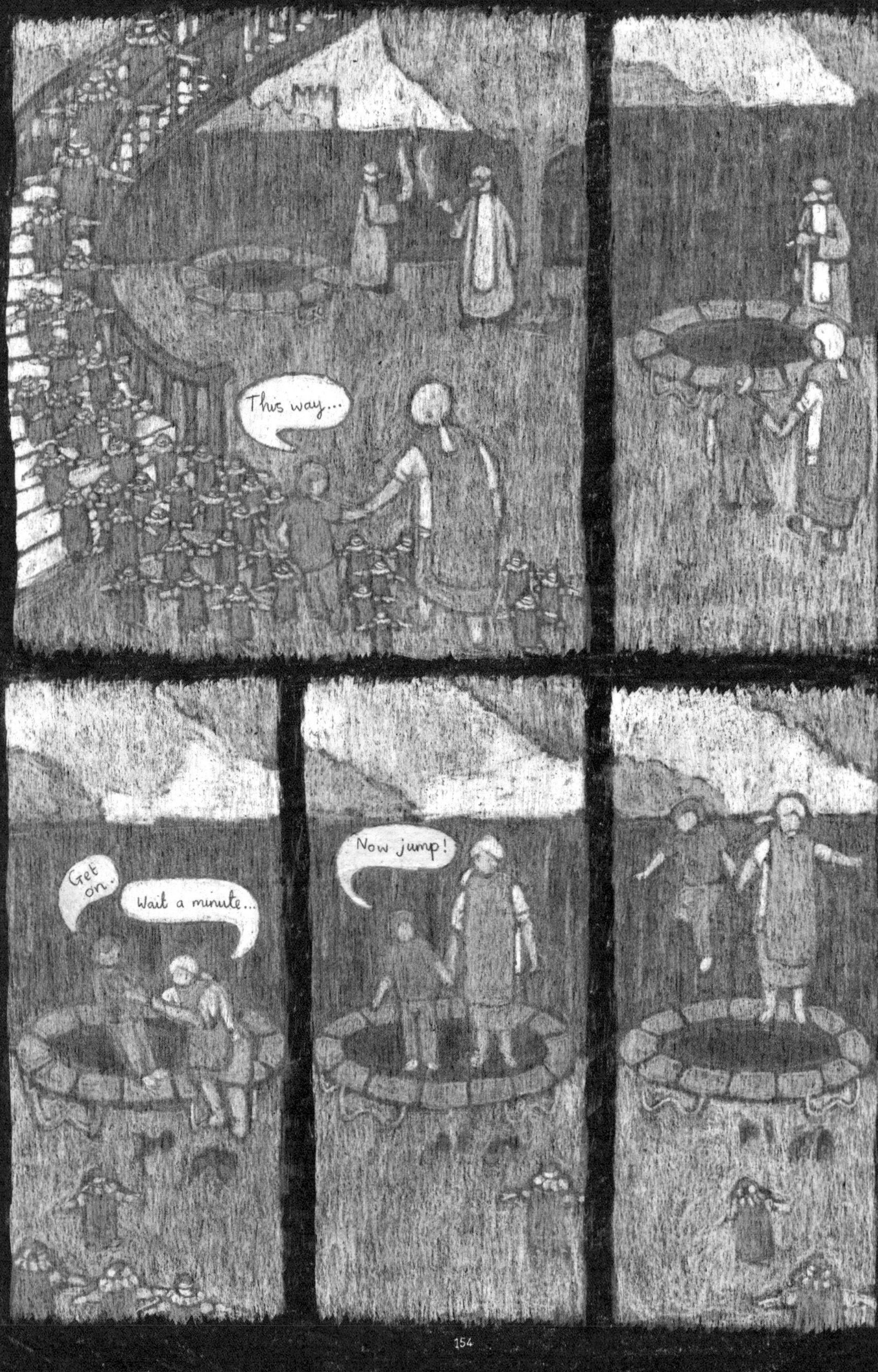
This way...
Get on.
Wait a minute...
Now jump!

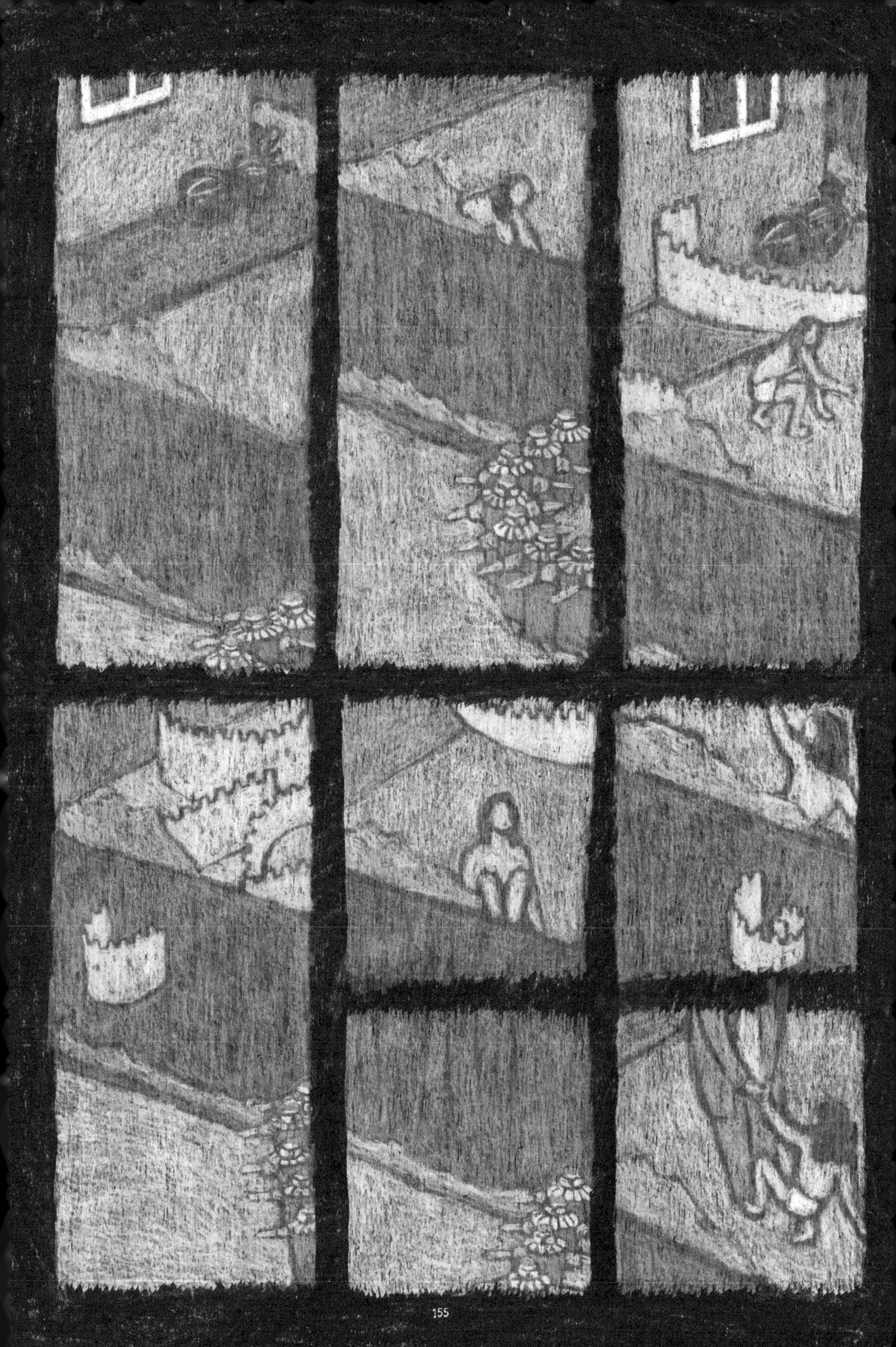

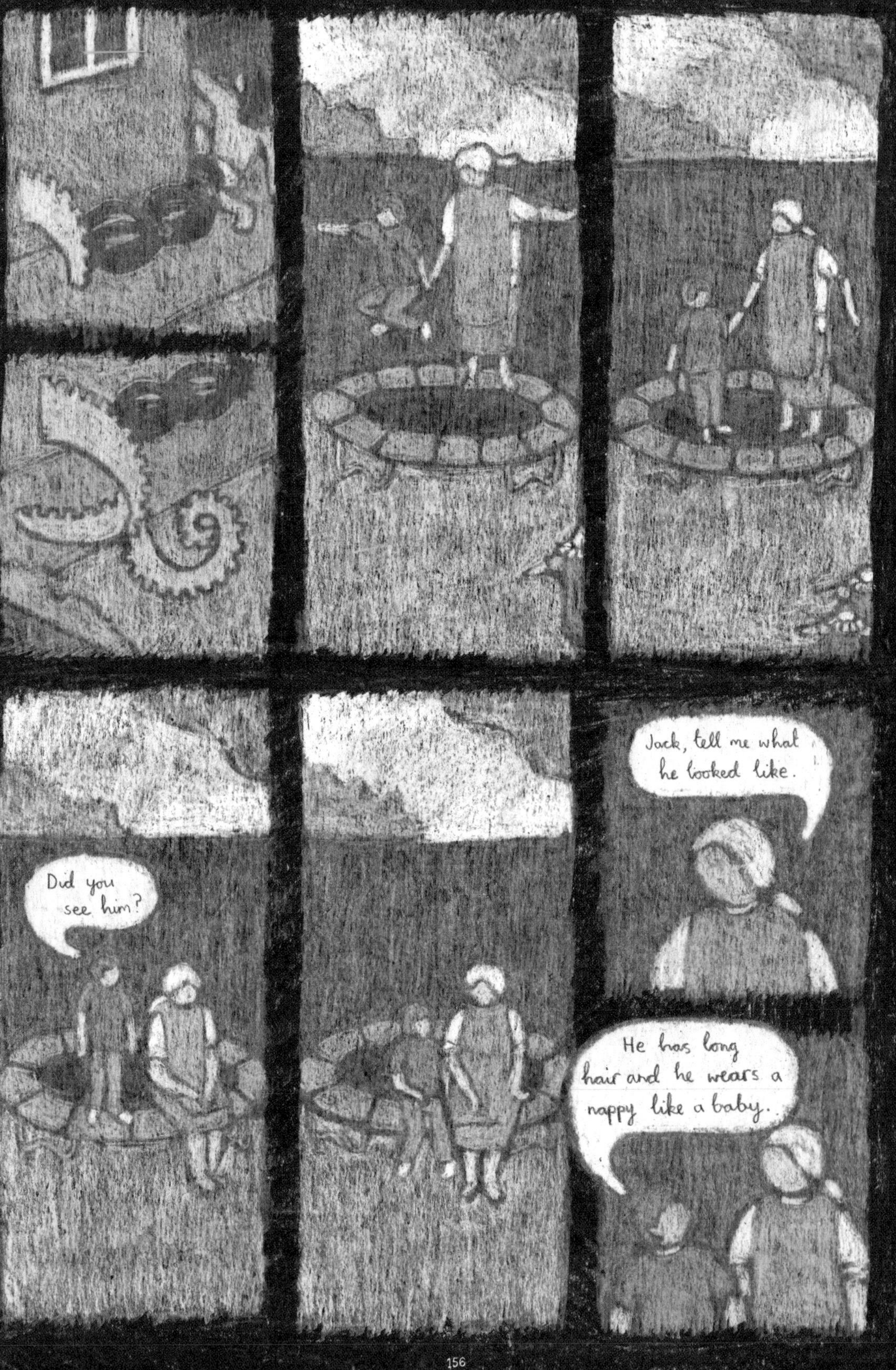
Did you see him?
Jack, tell me what he looked like.
He has long hair and he wears a nappy like a baby.

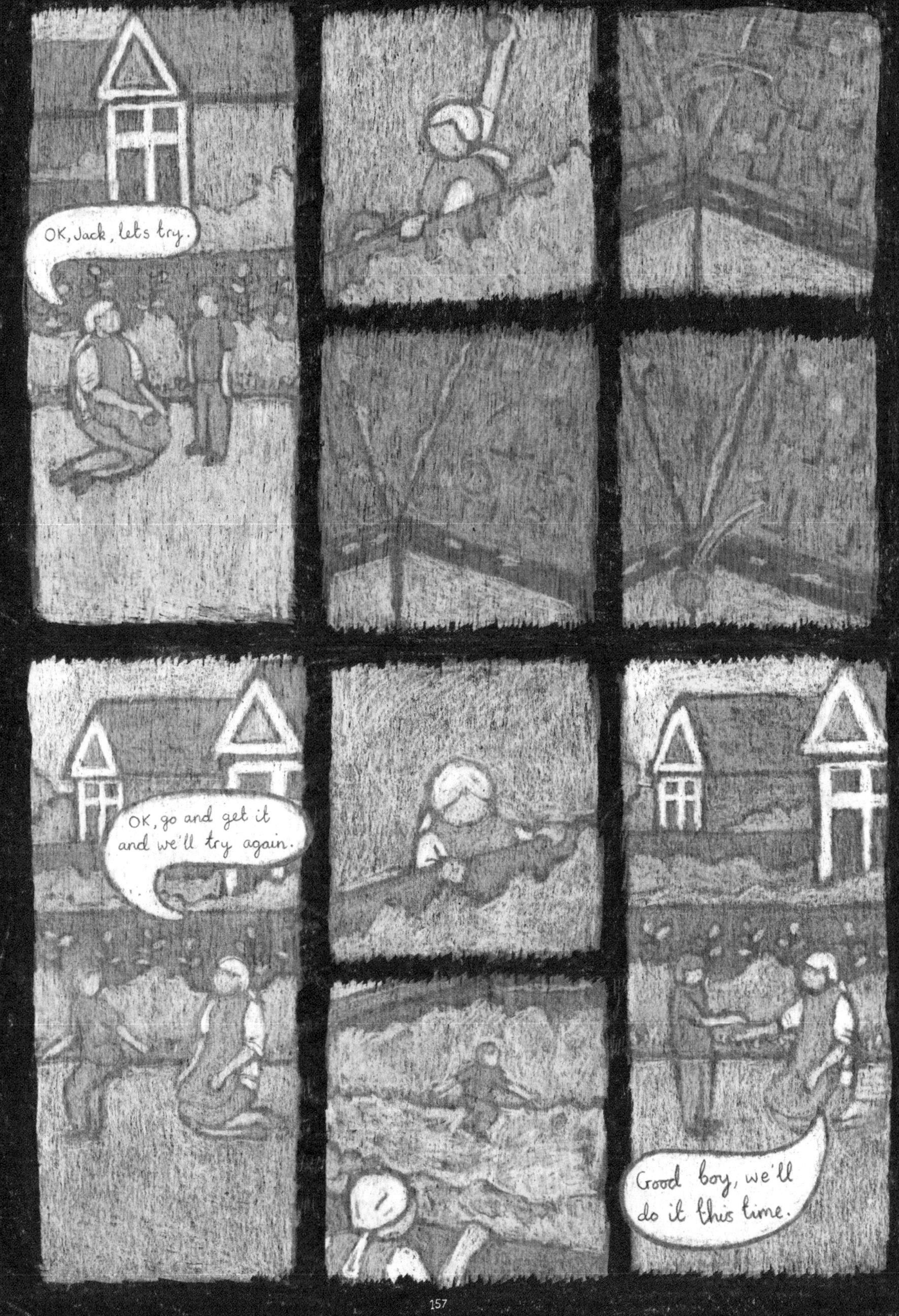
OK, Jack, lets try.
OK, go and get it and we'll try again.
Good boy, we'll do it this time.

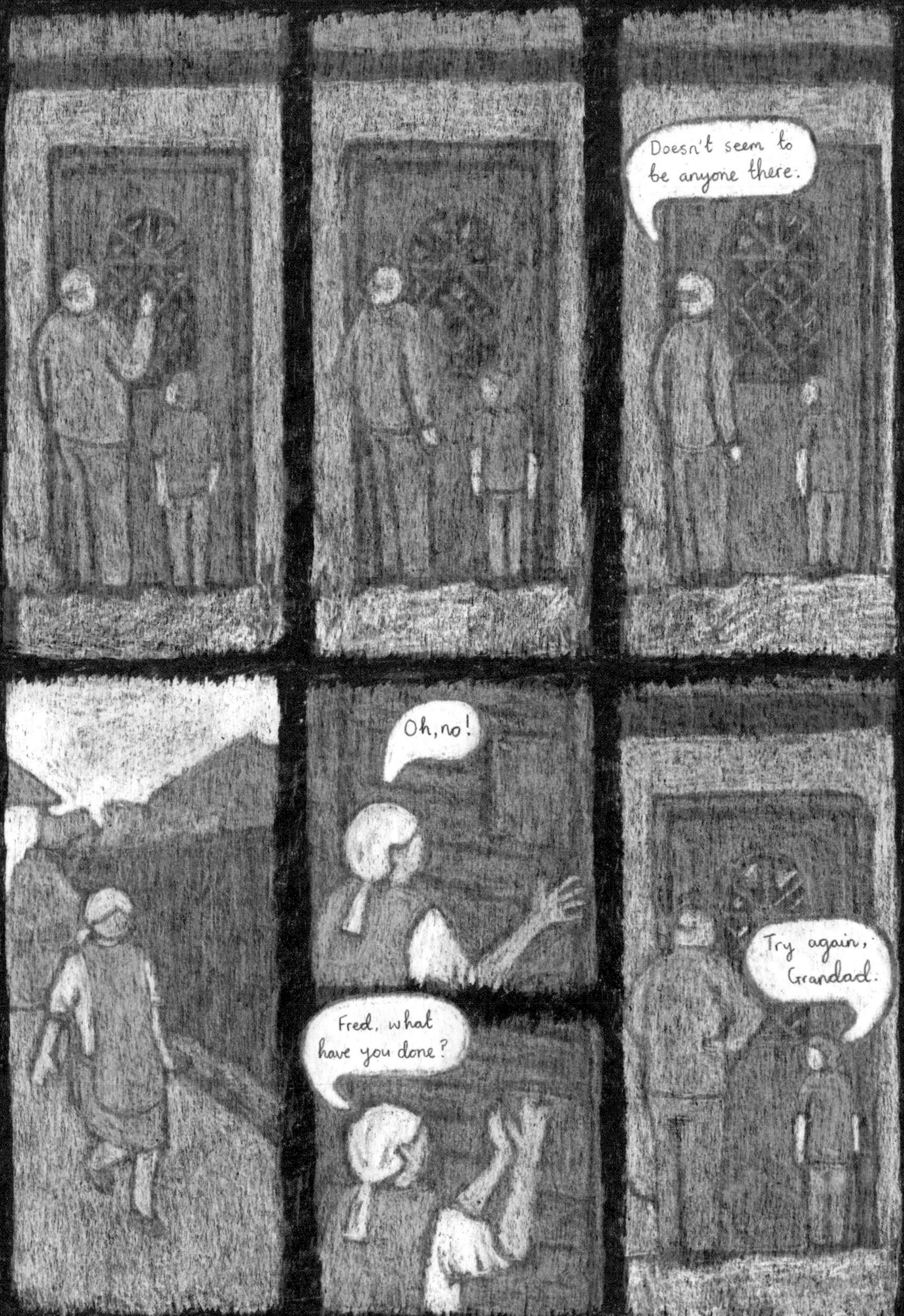
Doesn't seem to be anyone there.
Oh, no!
Fred, what have you done?
Try again, Grandad.

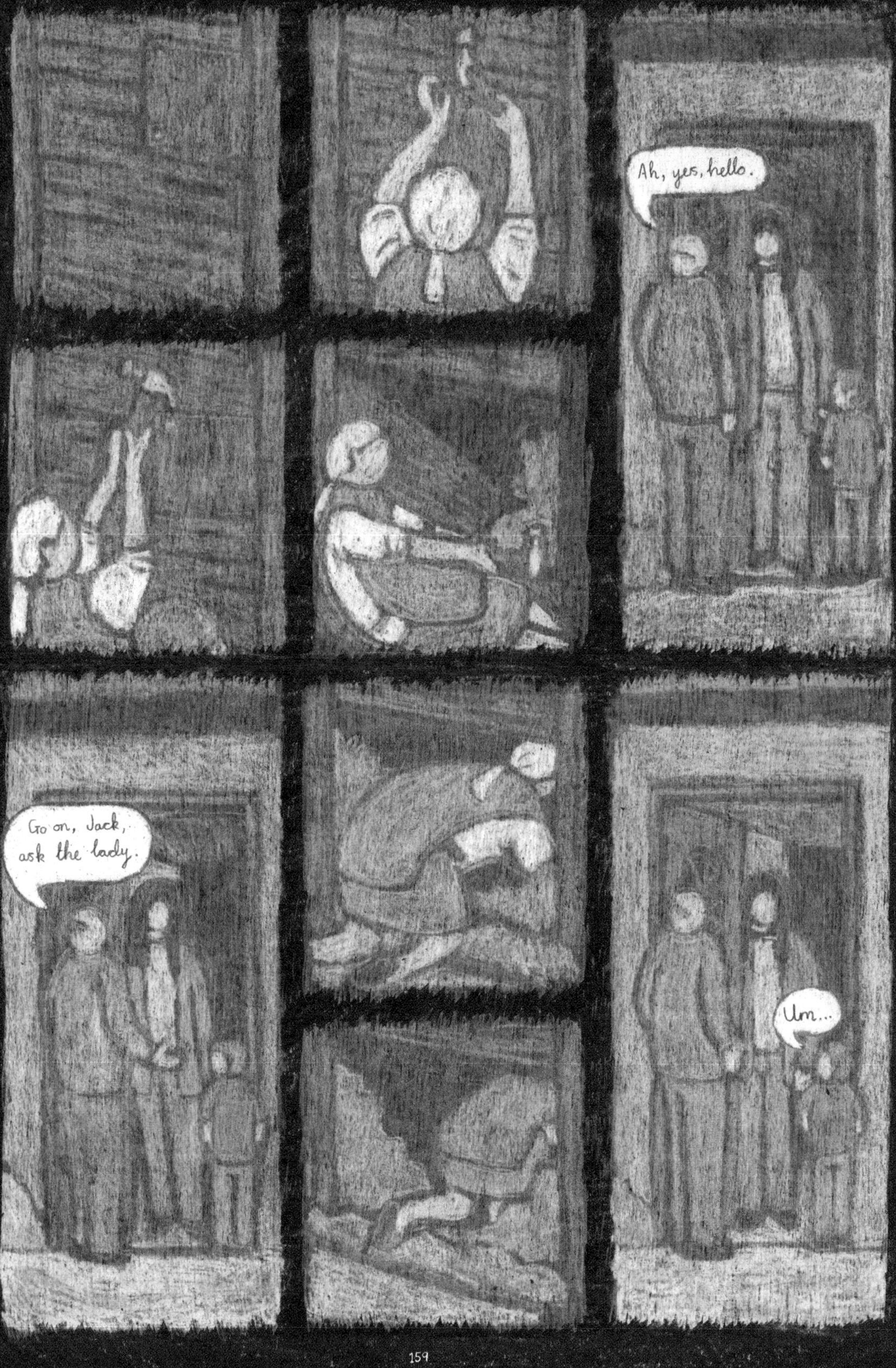
Ah, yes, hello.
Go on, Jack, ask the lady.
Um...

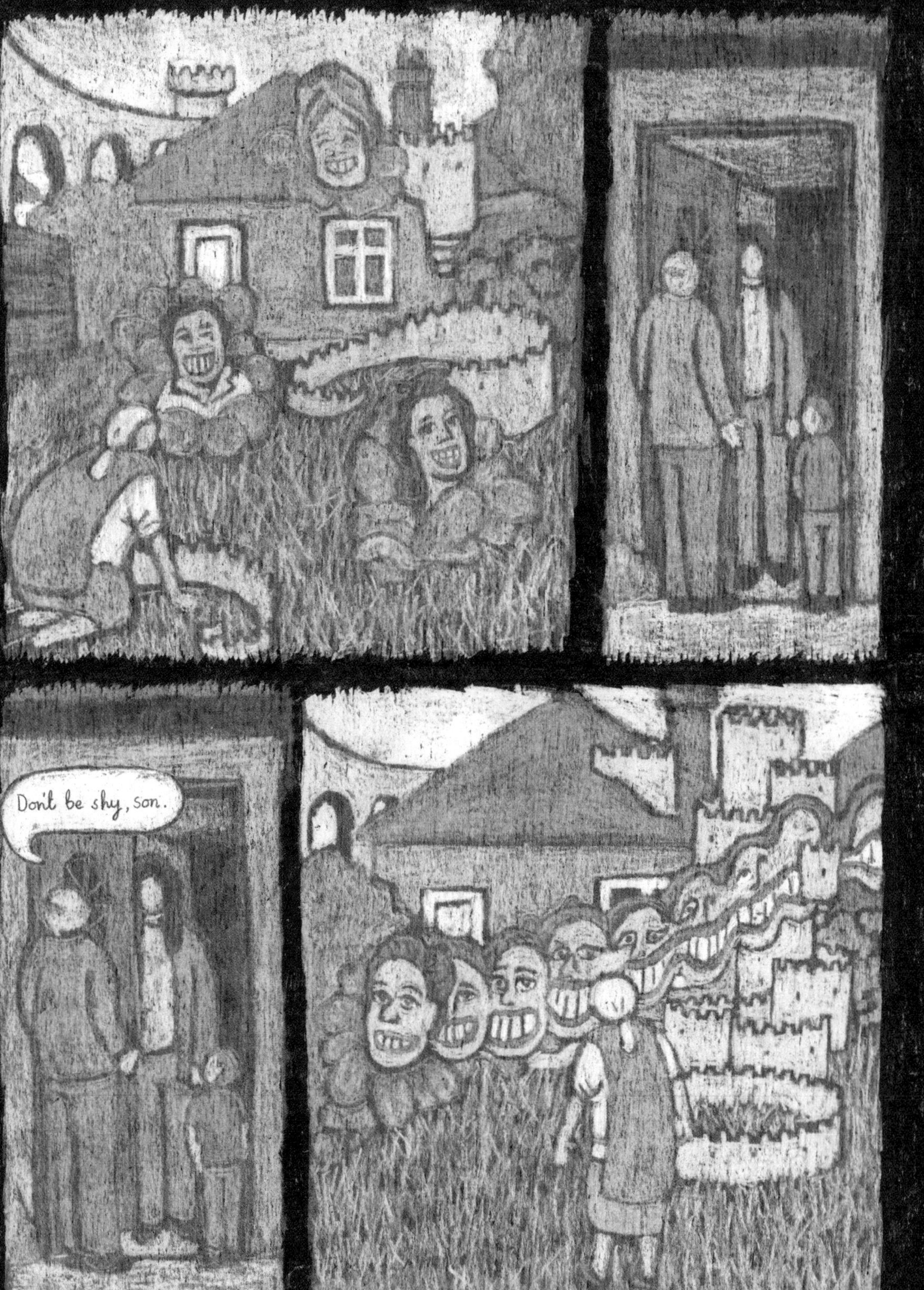
Don't be shy, son.

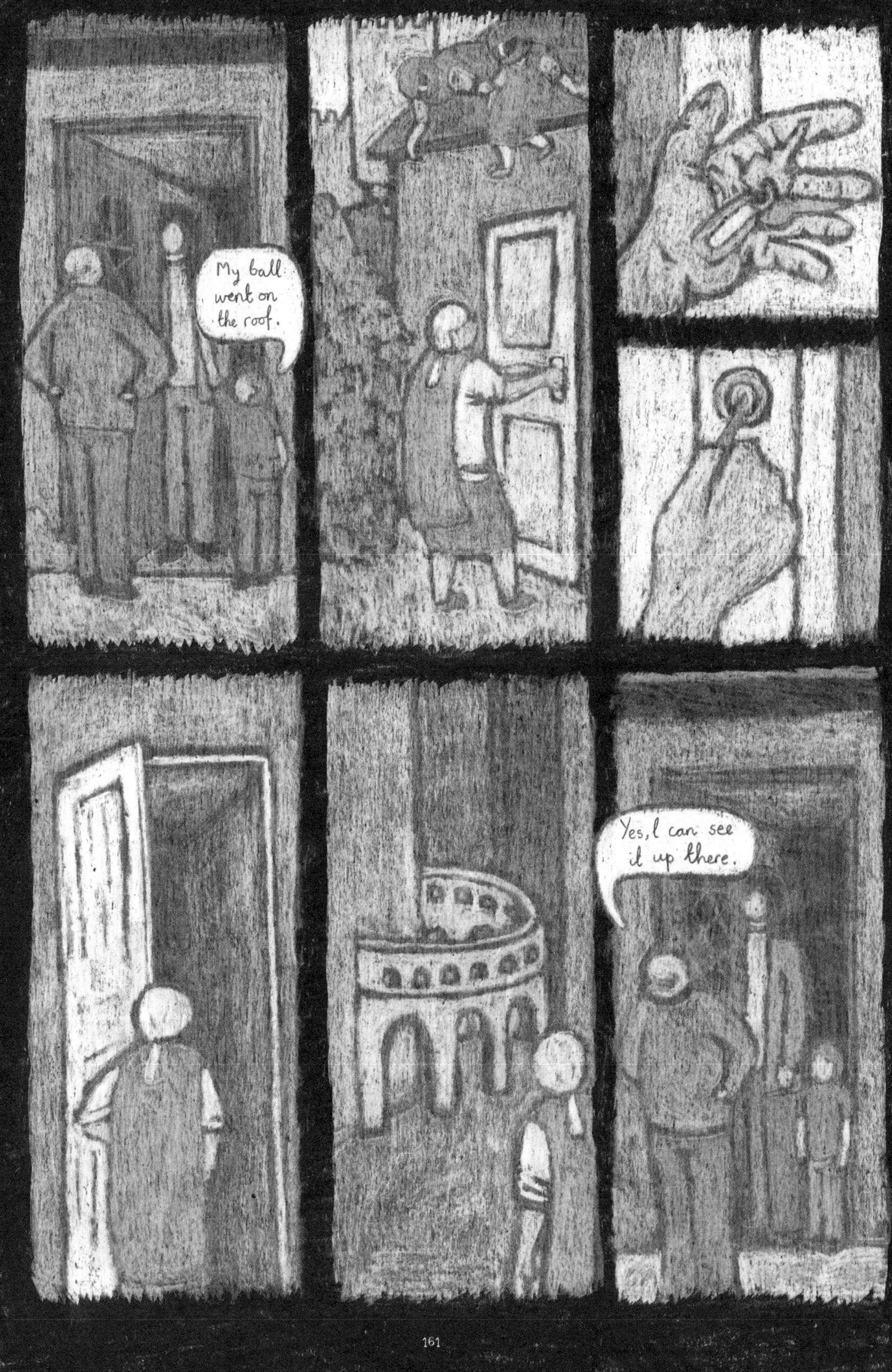
My ball went on the roof.
Yes, I can see it up there.

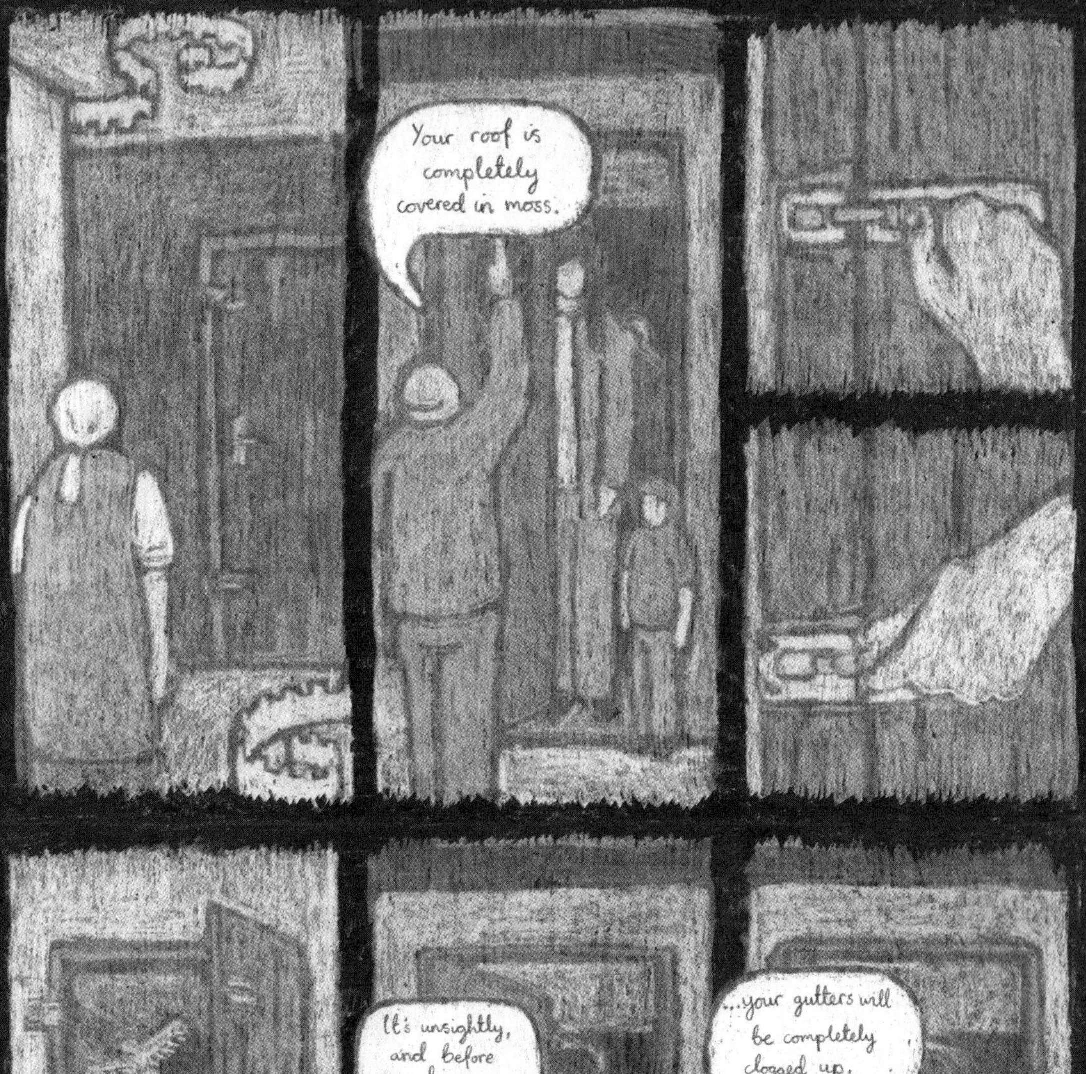
Your roof is completely covered in moss.
It's unsightly, and before you know what's what...
...your gutters will be completely clogged up.
yoooooaaw

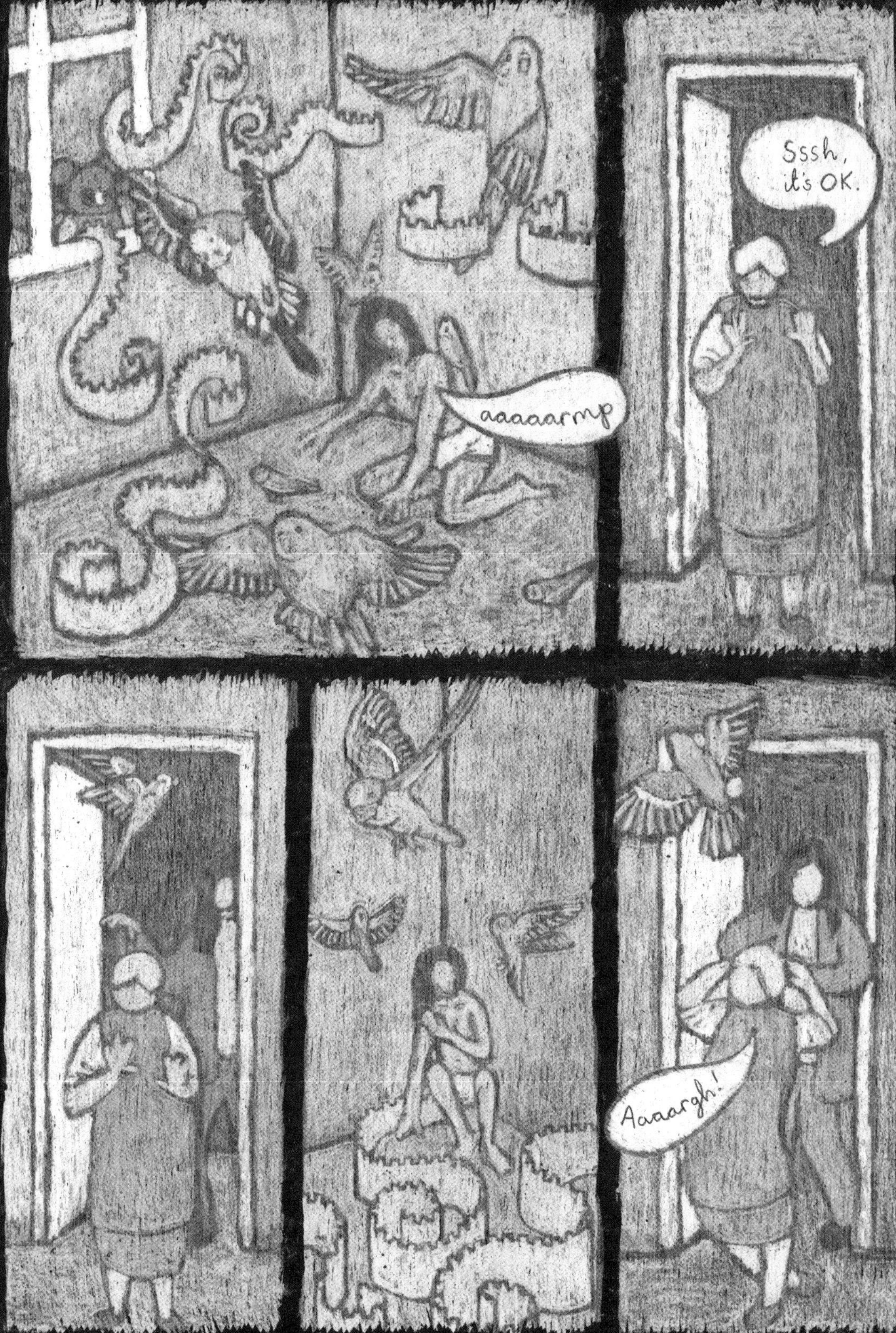
aaaaarmp
Sssh, it's OK.
Aaaargh!

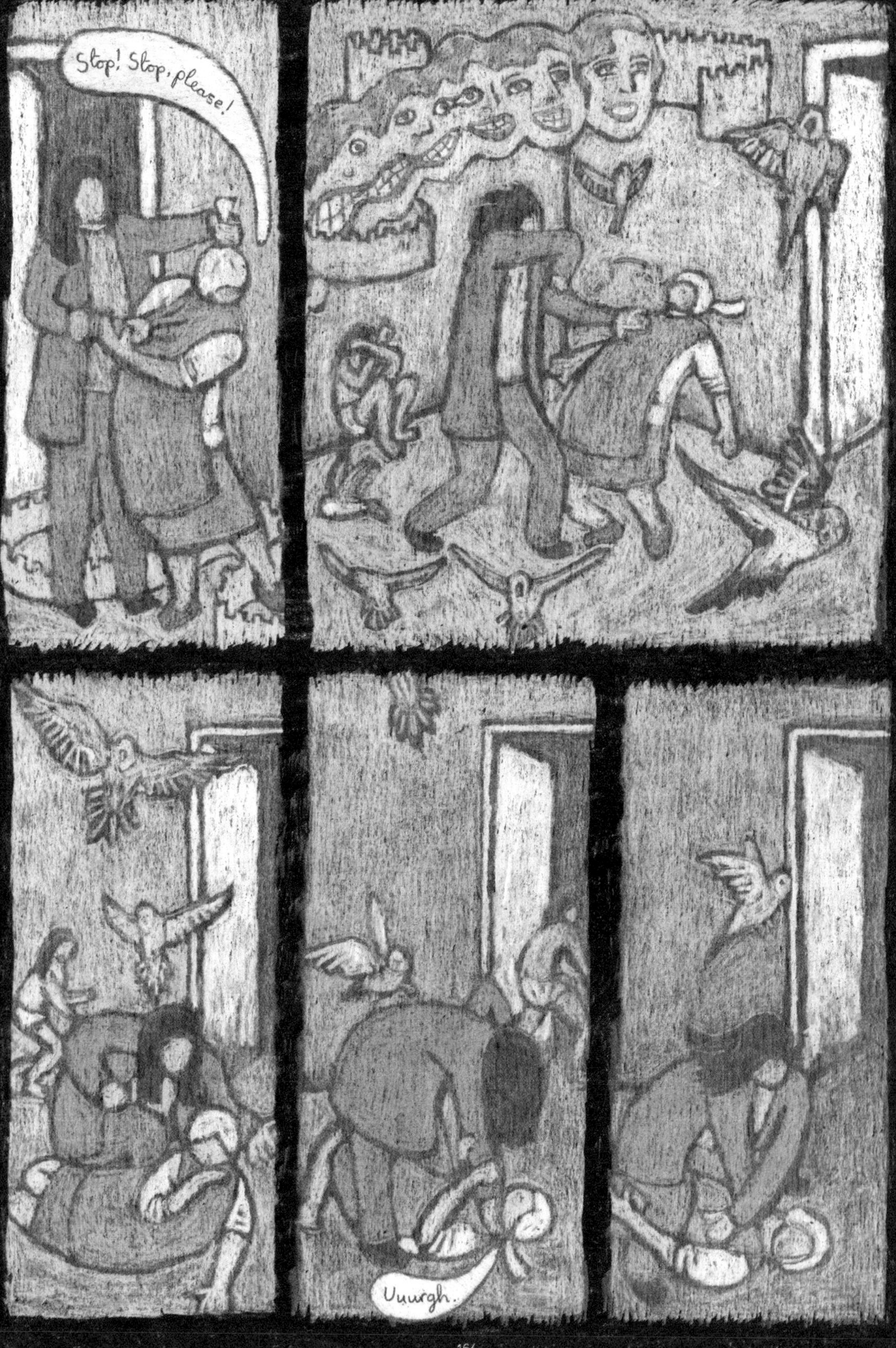
Stop! Stop, please!
Uuurgh..

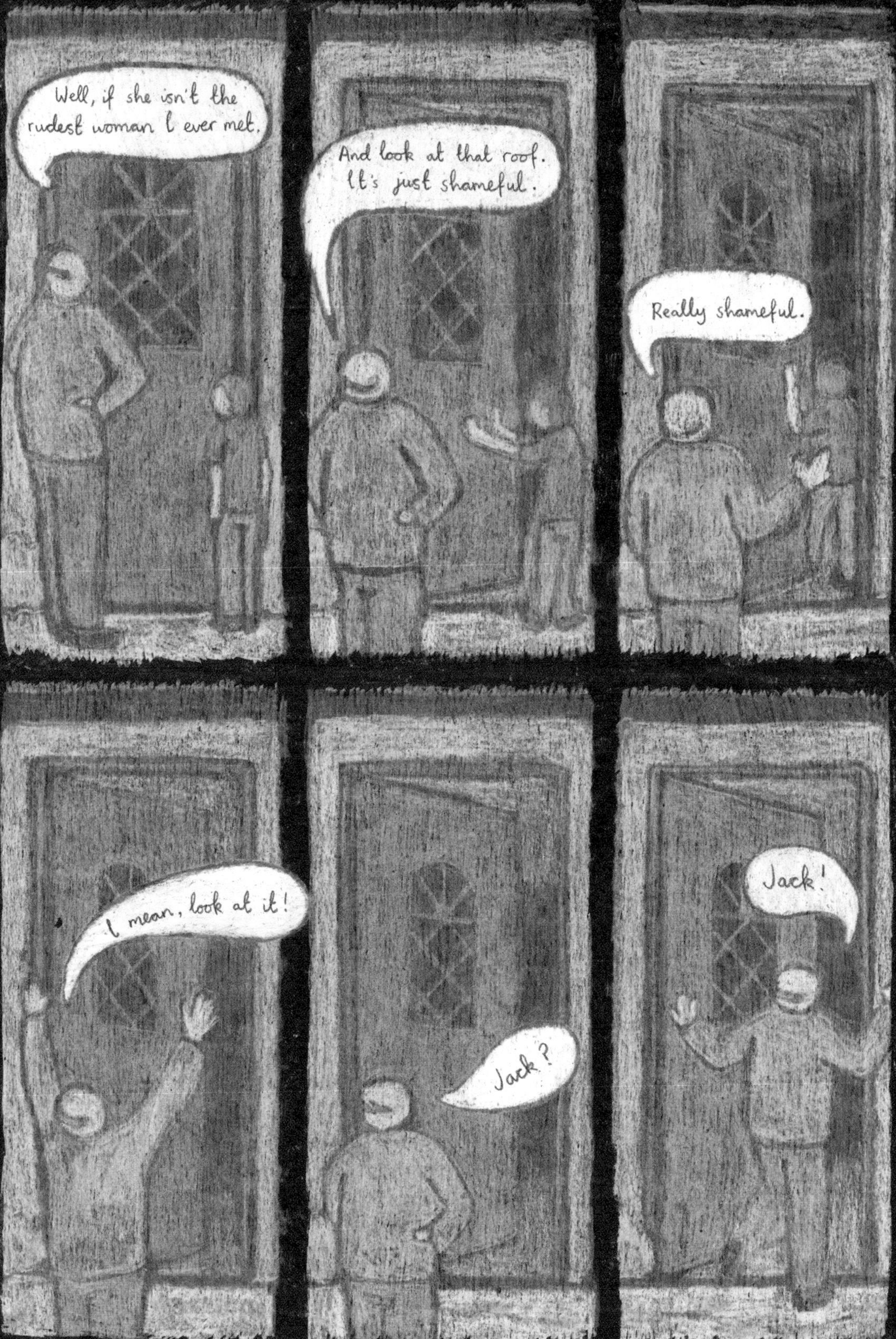
Well, if she isn't the rudest woman I ever met.
And look at that roof. It's just shameful.
Really shameful.
I mean, look at it!
Jack?
Jack!

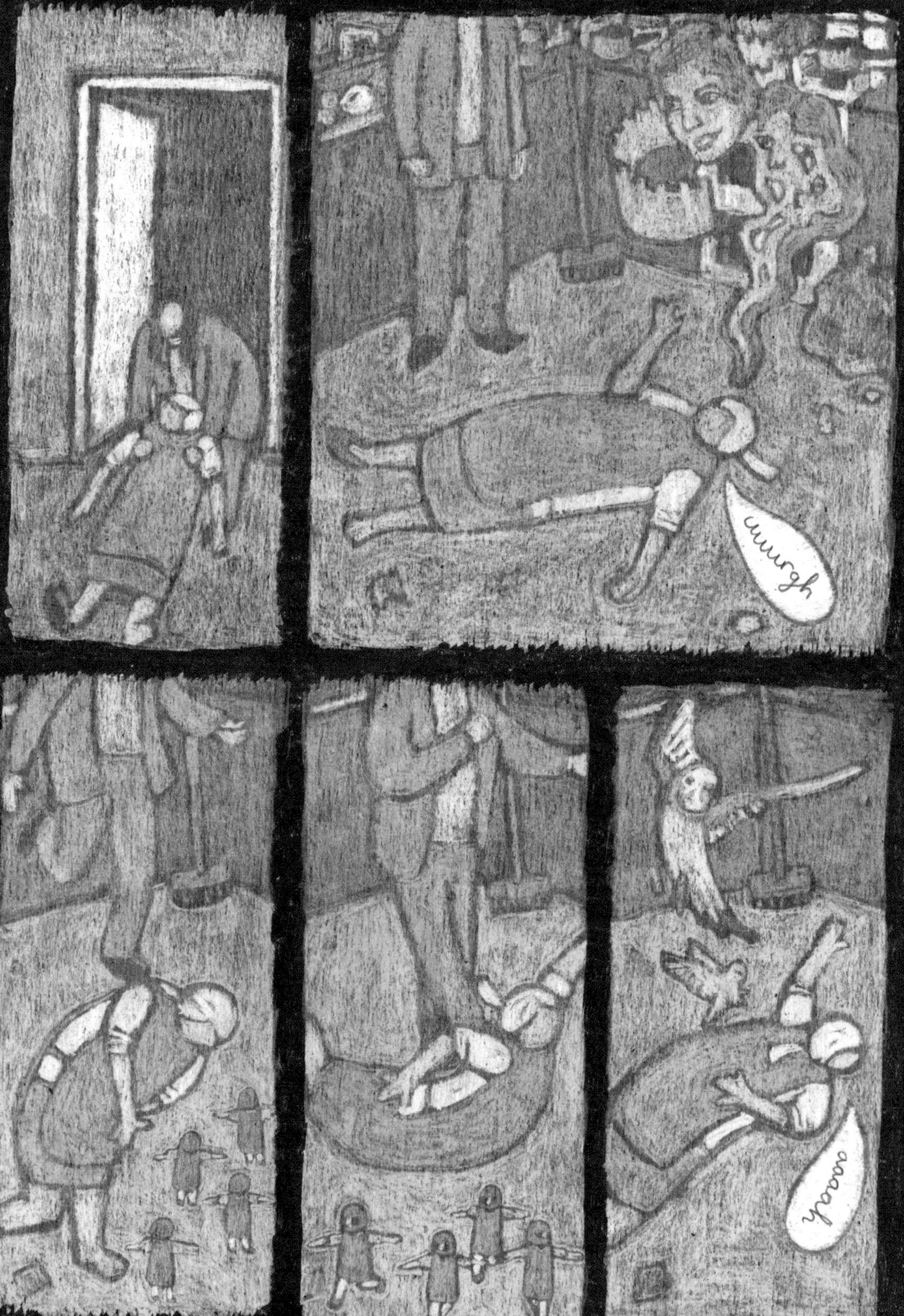
uuurgh
aaaah

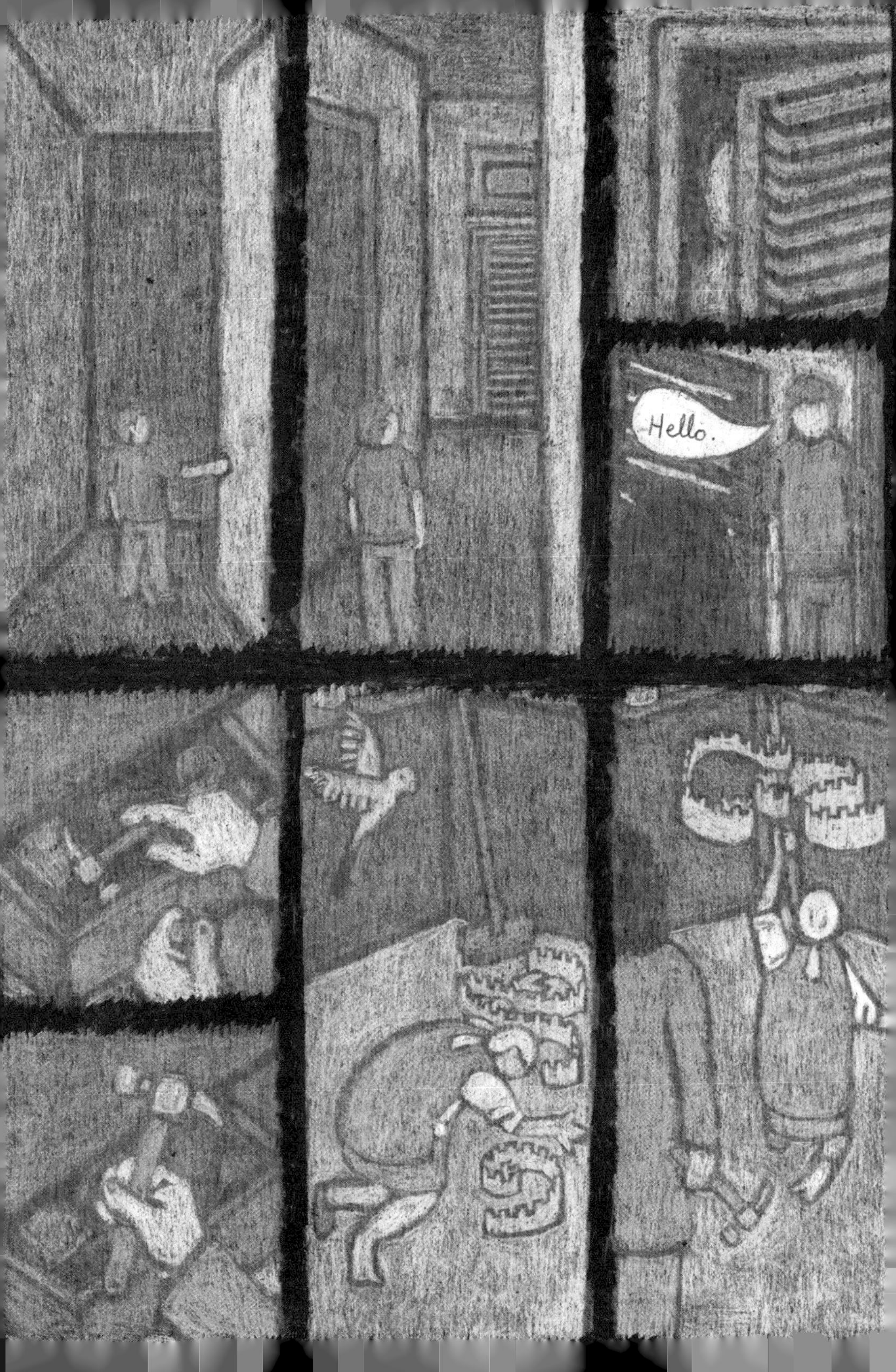
Hello.

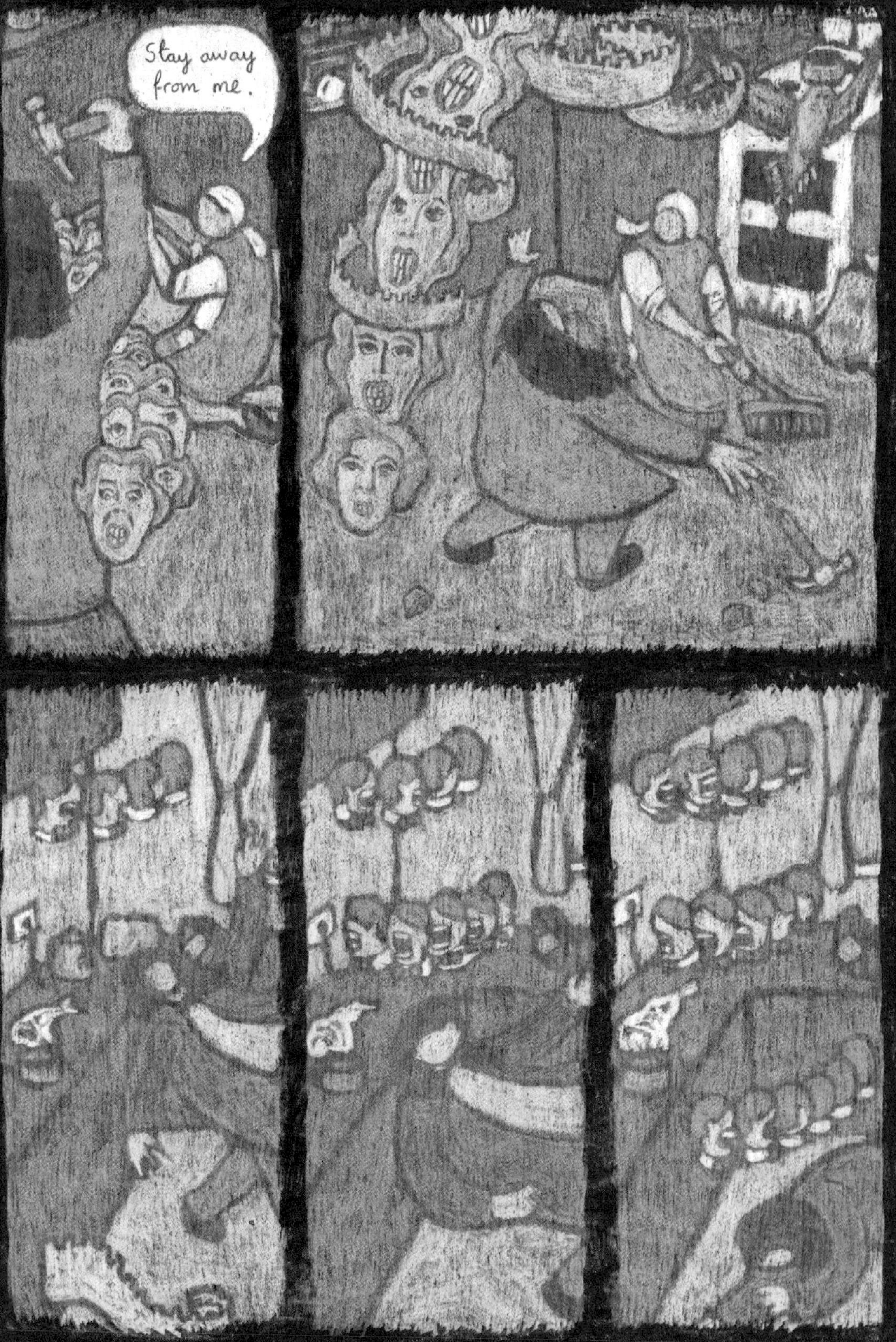
Stay away from me.

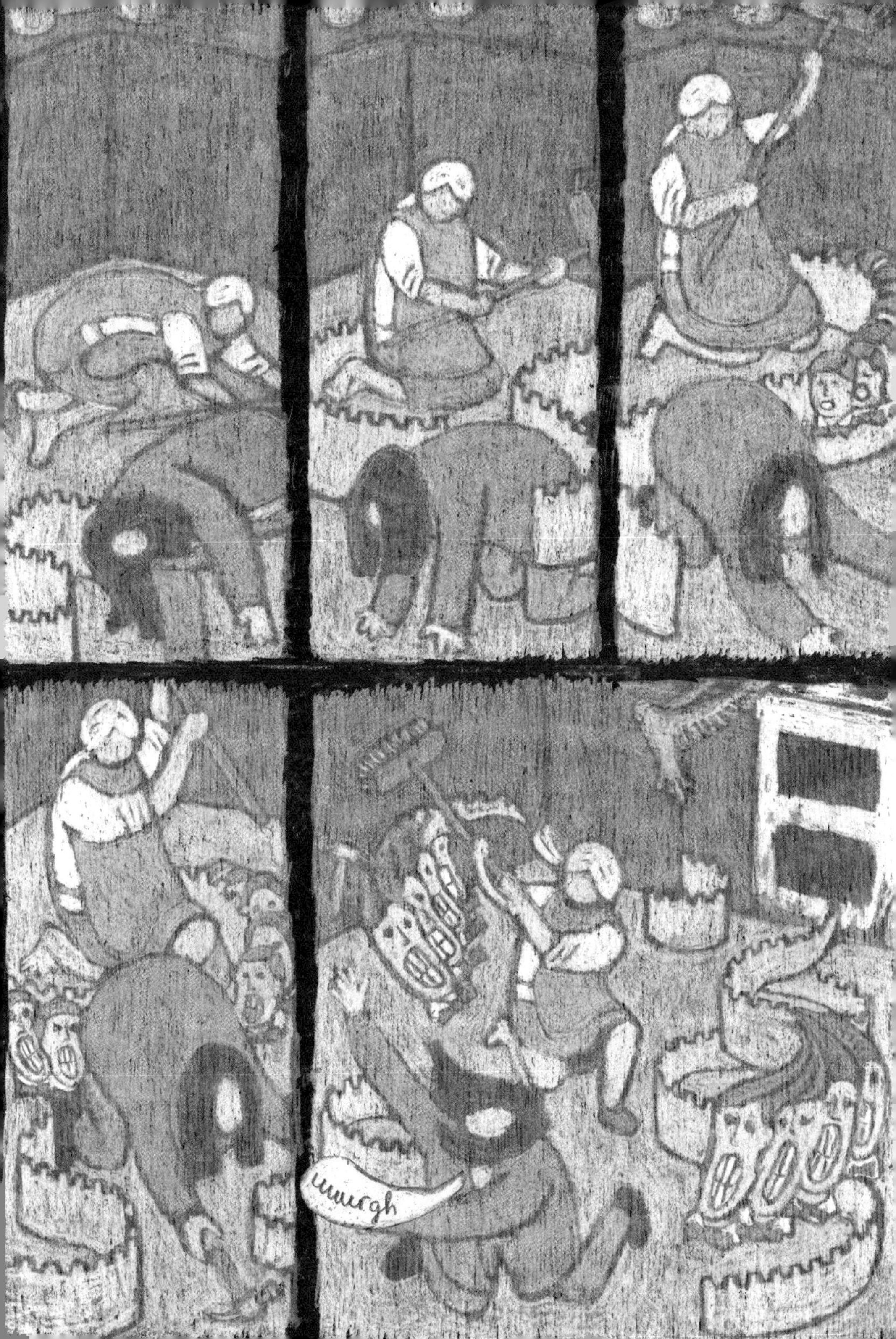
uuurgh

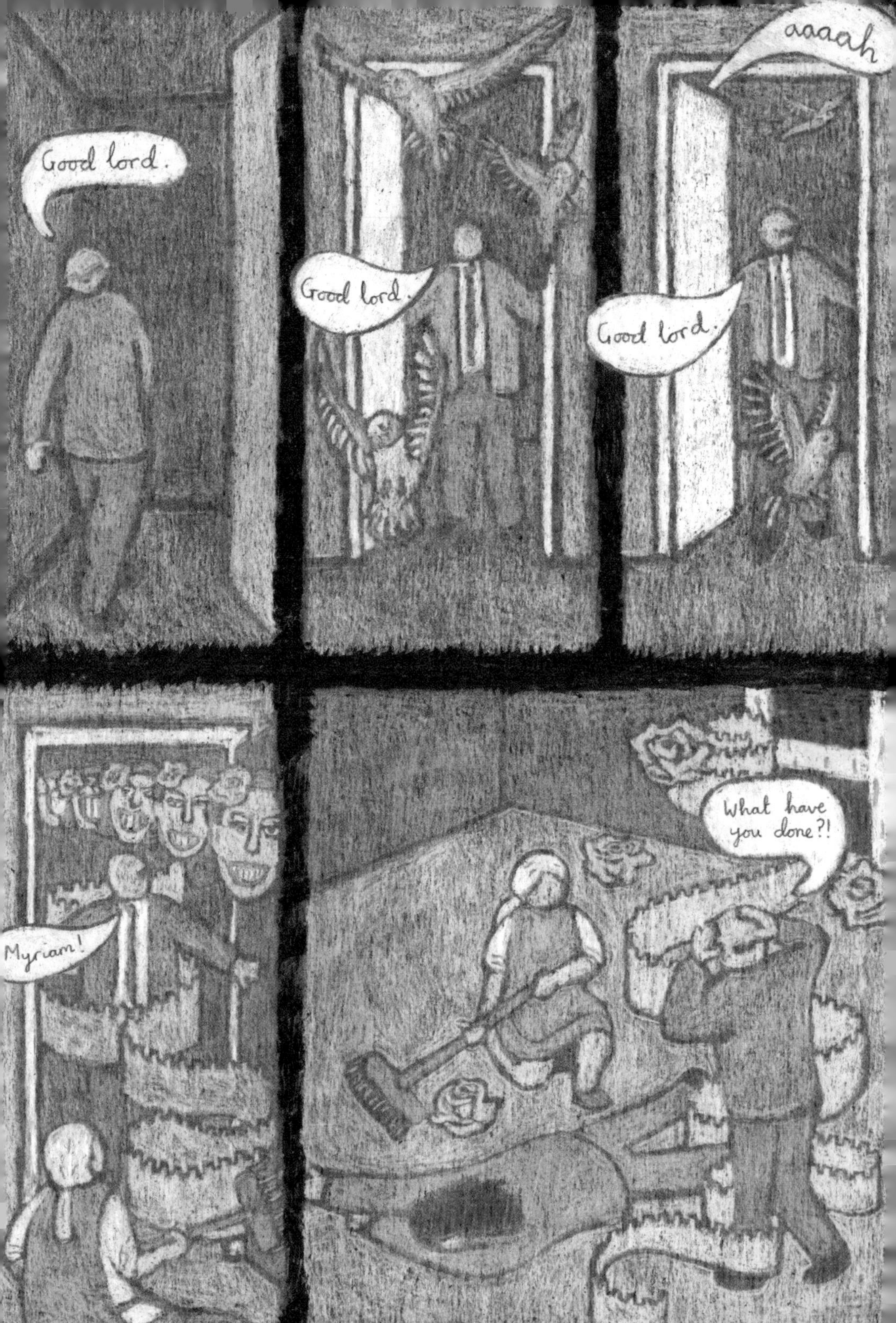
Good lord.
Good lord.
aaaah
Good lord.
Myriam!
What have you done?!

Come on.
Come on!

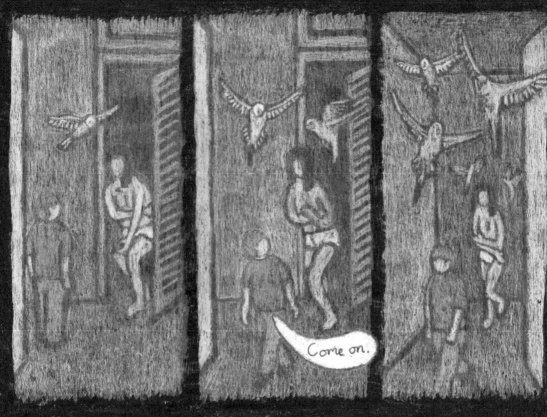

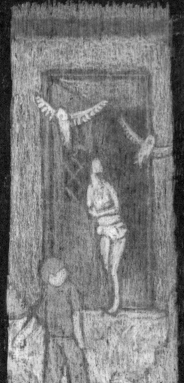

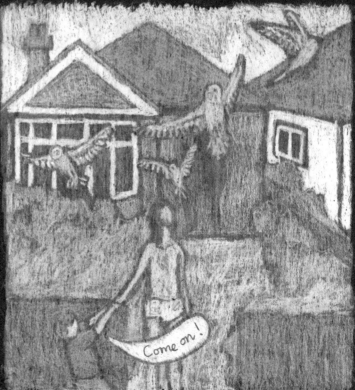

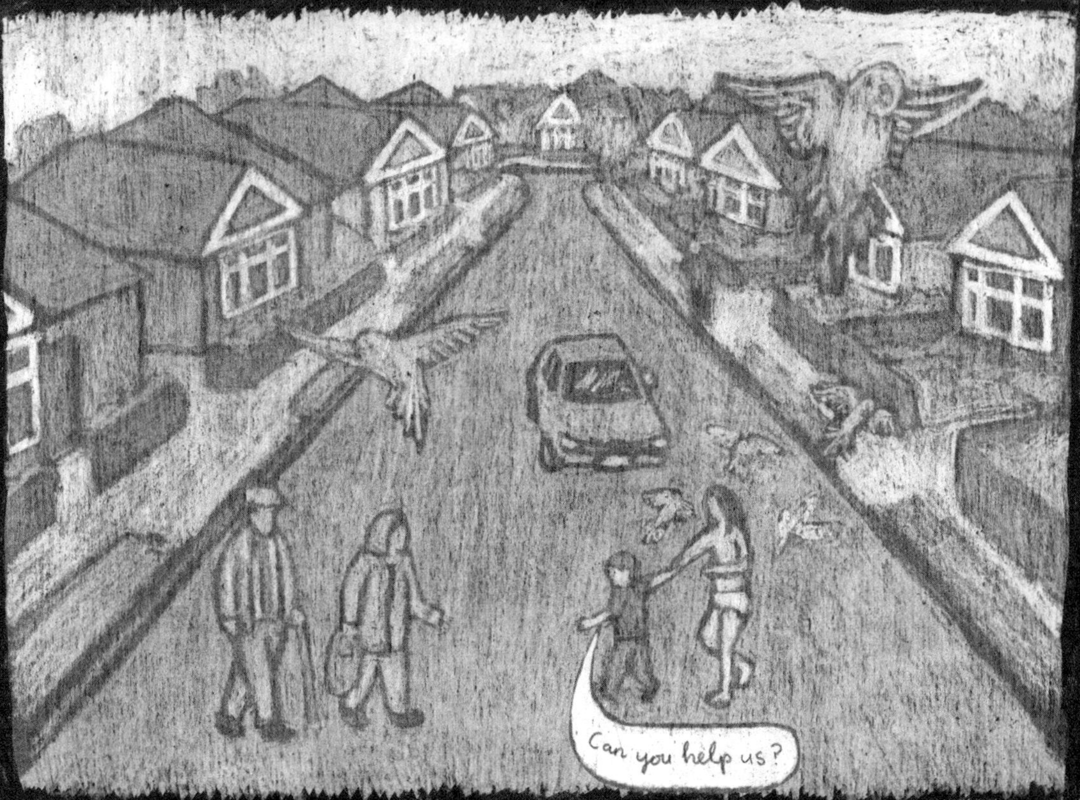
Can you help us?

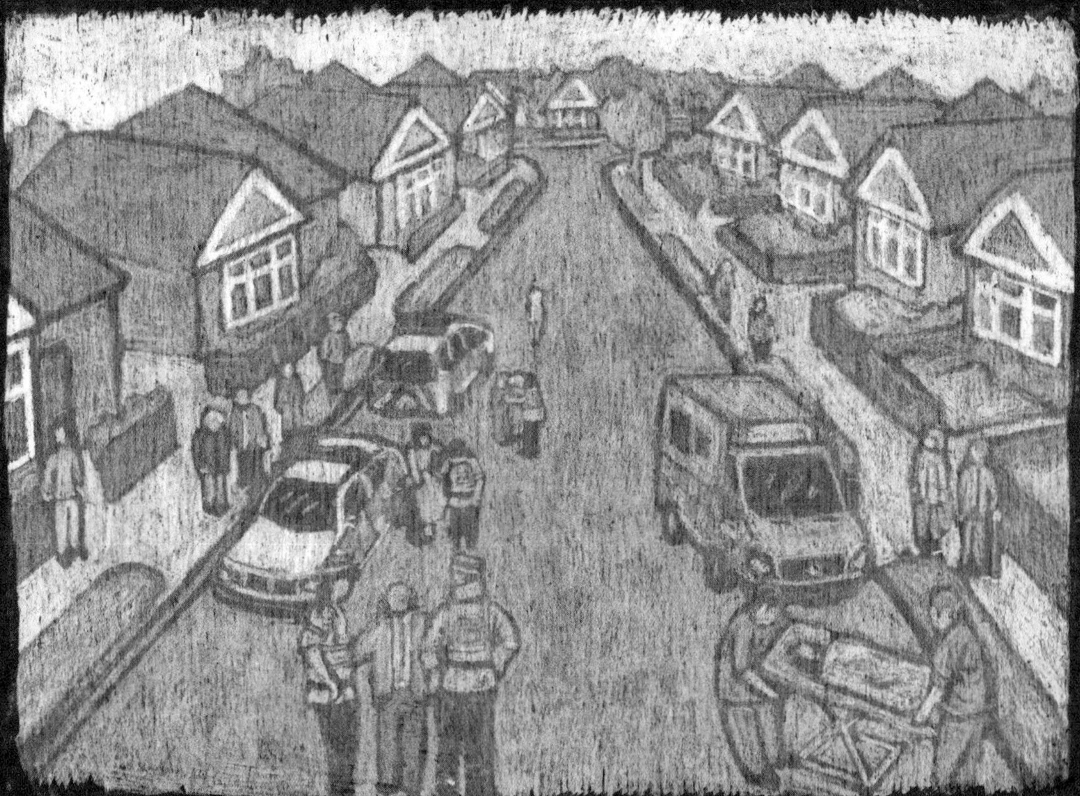

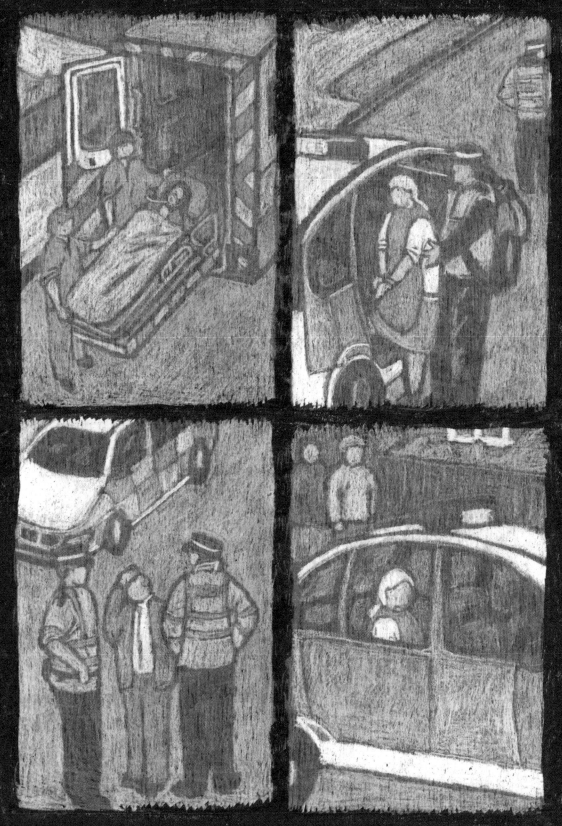

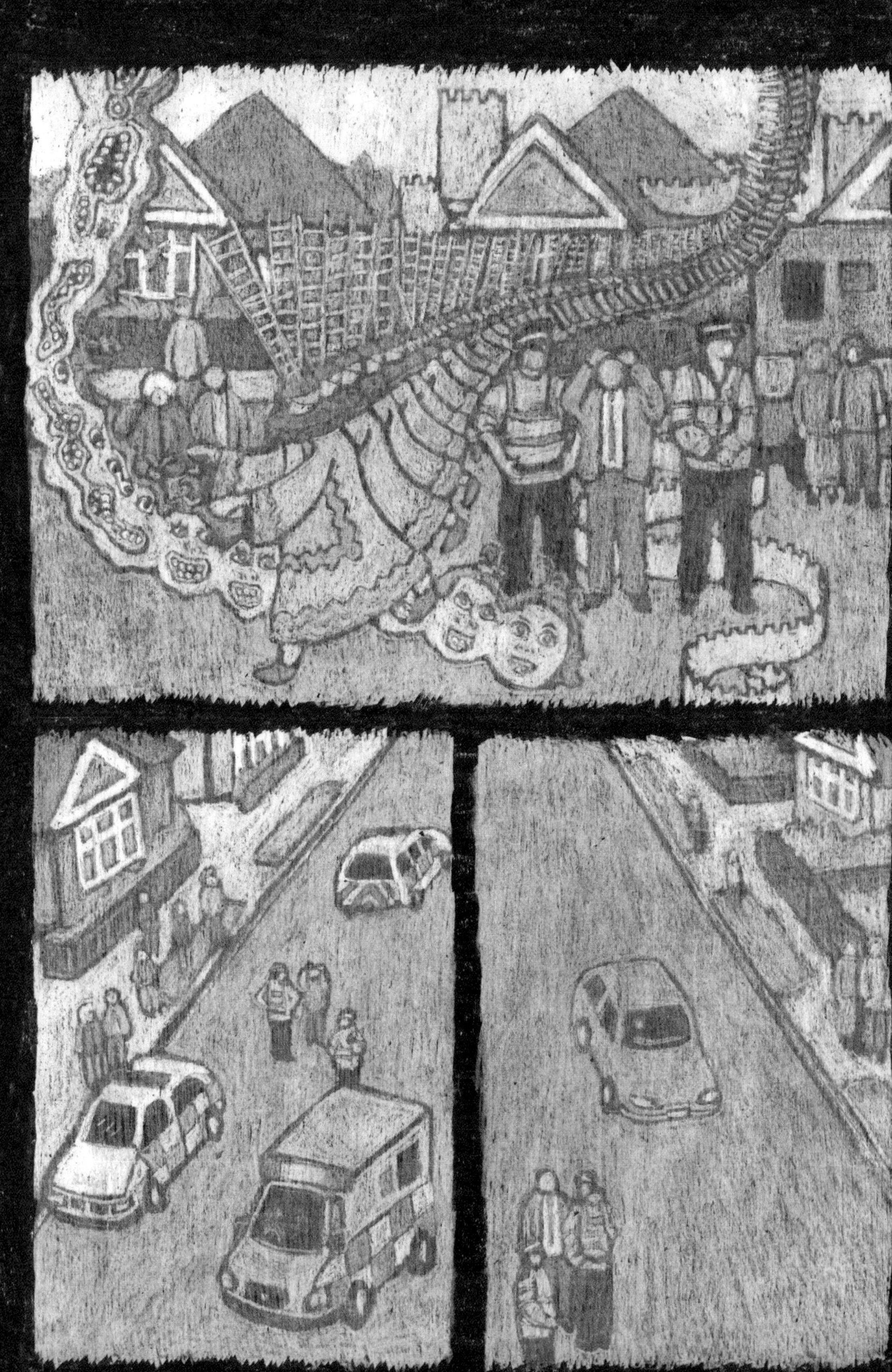

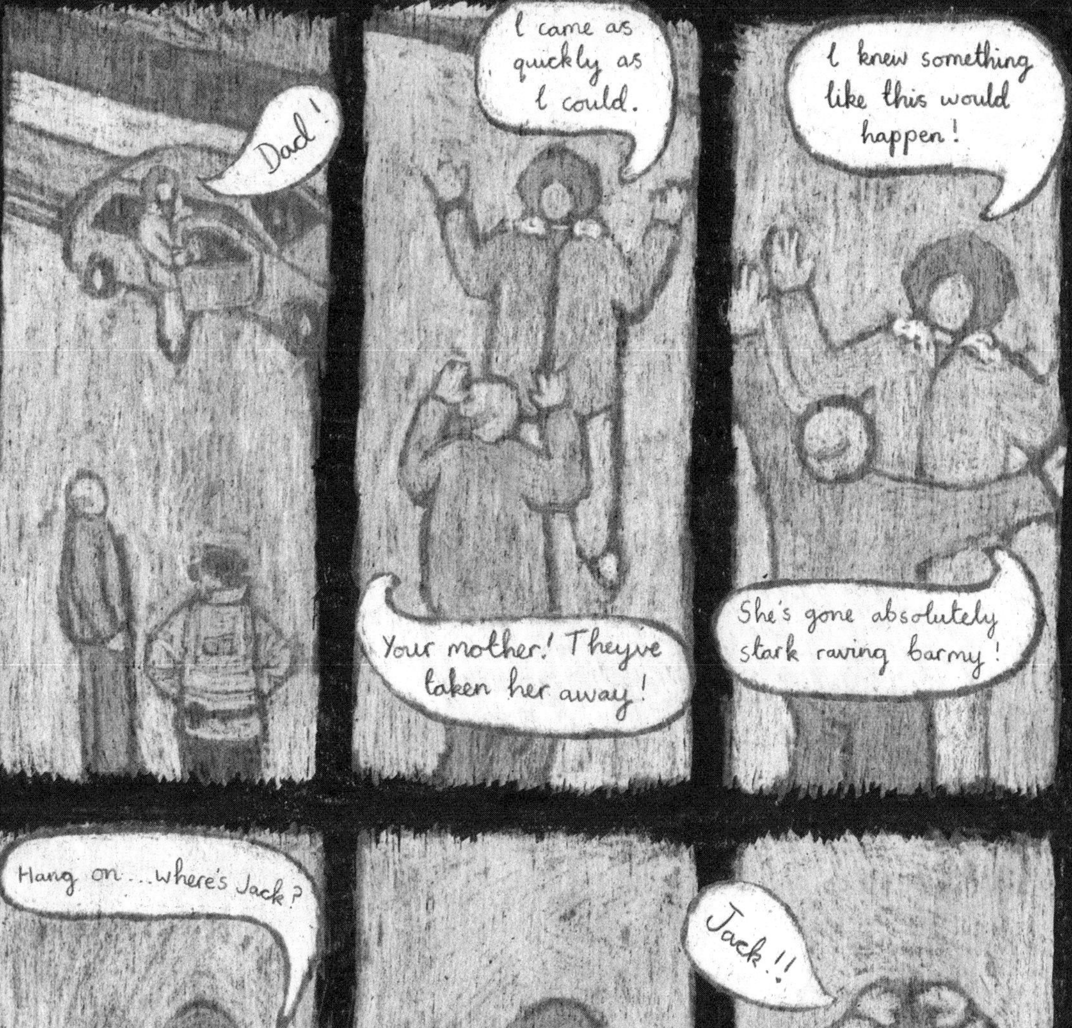
Dad!
I came as quickly as I could.
Your mother! They've taken her away!
I knew something like this would happen!
She's gone absolutely stark raving barmy!
Hang on...where's Jack?
Jack!!
Ah-erm...

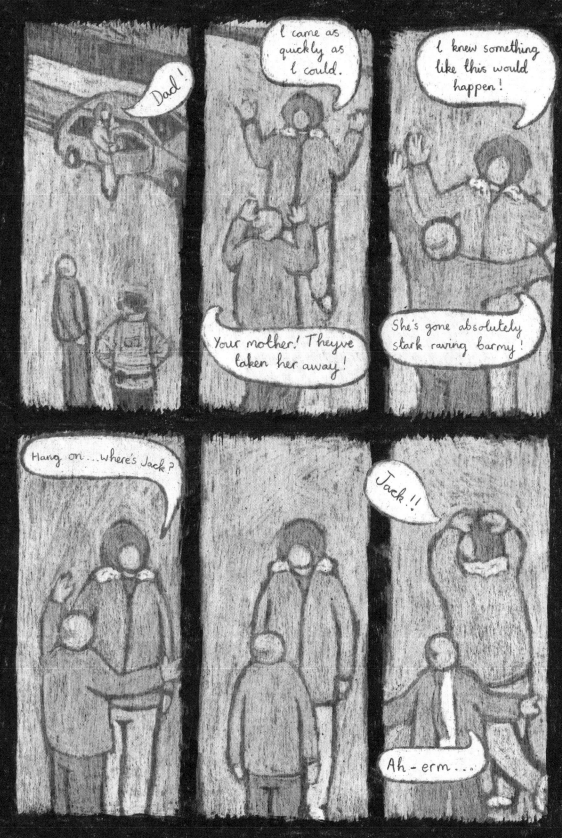

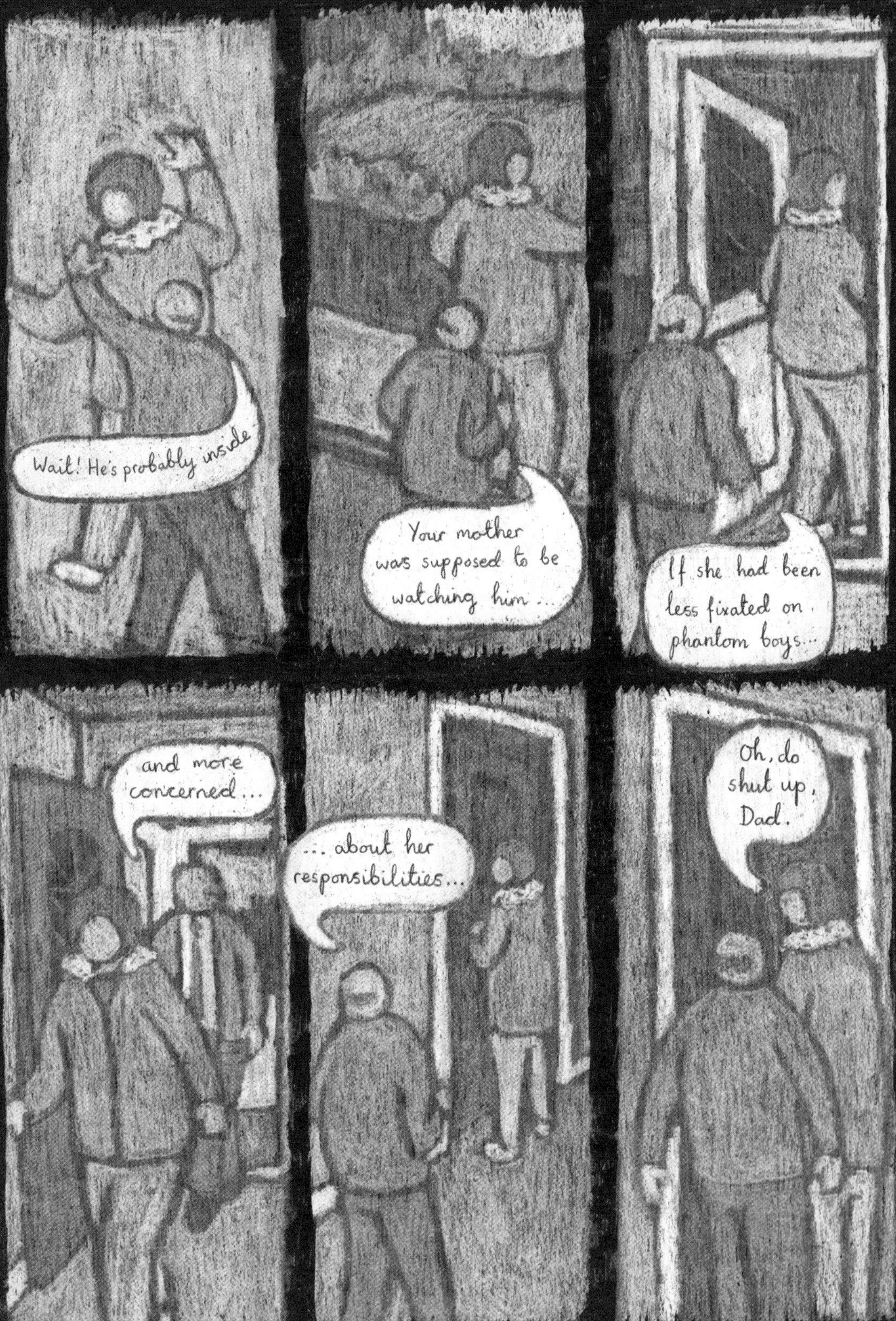
Wait! He's probably inside
Your mother was supposed to be watching him...
If she had been less fixated on phantom boys...
and more concerned...
... about her responsibilities...
Oh, do shut up, Dad.

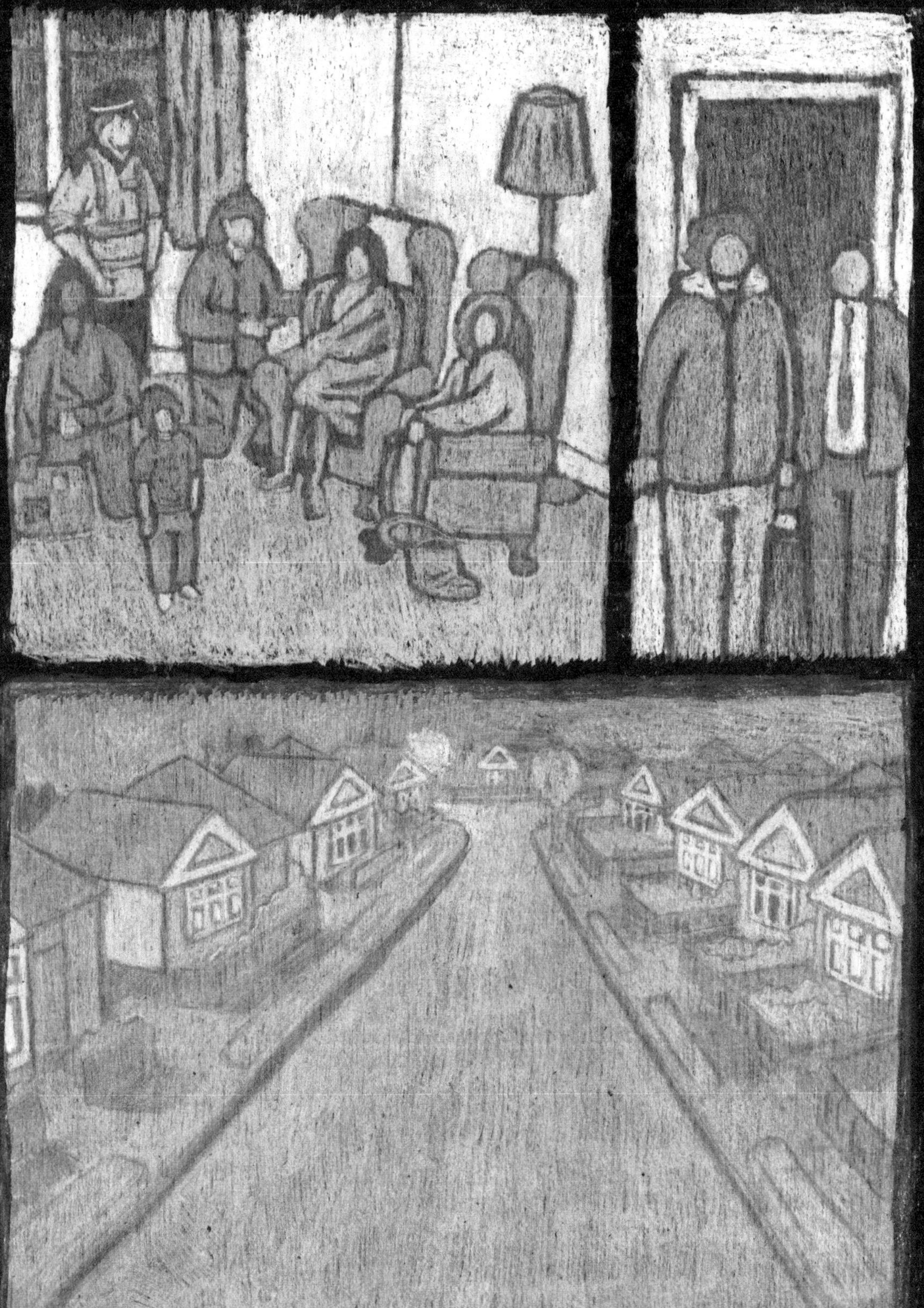

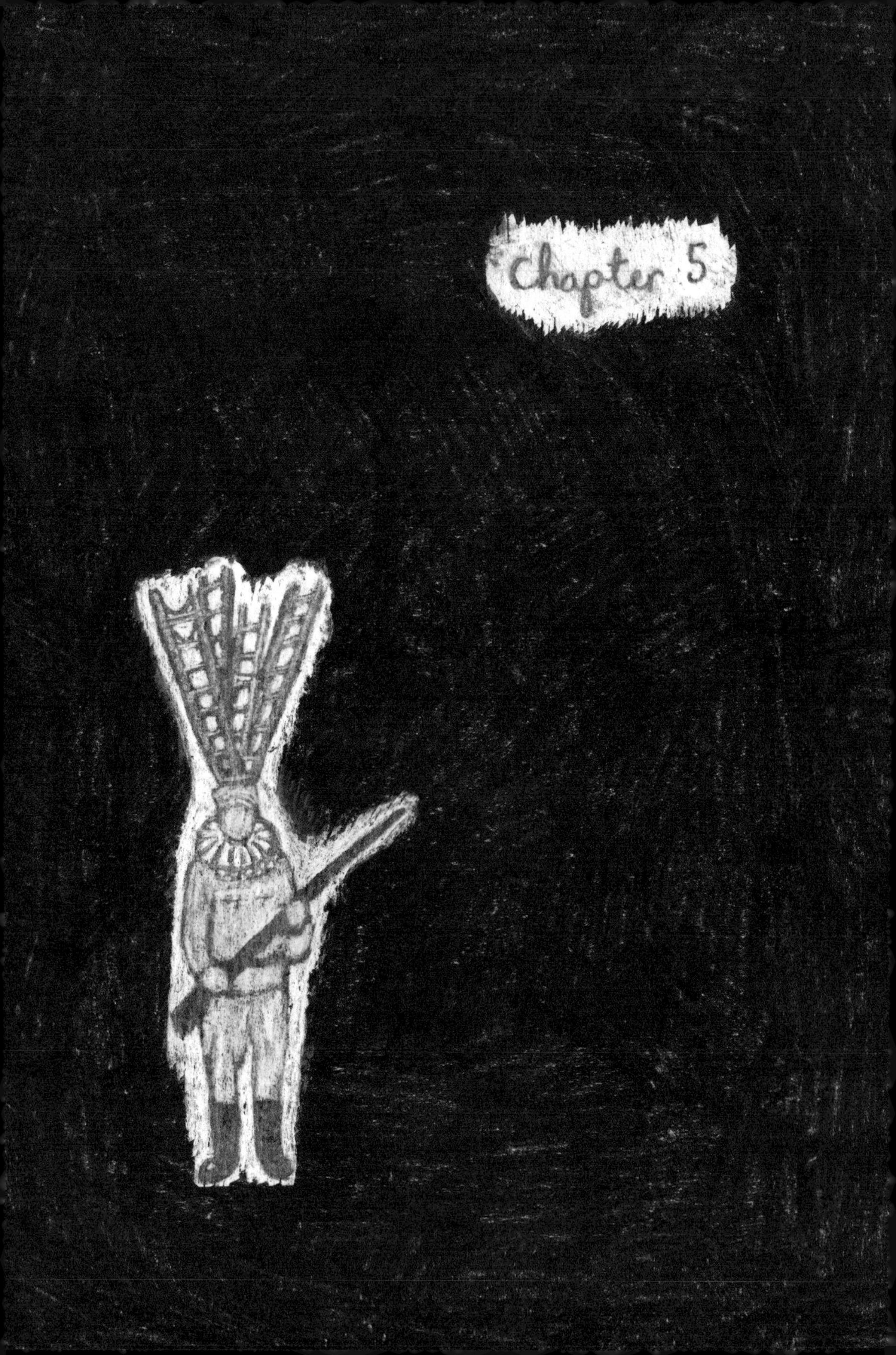
Chapter 5

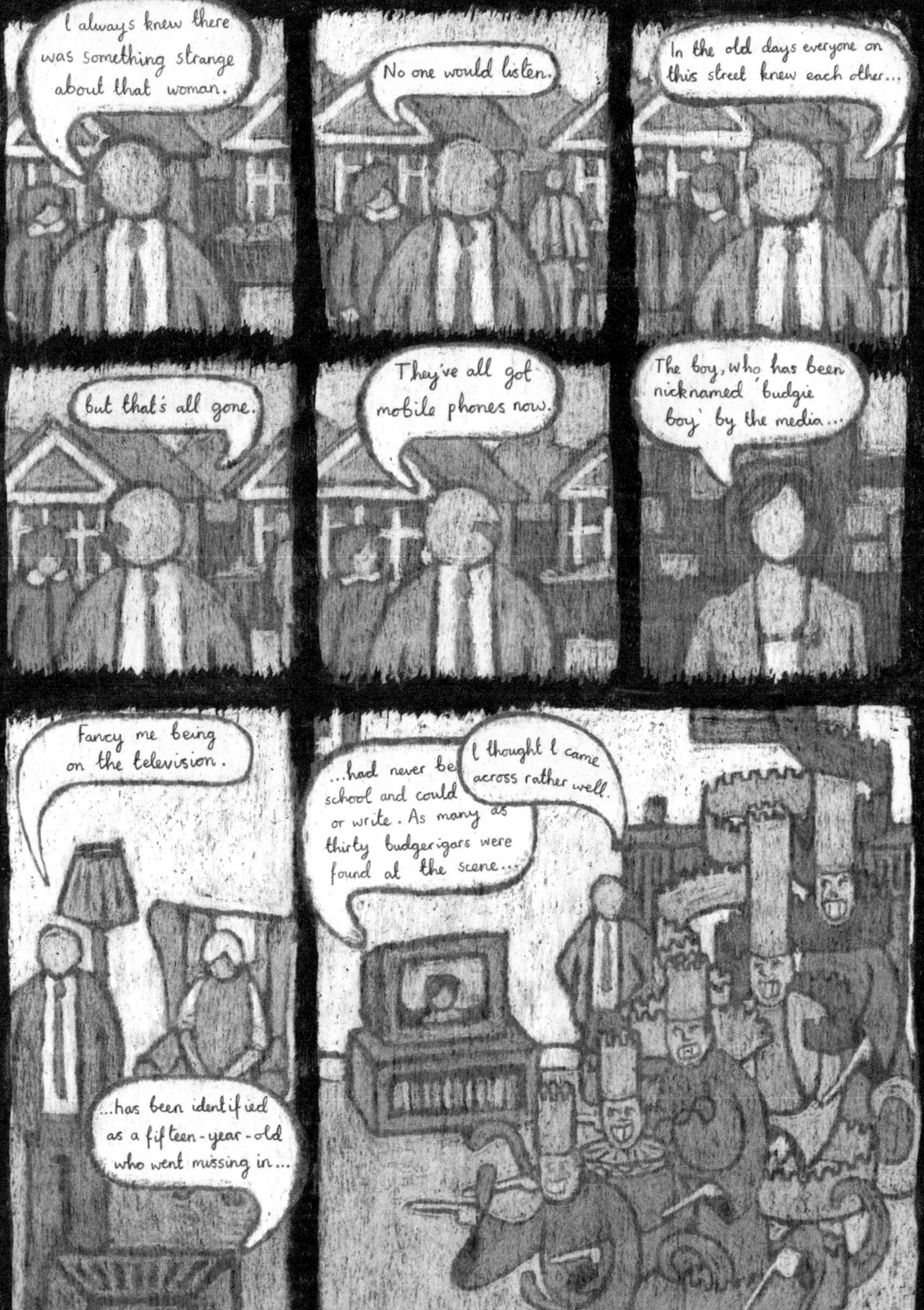

I always knew there was something strange about that woman.
No one would listen.
In the old days everyone on this street knew each other...
but that's all gone.
They've all got mobile phones now.
The boy, who has been nicknamed 'budgie boy' by the media...
Fancy me being on the television.
...has been identified as a fifteen-year-old who went missing in...
...had never be school and could or write. As many as thirty budgerigars were found at the scene...
I thought I came across rather well.

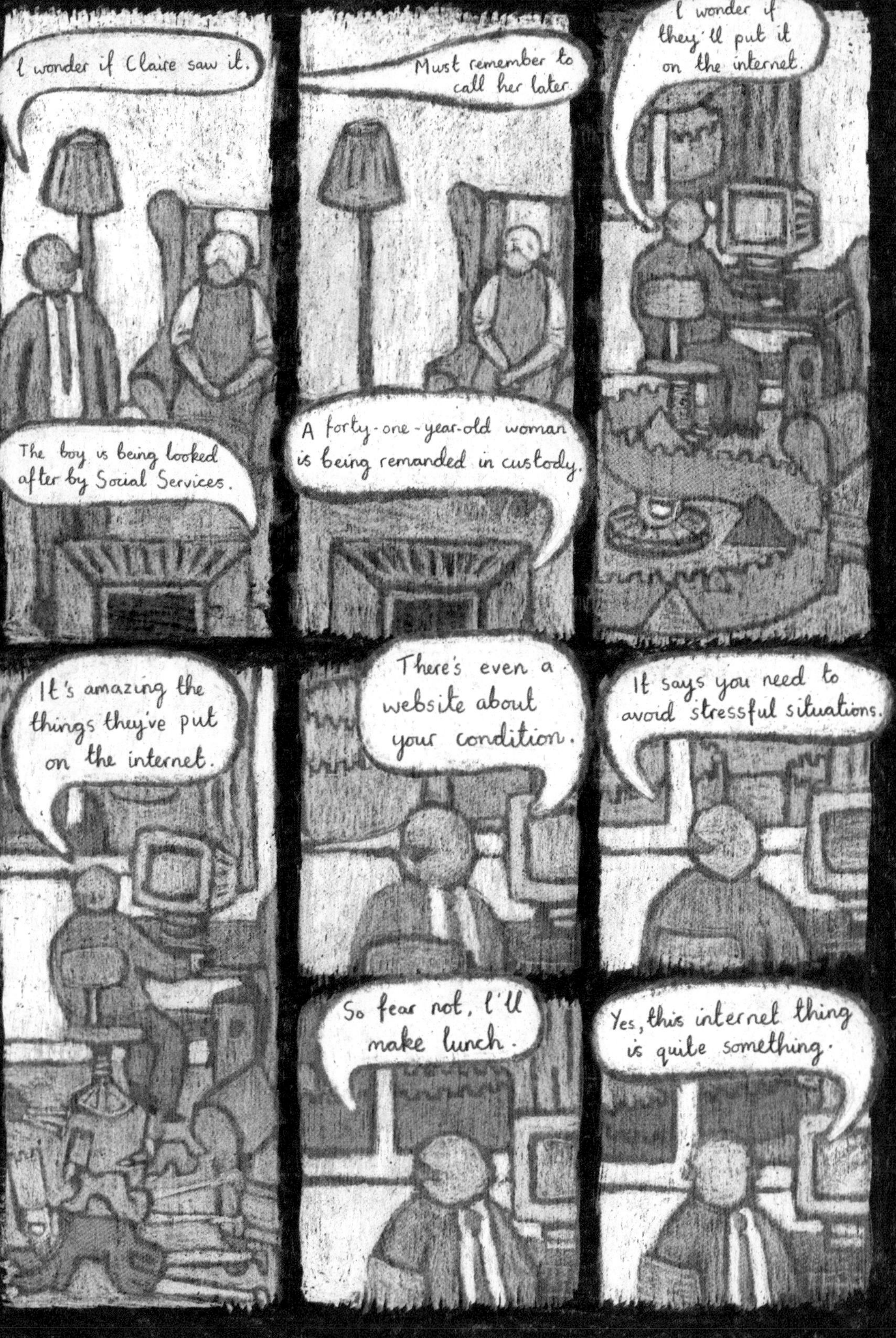
I wonder if Claire saw it.
The boy is being looked after by Social Services.
Must remember to call her later.
A forty-one-year-old woman is being remanded in custody.
I wonder if they'll put it on the internet.
It's amazing the things they've put on the internet.
There's even a website about your condition.
So fear not, I'll make lunch.
It says you need to avoid stressful situations.
Yes, this internet thing is quite something.

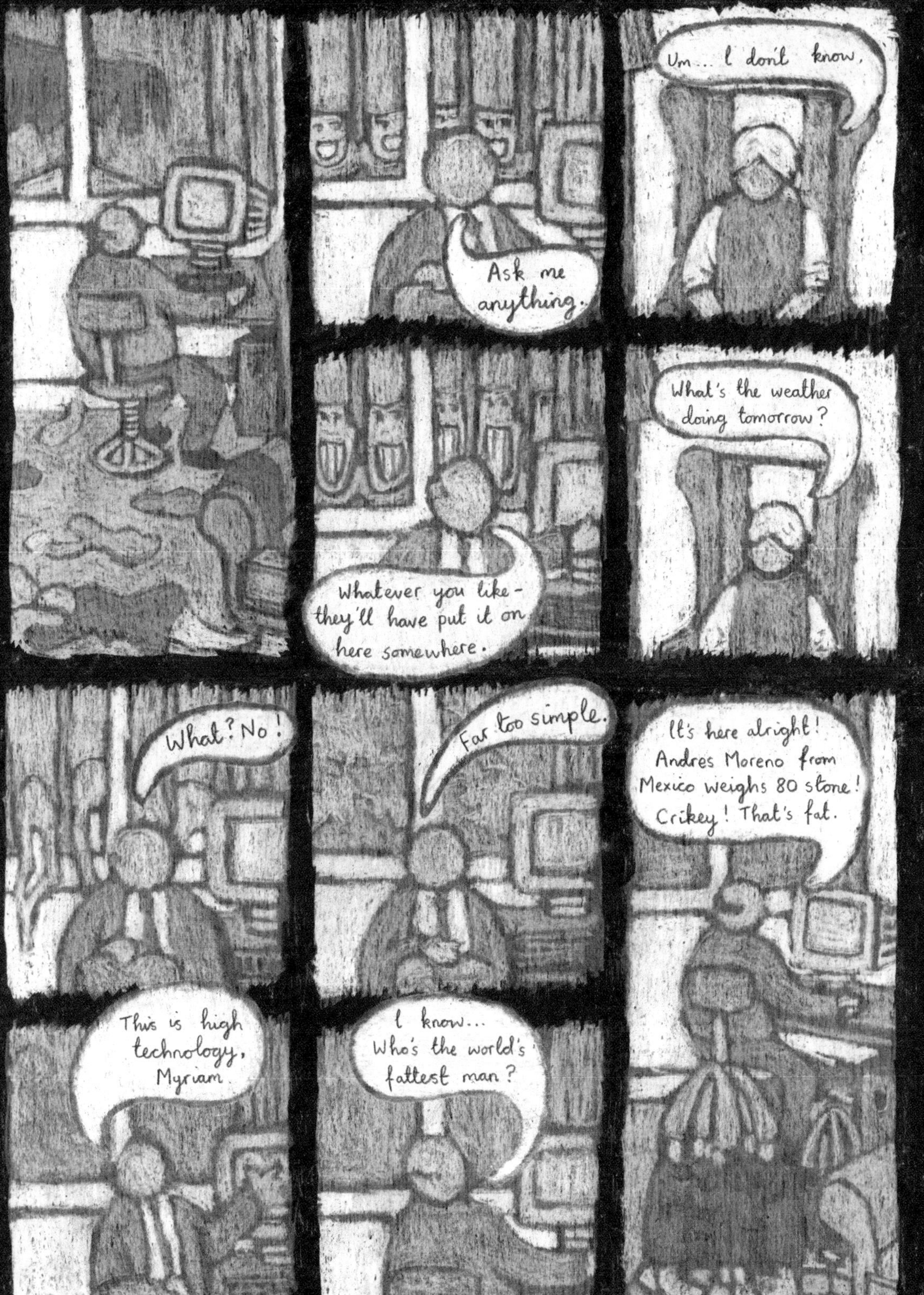
Ask me anything.
Um... I don't know.
Whatever you like - they'll have put it on here somewhere.
What's the weather doing tomorrow?
What? No!
Far too simple.
It's here alright! Andres Moreno from Mexico weighs 80 stone! Crikey! That's fat.
This is high technology, Myriam
I know... Who's the world's fattest man?

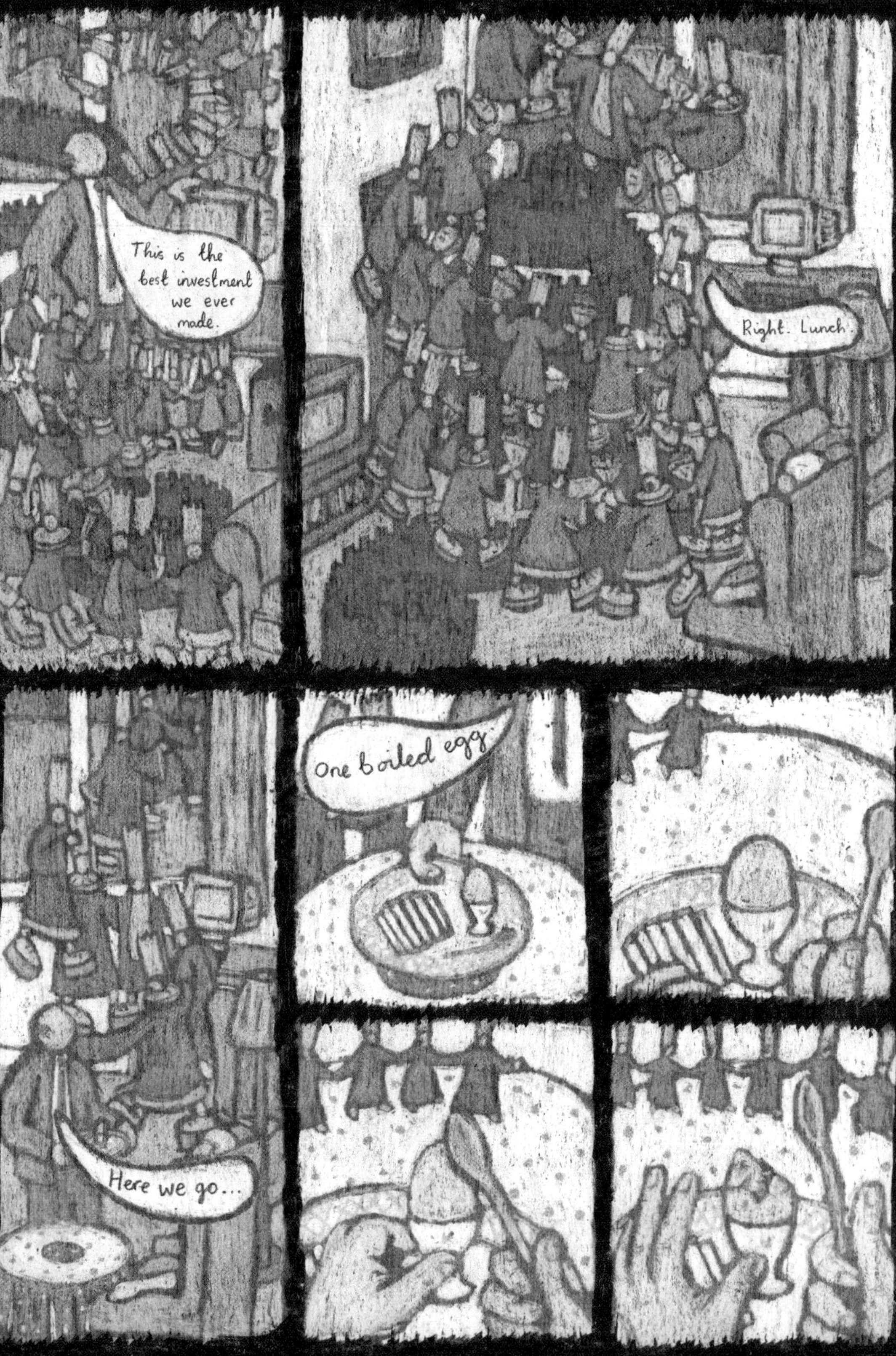
This is the best investment we ever made.
Right. Lunch.
Here we go...
One boiled egg.

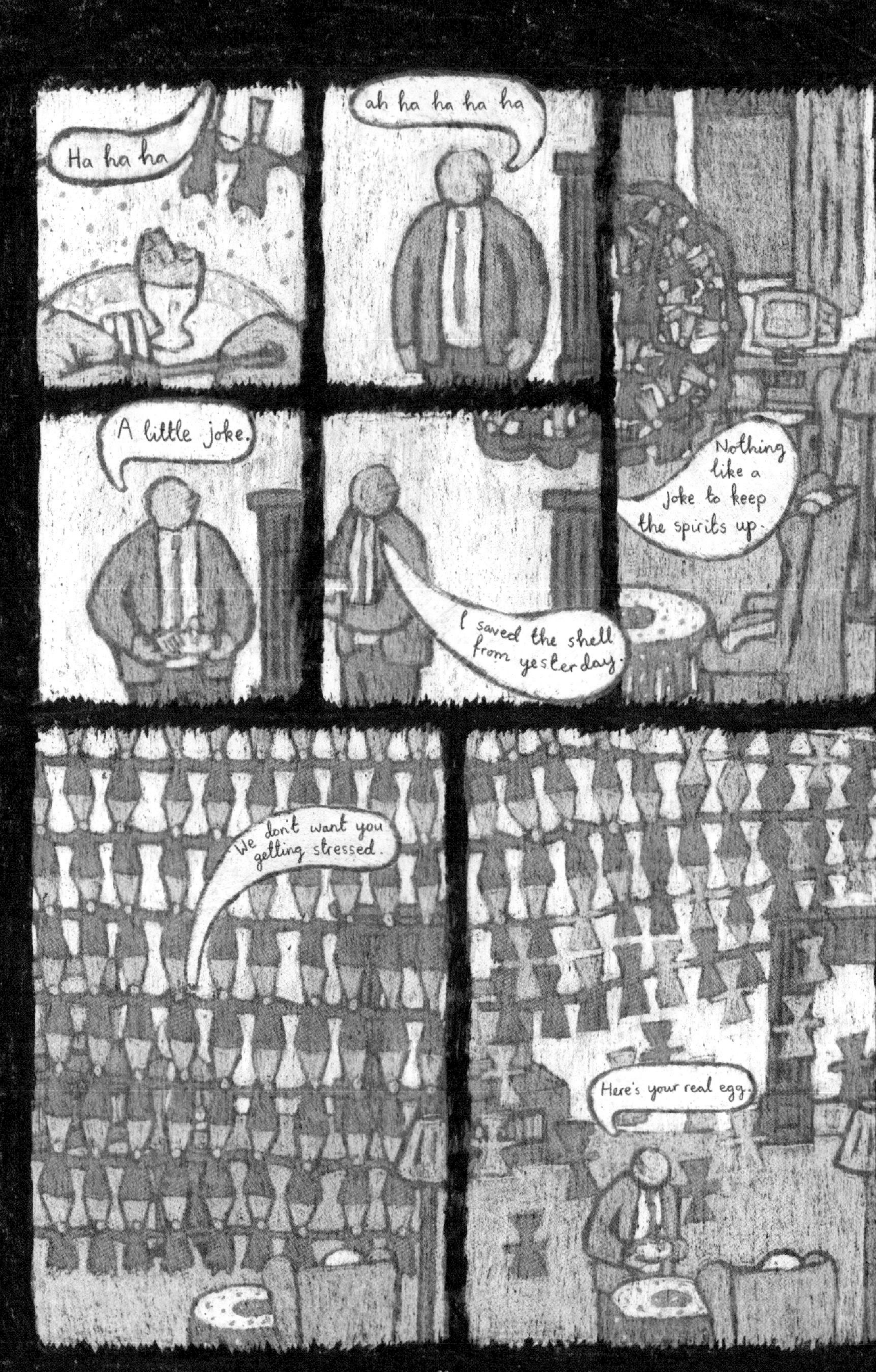
Ha ha ha
ah ha ha ha ha
A little joke.
I saved the shell from yesterday.
Nothing like a joke to keep the spirits up.
We don't want you getting stressed.
Here's your real egg.

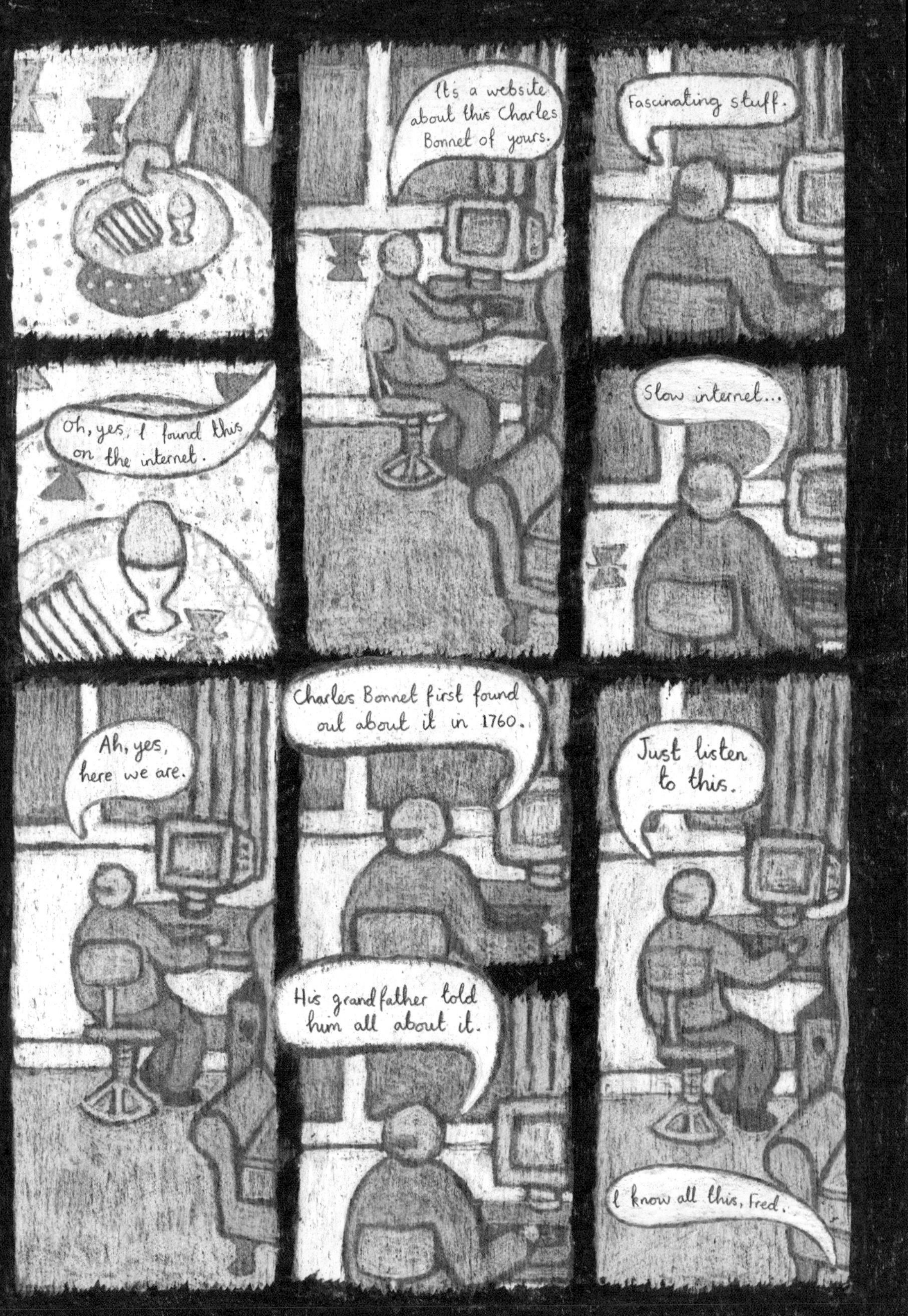
It's a website about this Charles Bonnet of yours.
Fascinating stuff.
Oh, yes, I found this on the internet.
Slow internet...
Ah, yes, here we are.
Charles Bonnet first found out about it in 1760.
His grandfather told him all about it.
Just listen to this.
I know all this, Fred.

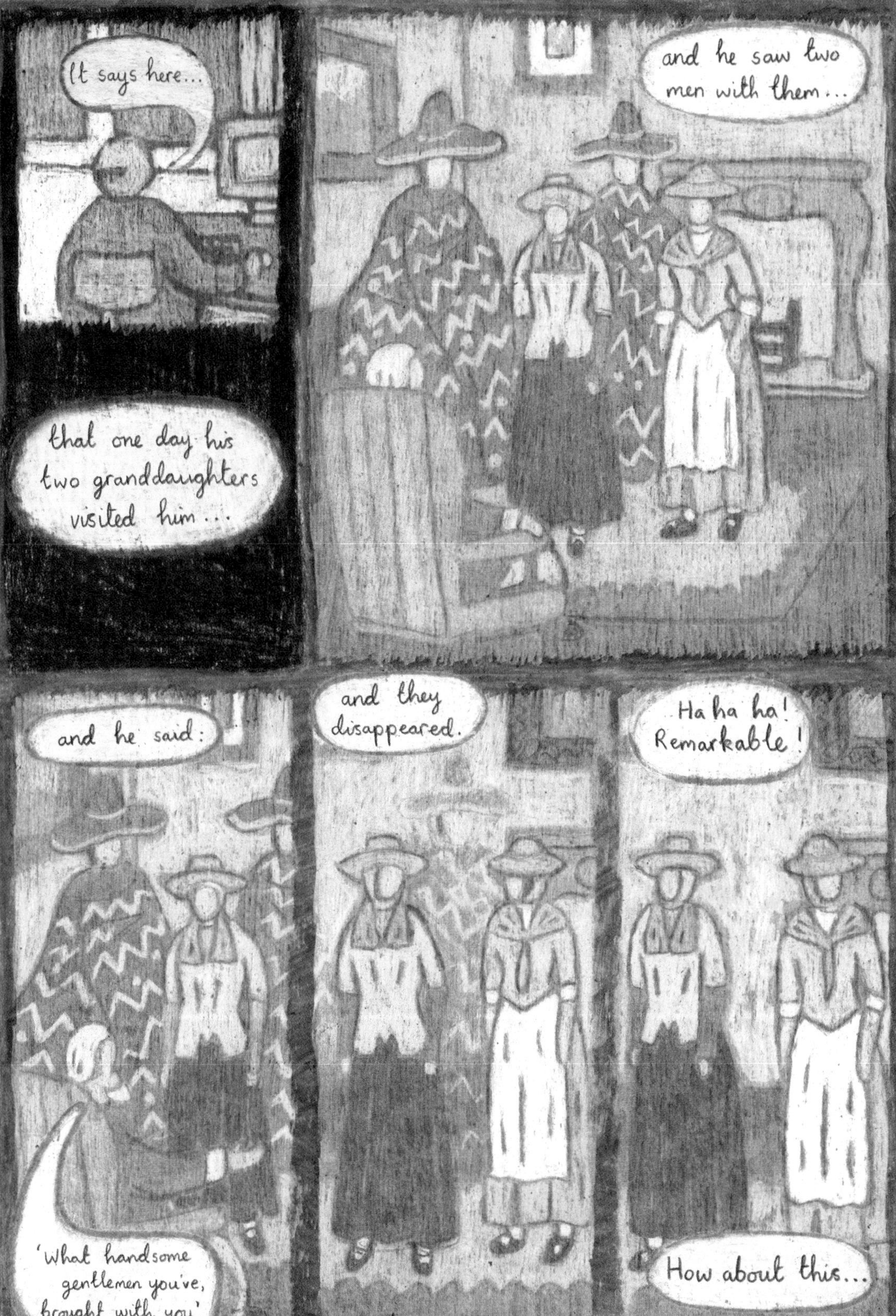

It says here...
that one day his two granddaughters visited him...
and he saw two men with them...
and he said:
'What handsome gentlemen you've brought with you',
and they disappeared.
Ha ha ha! Remarkable!
How about this...

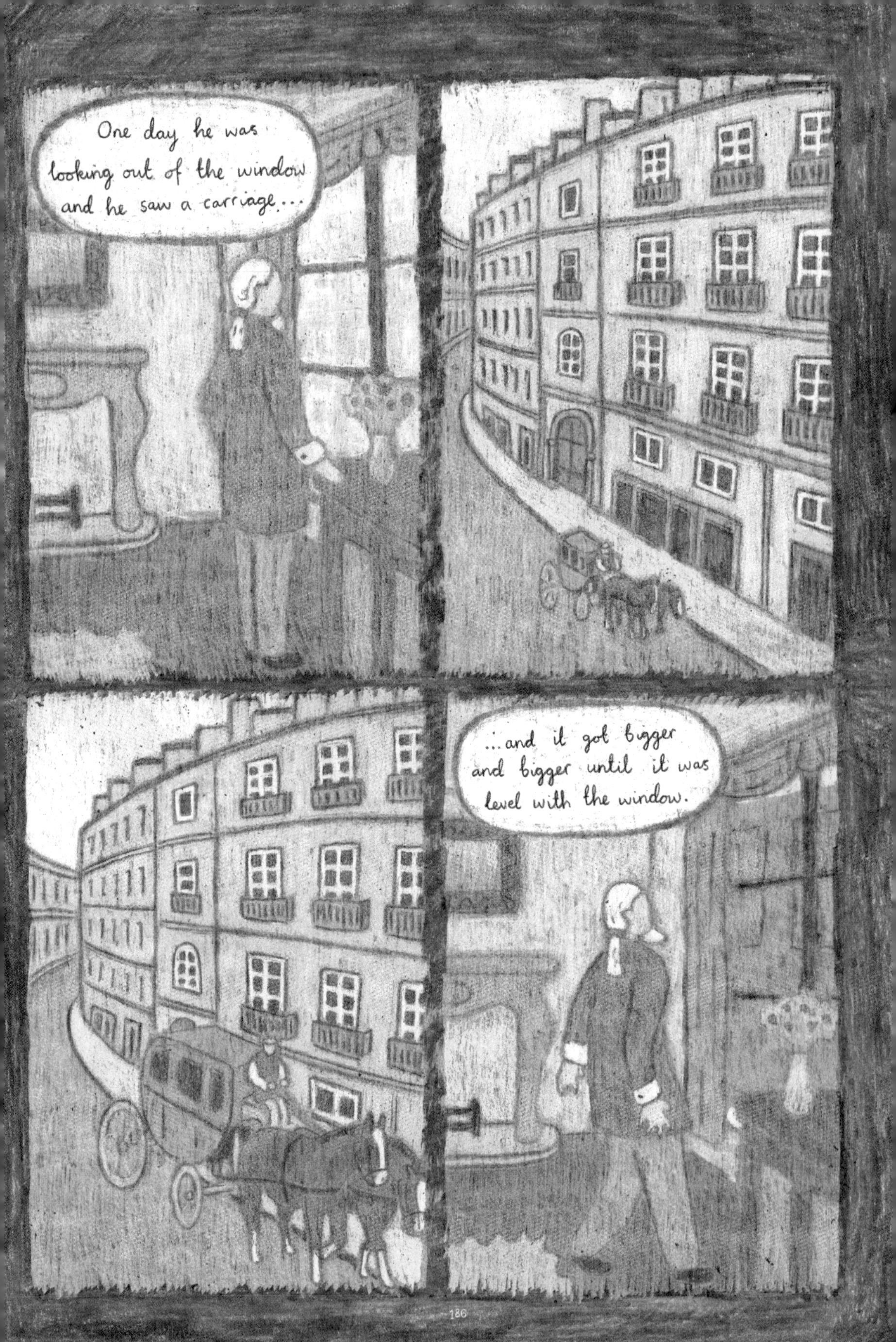
One day he was looking out of the window and he saw a carriage...
...and it got bigger and bigger until it was level with the window.

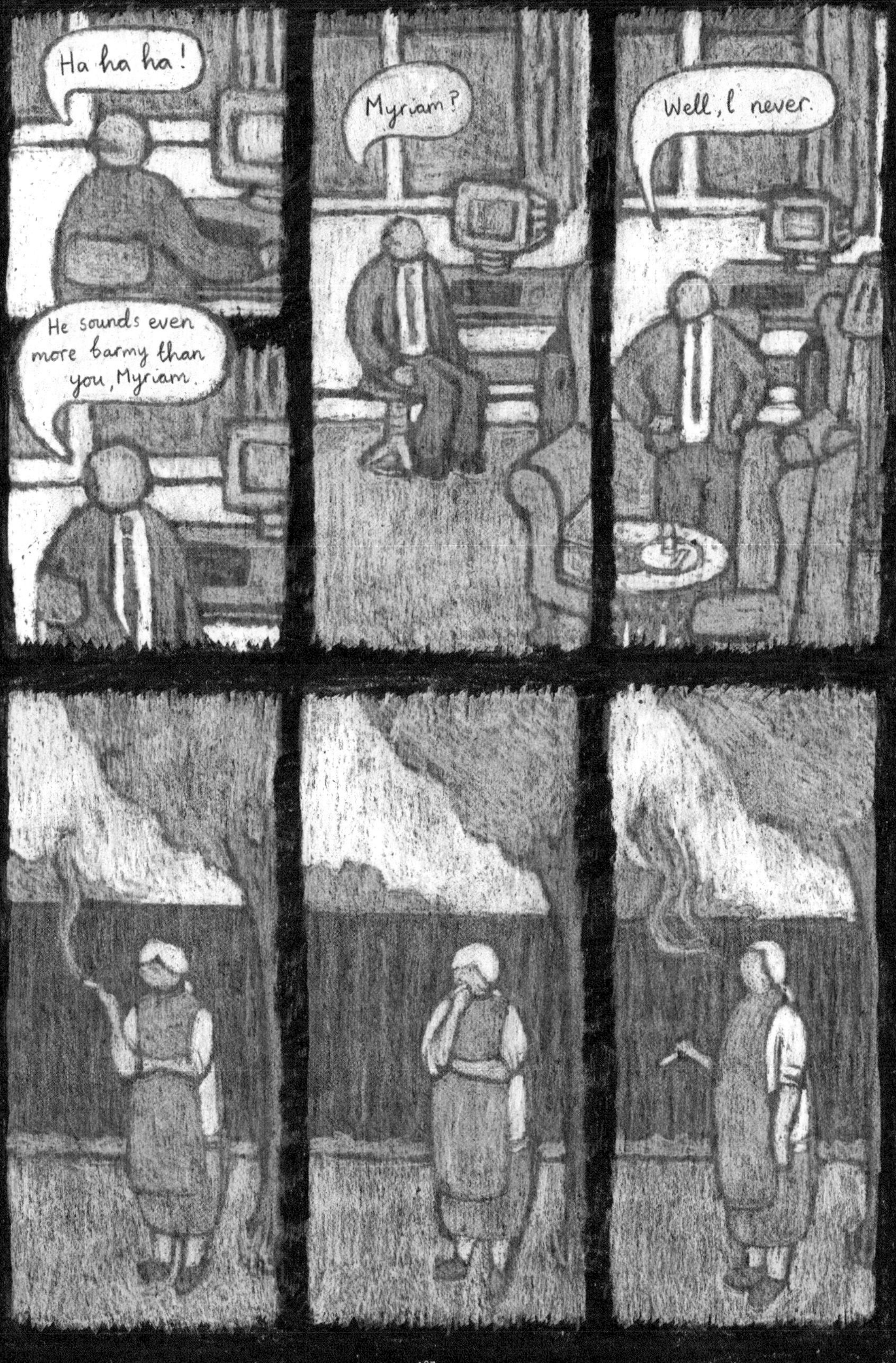
Ha ha ha!
He sounds even more barmy than you, Myriam.
Myriam?
Well, I never.

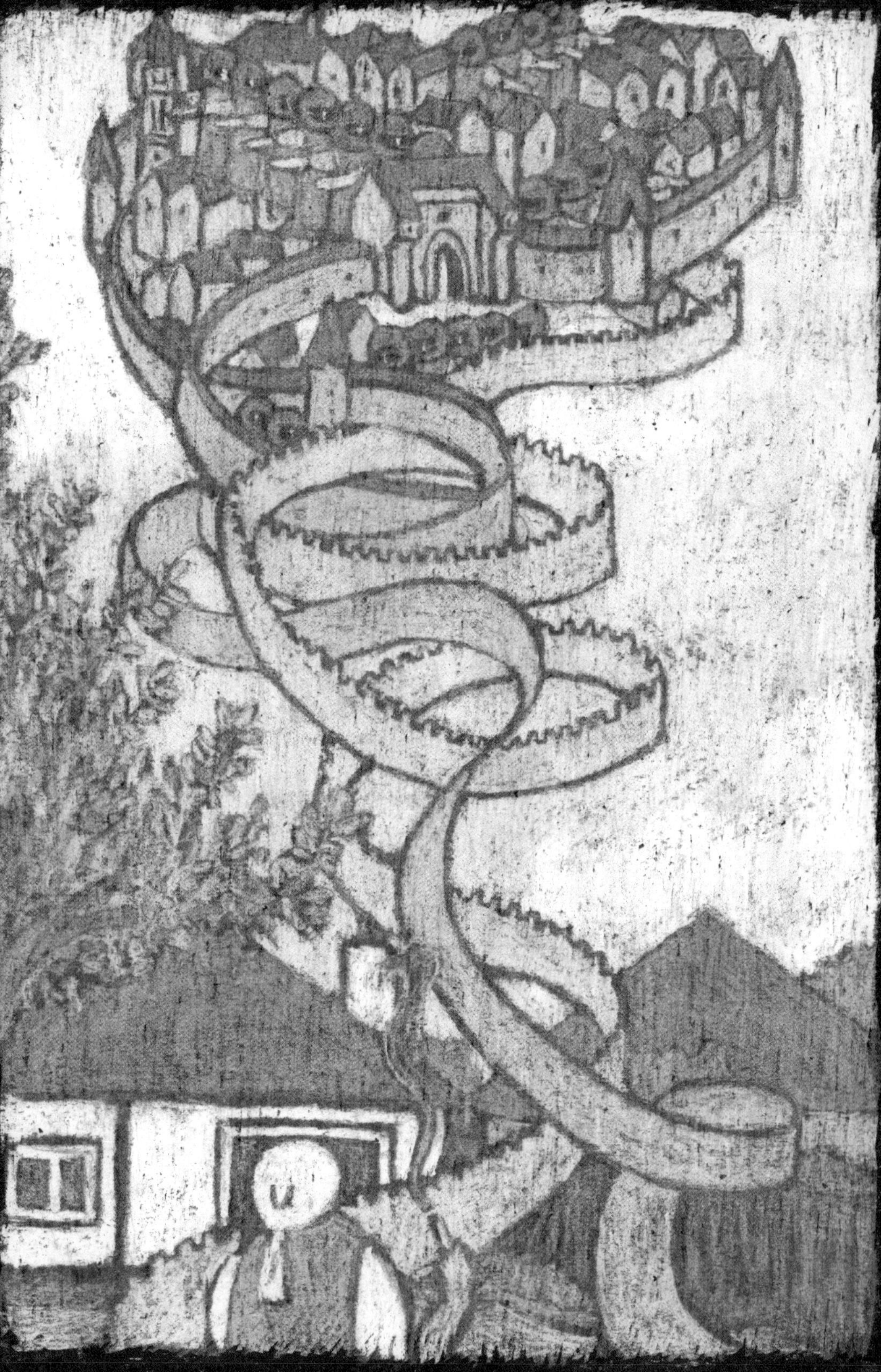

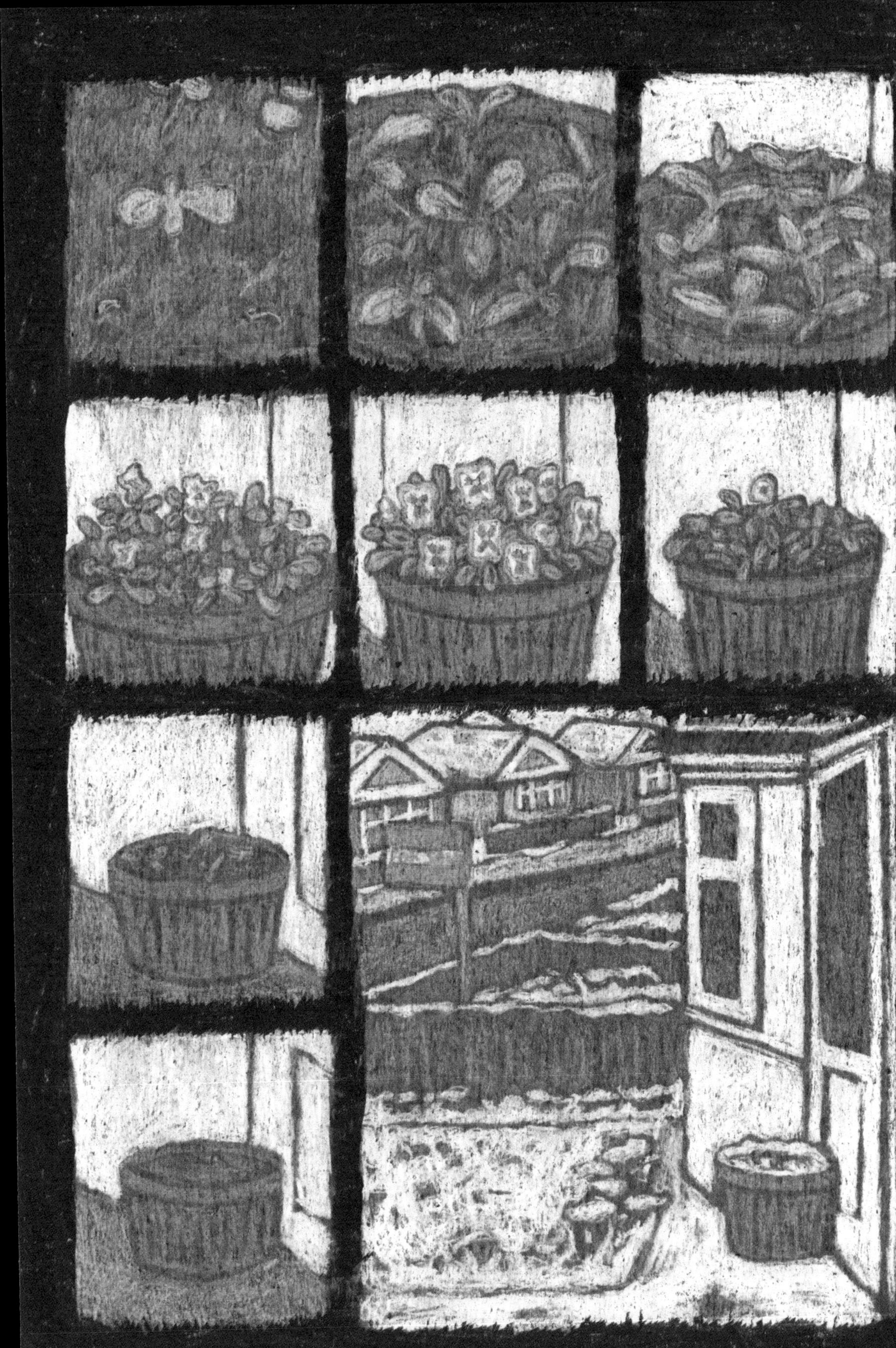

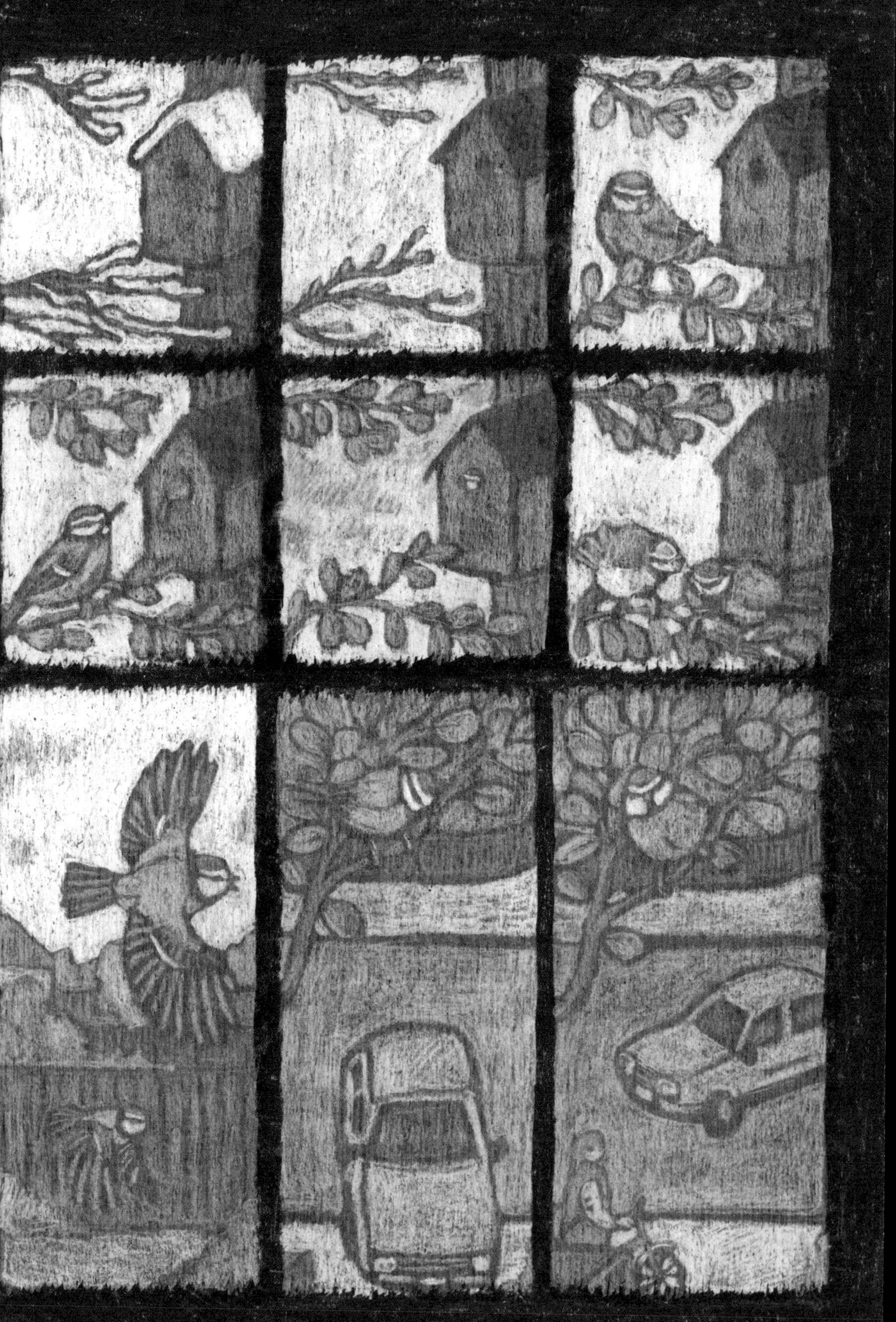

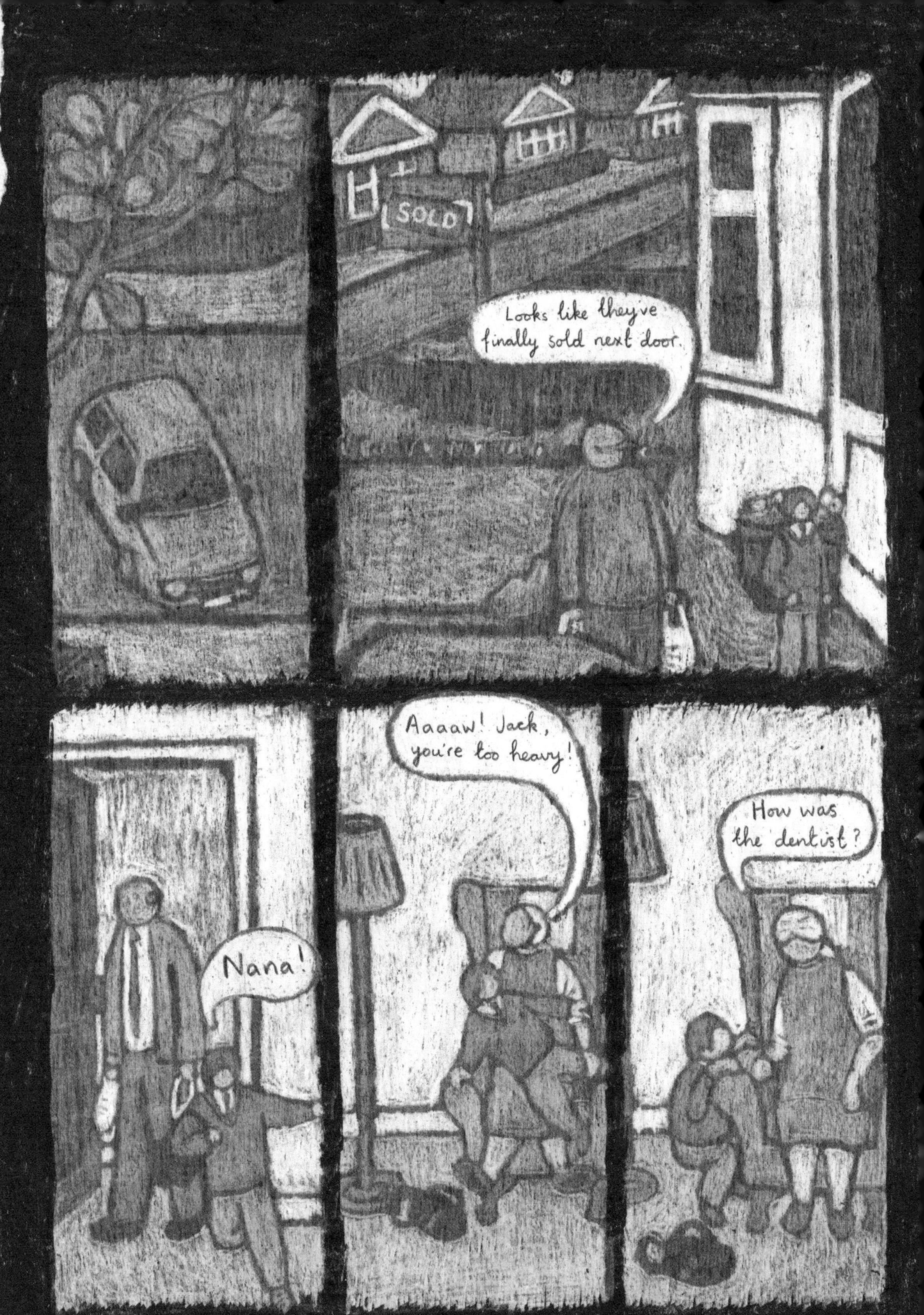
SOLD
Looks like they've finally sold next door.
Nana!
Aaaaw! Jack, you're too heavy!
How was the dentist?

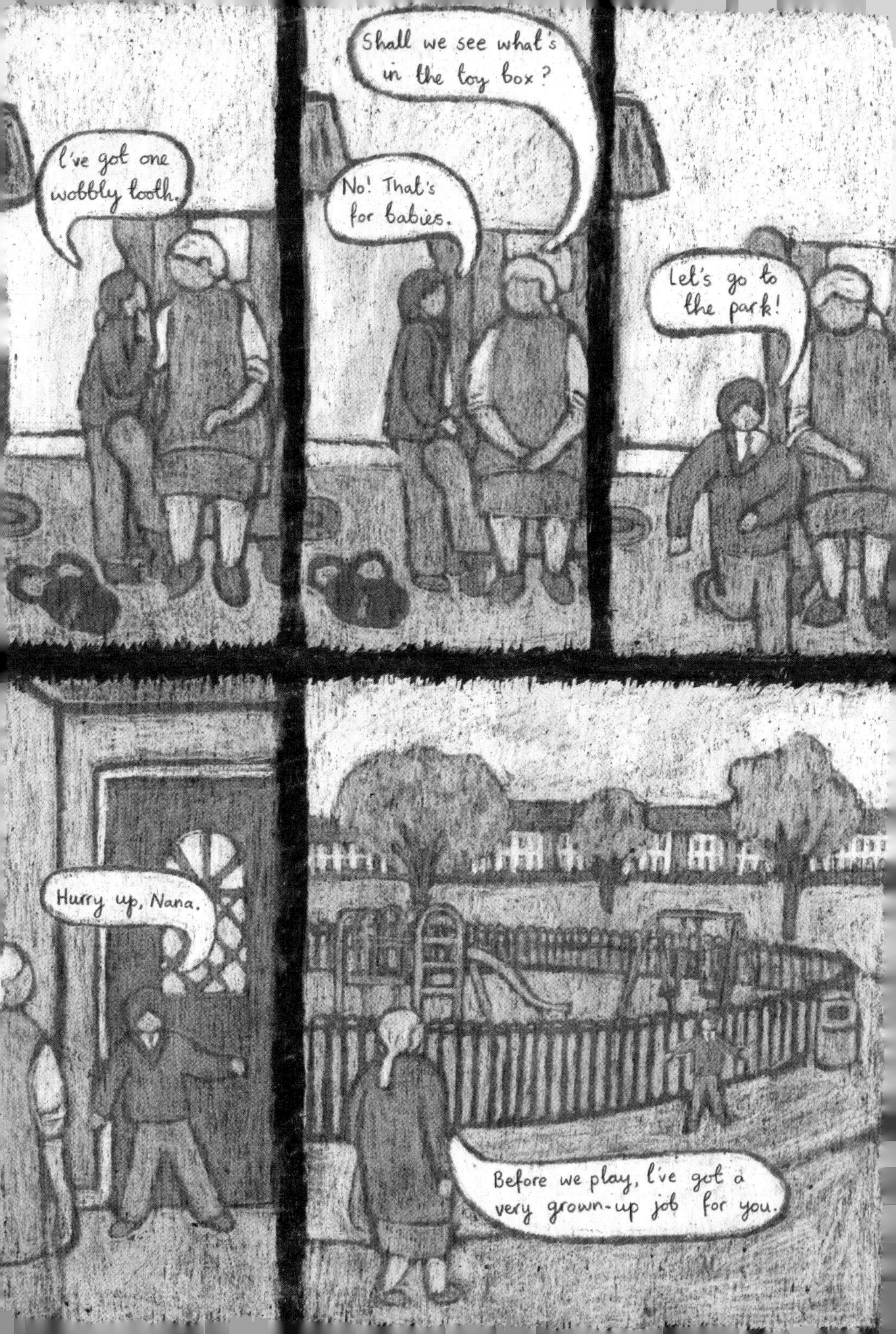
I've got one wobbly tooth.
Shall we see what's in the toy box?
No! That's for babies.
Let's go to the park!
Hurry up, Nana.
Before we play, I've got a very grown-up job for you.

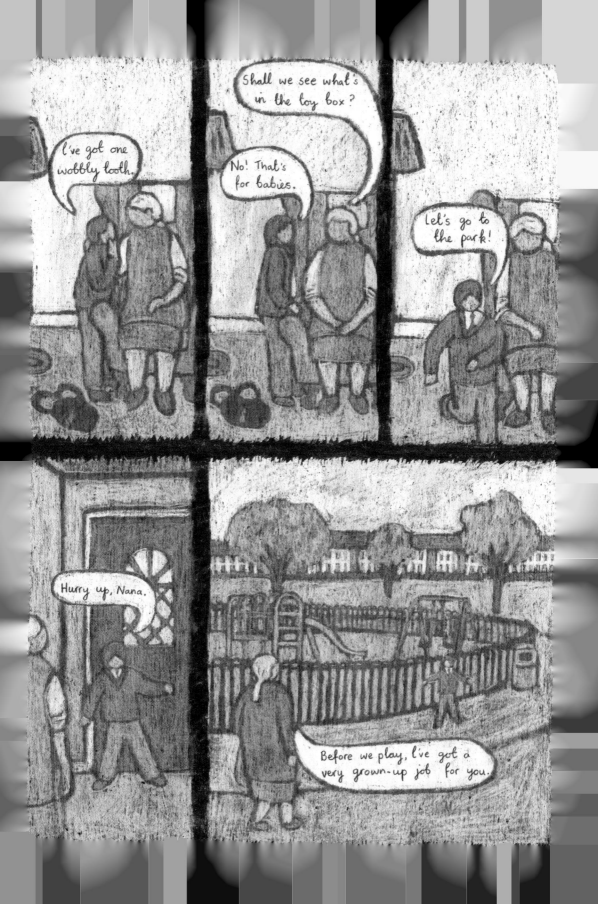

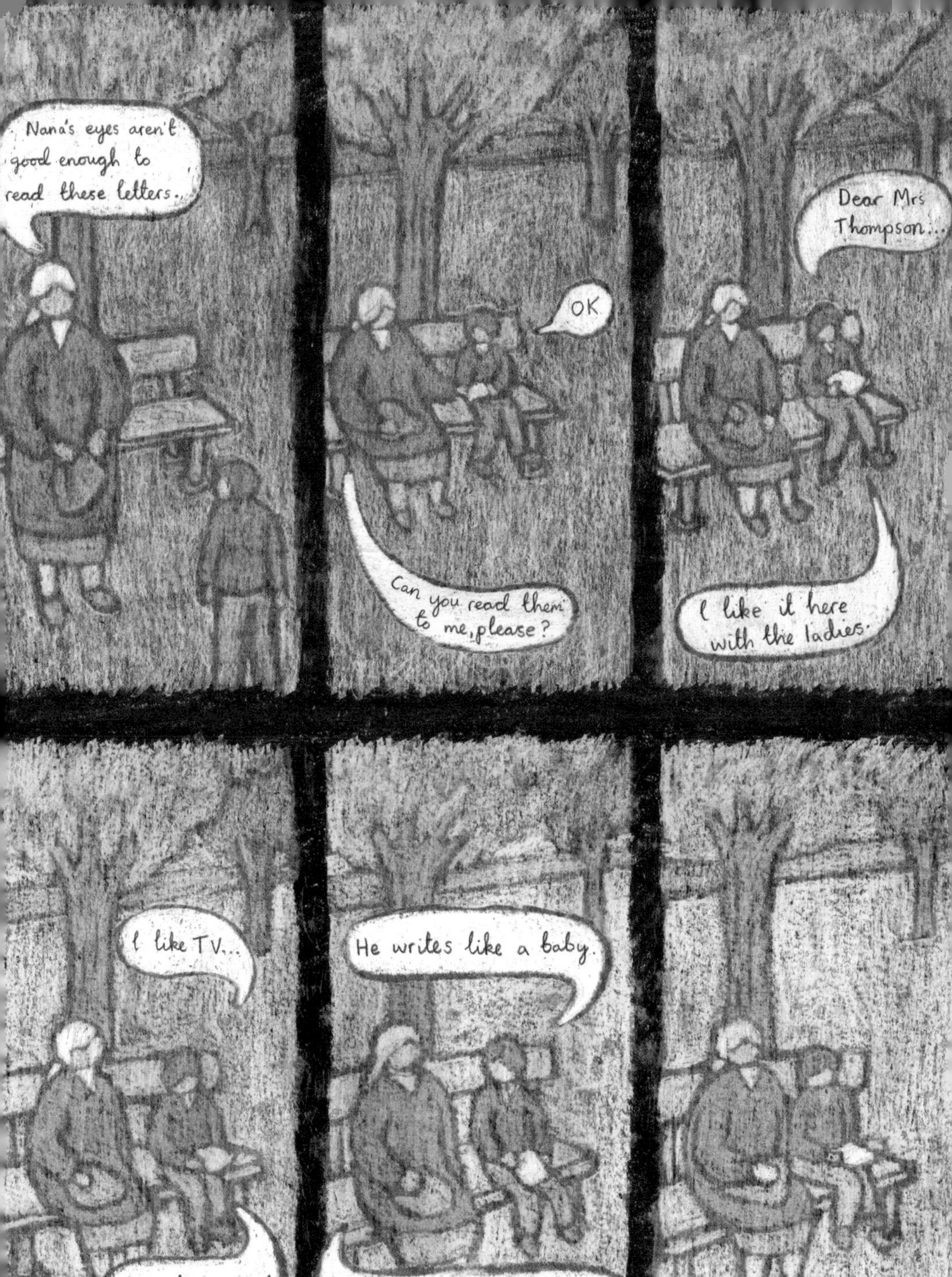
Nana's eyes aren't good enough to read these letters...
Can you read them to me, please?
OK
Dear Mrs Thompson...
I like it here with the ladies.
I like TV...
story time and nature time.
He writes like a baby.
He hasn't been learning as long as you have...

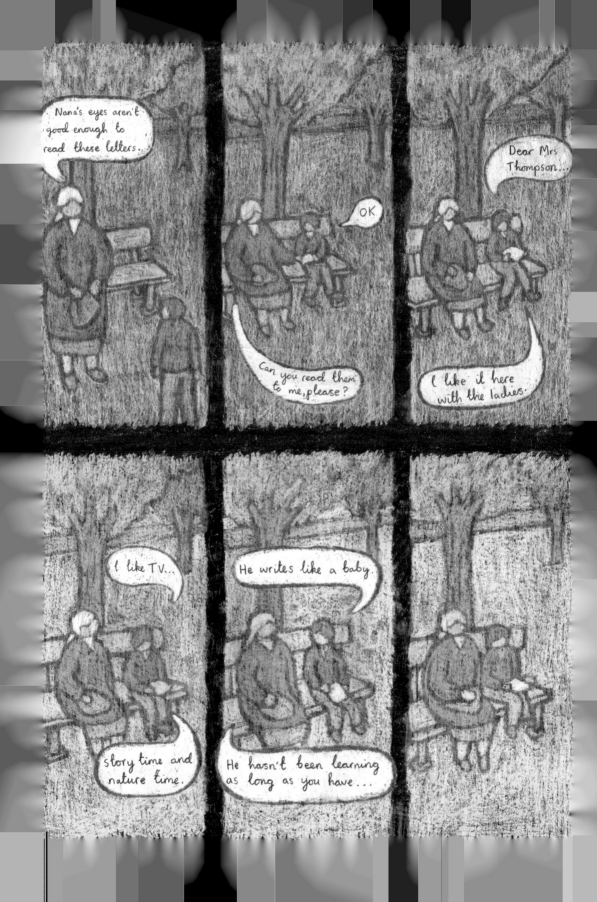

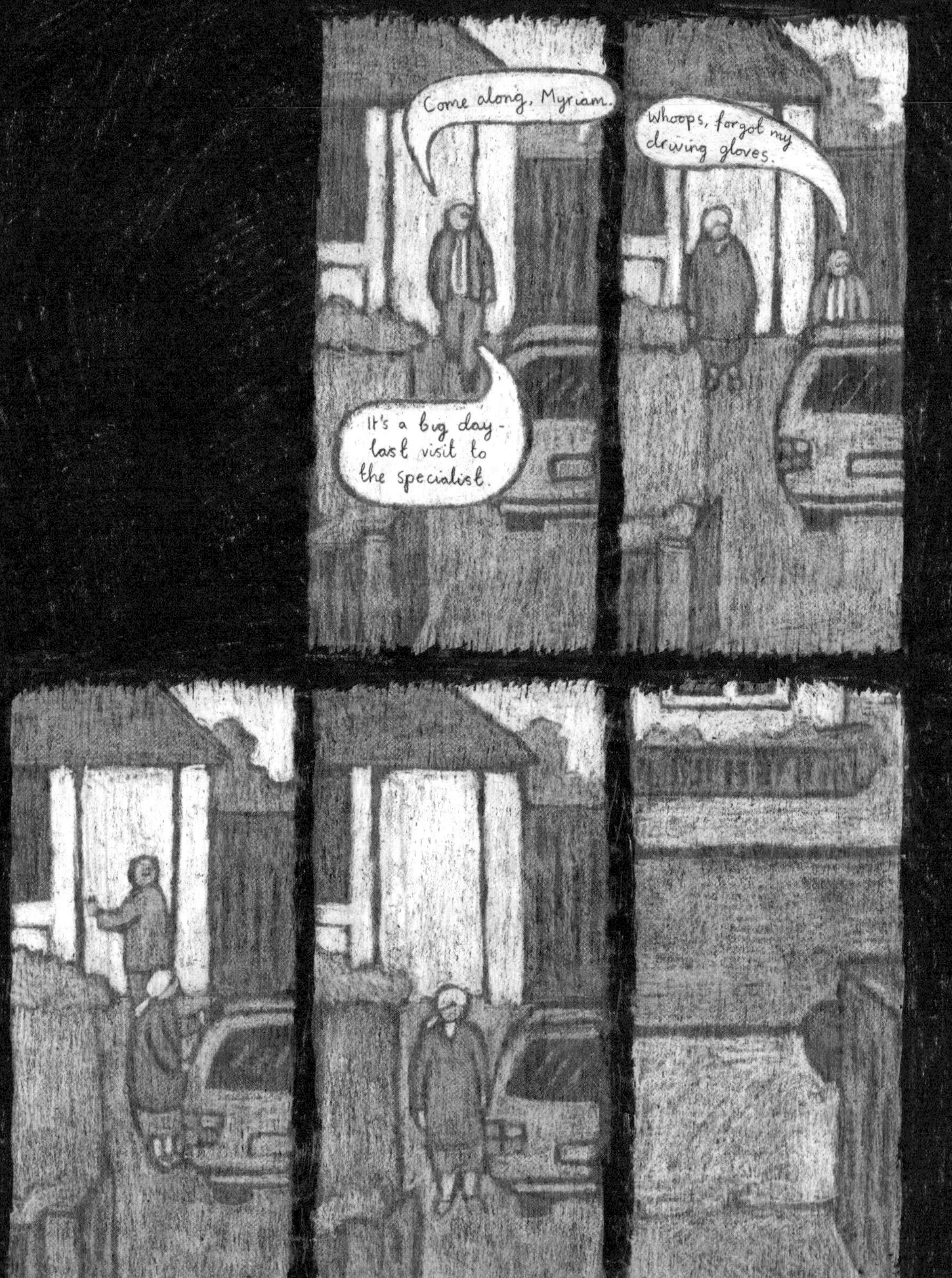
Come along, Myriam.
It's a big day-last visit to the specialist.
Whoops, forgot my driving gloves.

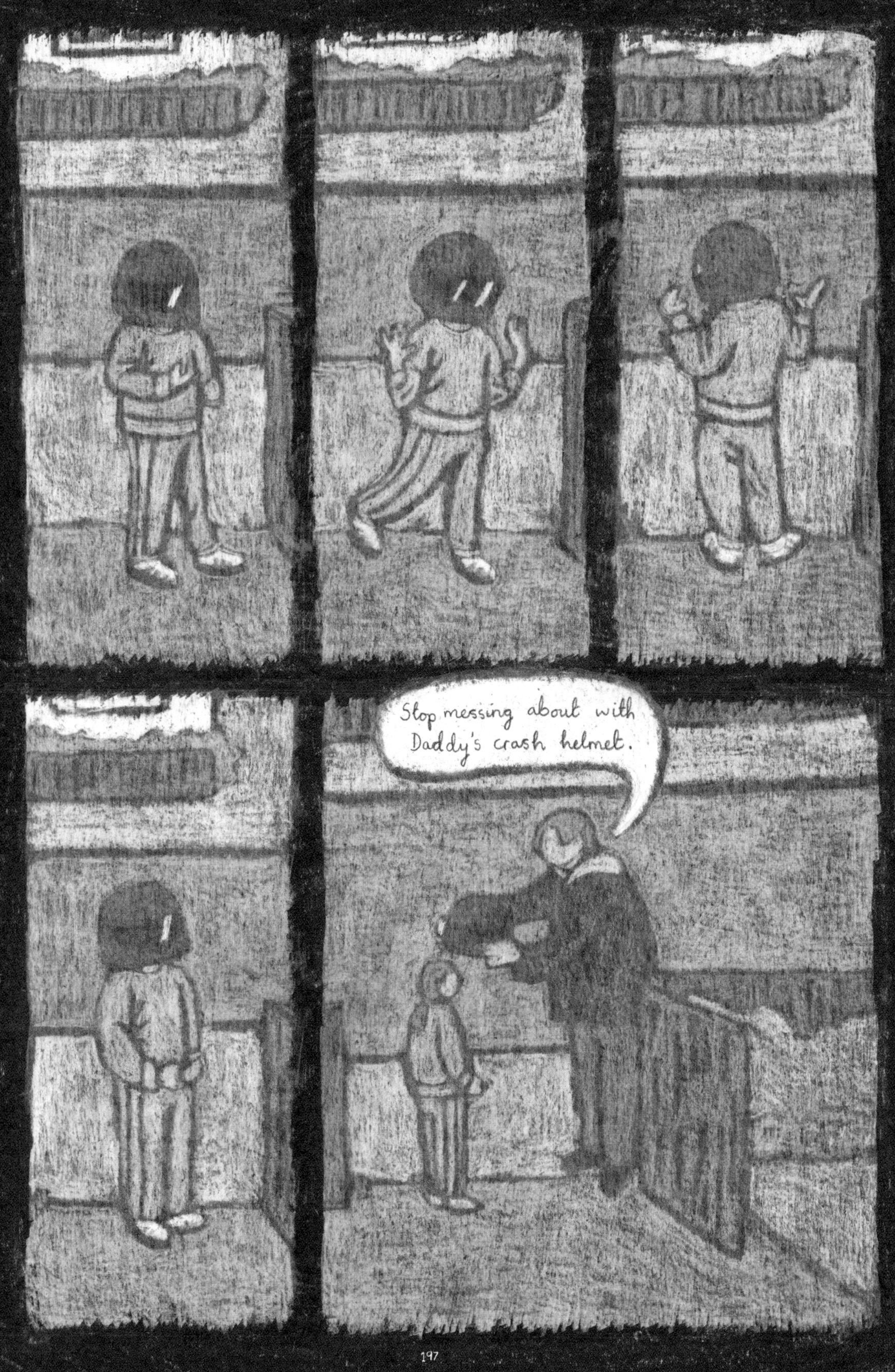
Stop messing about with Daddy's crash helmet.

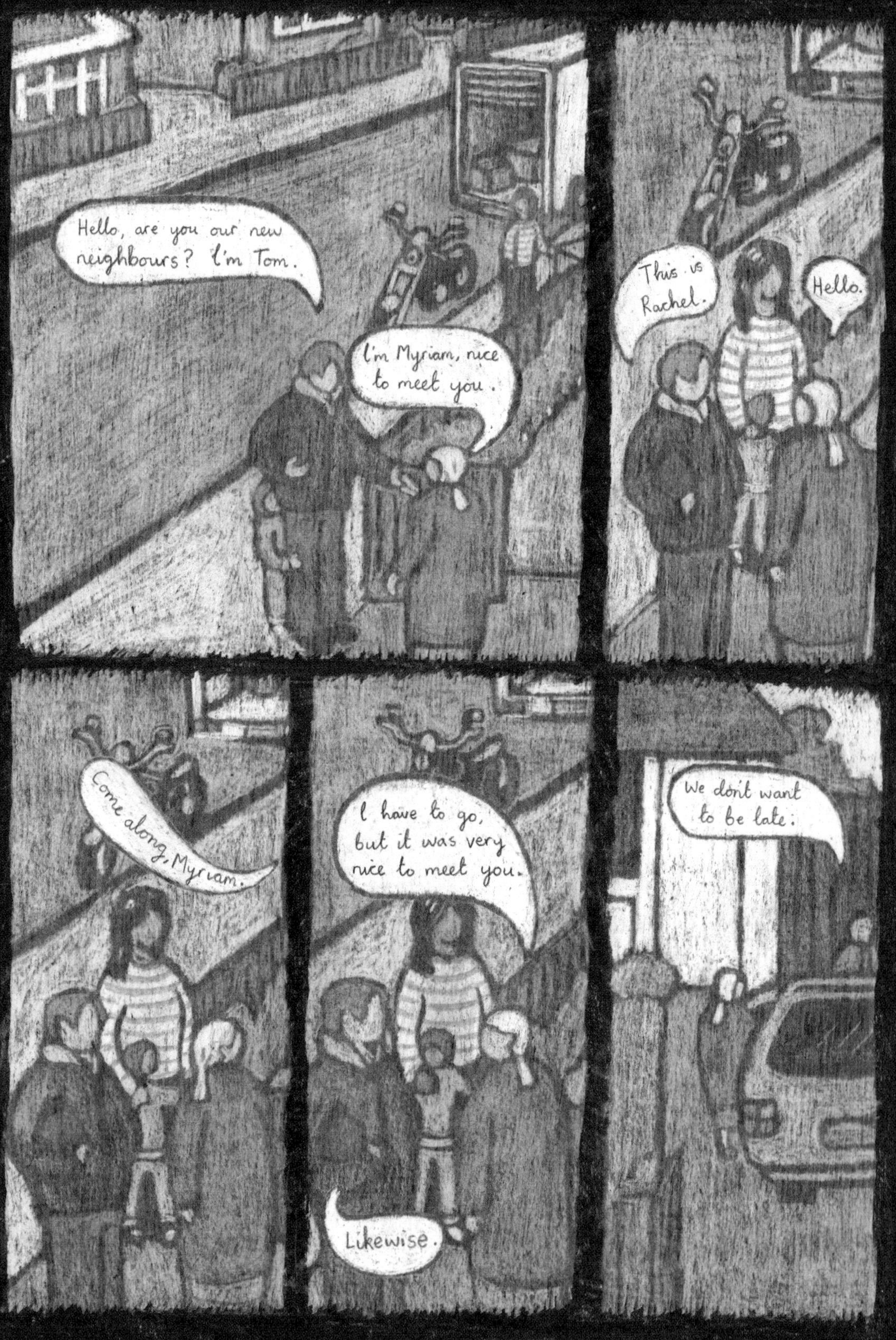
Hello, are you our new neighbours? I'm Tom.
I'm Myriam, nice to meet you.
This is Rachel.
Hello.
Come along, Myriam.
I have to go, but it was very nice to meet you.
Likewise.
We don't want to be late.

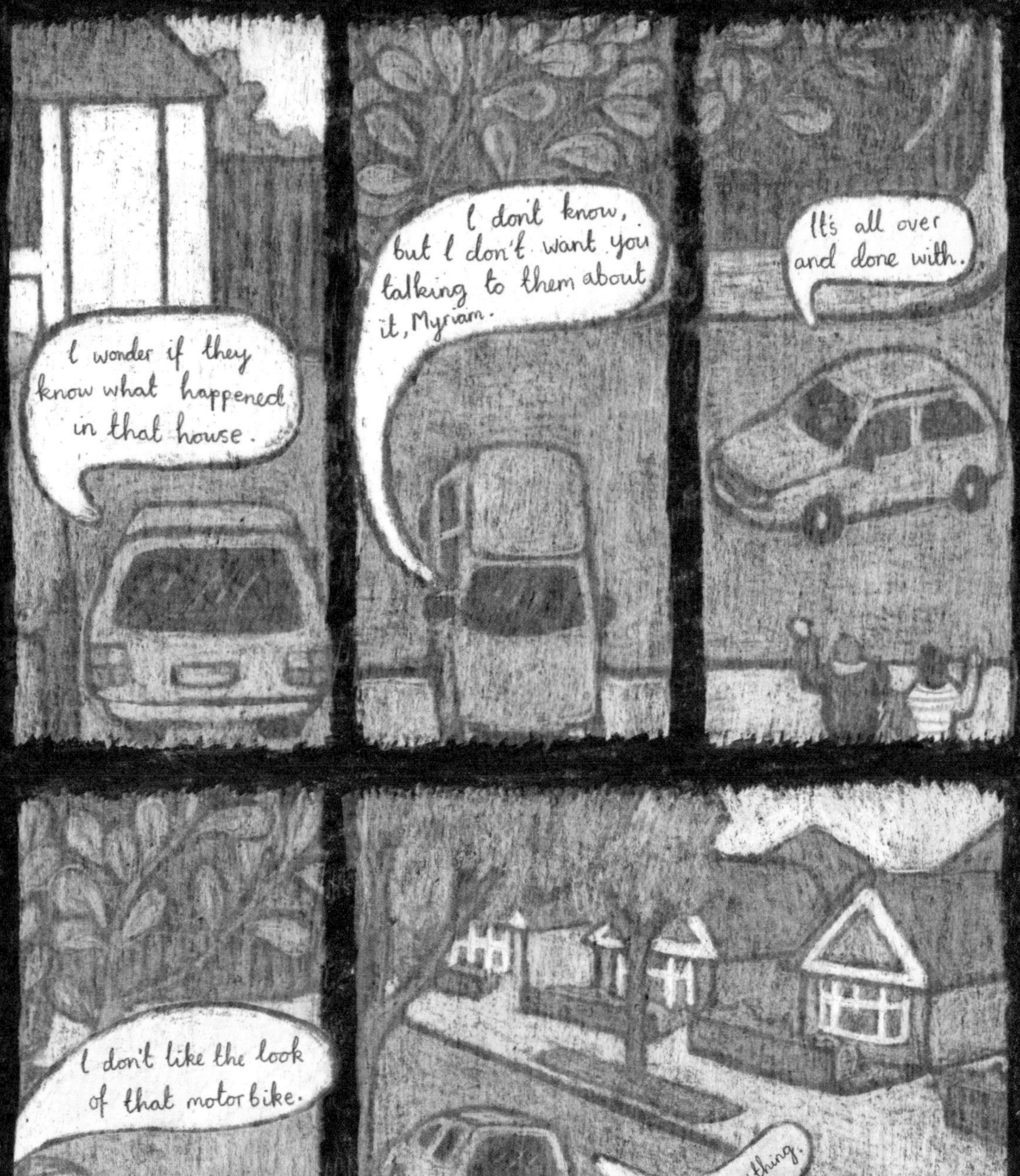
I wonder if they know what happened in that house.
I don't know, but I don't want you talking to them about it, Myriam.
It's all over and done with.
I don't like the look of that motorbike.
Noisy bloomin' thing.

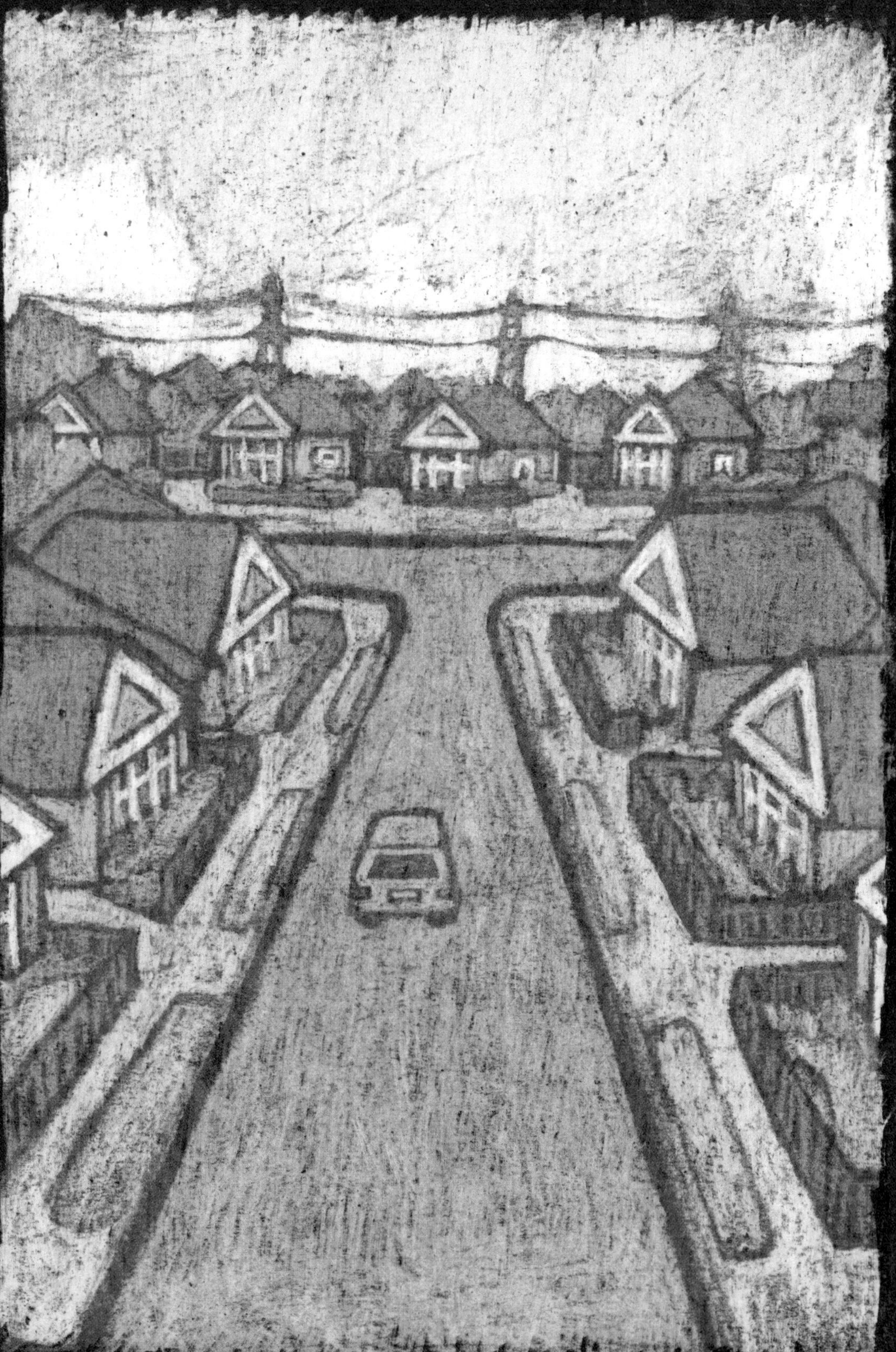

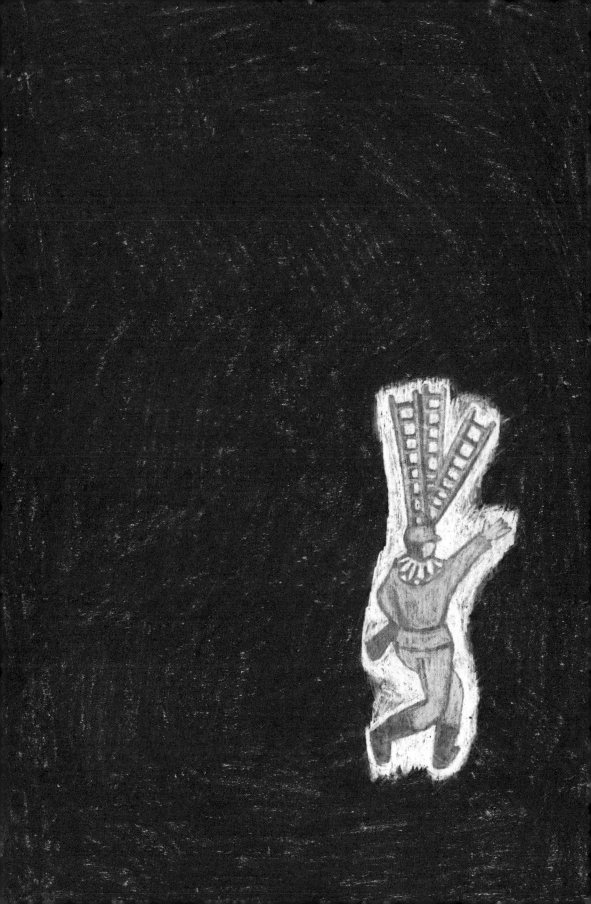

Charles Bonnet Syndrome (CBS) is a mysterious condition affecting those with deteriorating vision.

People with CBS experience complex hallucinations including cartoon characters, little people, strange buildings, figures wearing exotic and brightly coloured clothes, geometric patterns, colours, indecipherable writing, animals and bizarre vehicles.

While these visions are indistinguishable from reality, the person experiencing them remains emotionally disconnected, and can often discern what's real from what isn't by the sheer incongruity of the apparitions.

In many cases CBS goes undiagnosed because the sufferer is afraid to admit to them, thinking that what they are experiencing is a form of mental illness or dementia.

However, in most cases they are mentally healthy people who've lost most or all of their eyesight.

For more information, visit www.charlesbonnetsyndrome.uk

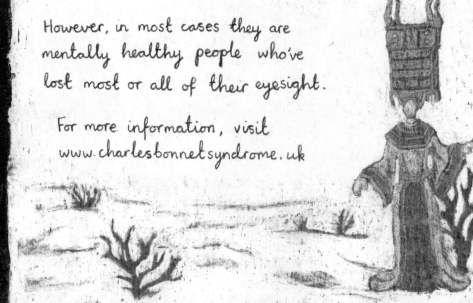

Acknowledgements

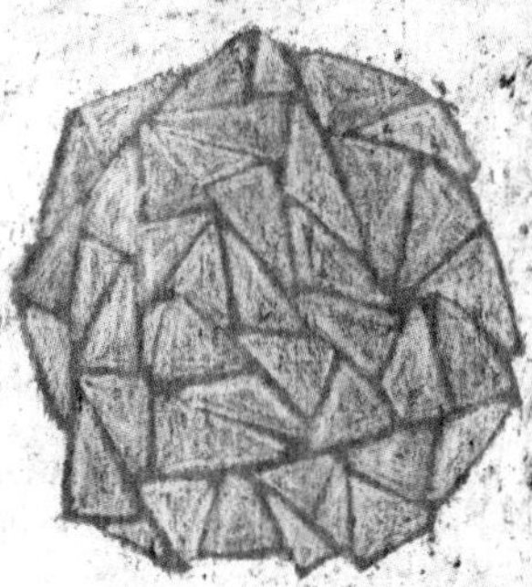

Big thanks to my friends and family for their support over the years and to everyone in the U.K. comics community.

Special thanks to Steve Tillotson, Andy Brookes, Emma Simpson, Lando, Amber Hsu, Nicola Streeten, Corinne Pearlman and everyone at Myriad.

I would also like to thank Dr Dominic ffytche for his invaluable help and expertise concerning Charles Bonnet Syndrome.

Supported using public funding by Arts Council England.

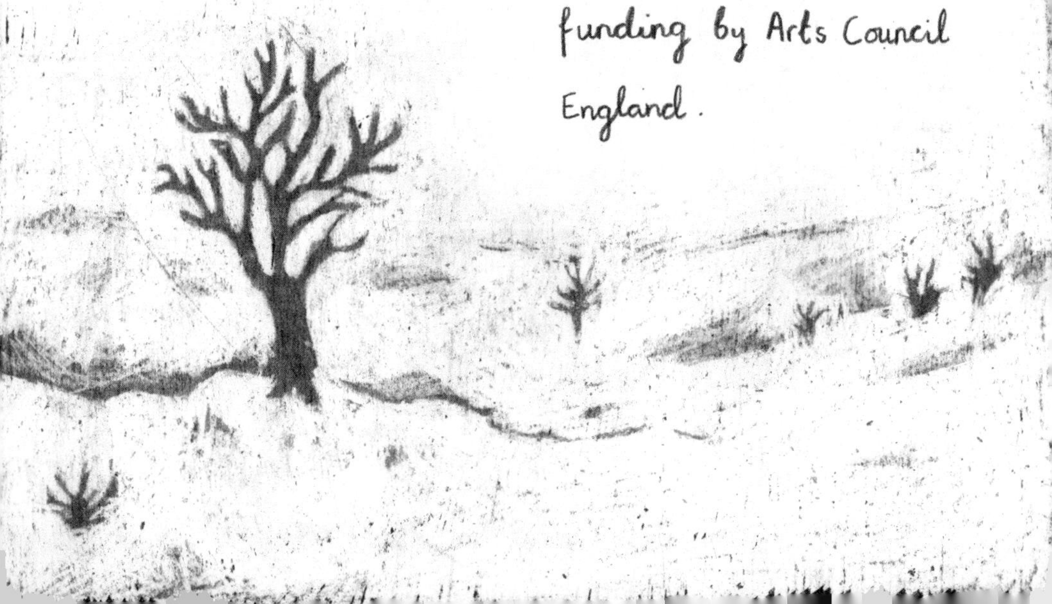

ALSO BY GARETH BROOKES

THE BLACK PROJECT
Gareth Brookes

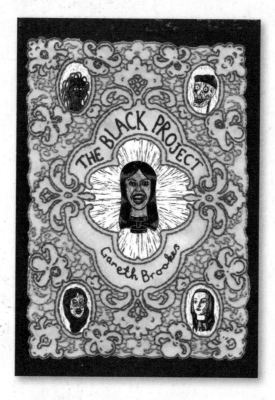

Praise for *The Black Project*

'Like Cath Kidston embroidering for David Lynch.'
Herald

'Exquisite, excruciating and exceptional...
a landmark, once read, not easily forgotten.'
Paul Gravett

'Clandestine first love with a papier-mâché twist is the order of the day in this remarkable debut... the perfect entry point into the wicked whimsy of [Brookes's] creative mind.'
Andy Oliver, Broken Frontier

'Really unsettling, genuinely creepy.'
Richard Bruton, Forbidden Planet

'Truly incredible with his first book... genuinely unlike anything else happening in the graphic medium at the moment.'
We Love This Book

'Dark and funny and sad and moving and totally original.'
Stephen Collins

'One of the most powerful and distinctive graphic novels to come out in a long time – but brace yourself. It may make your skin crawl.'
Dylan Horrocks

'Utterly bizarre and quite brilliant.'
Steve Bell

'I enjoyed his weirdness.'
Will Self

GRAPHIC
MEDICINE

Taking Turns
Stories from HIV/AIDS Care Unit 371
MK Czerwiec

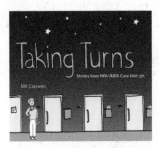

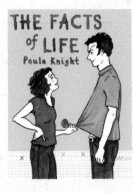

"Charts a remarkable episode in the history of medicine. It's a time of staggering loss but also remarkable change."
—Alison Bechdel, author of *Fun Home*

THE FACTS of LIFE
Paula Knight

"This is an intensely honest and personal book. . . . It makes you feel less alone."
—Victoria Macdonald, Channel 4 News (UK)

Hole in the Heart
Bringing Up Beth
HENNY BEAUMONT

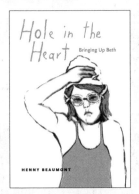

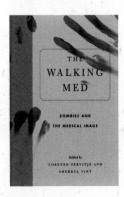

"*Hole in the Heart* packs a powerful emotional punch."
—Joanna Moorhead, *The Guardian*

THE WALKING MED
ZOMBIES AND THE MEDICAL IMAGE
Edited by
LORENZO SERVITJE AND SHERRYL VINT

"Ghastly smart stuff!"
—Colin Milburn, UC Davis

Dana Walrath
Aliceheimer's
Alzheimer's Through the Looking Glass

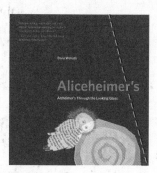

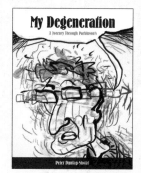

"A deeply moving, informative, and funny memoir by a woman watching her mother's descent into Alzheimer's disease."
—Roz Chast, author of *Can't We Talk About Something More Pleasant?*

My Degeneration
A Journey Through Parkinson's
Peter Dunlap-Shohl

"For patients, these irreverent archetypes validate their experiences. Clinicians, too, stand to gain a better appreciation of how they might appear to their patients."
—Arthur W. Frank, *Science*

THINGS
RETIREMENT
HOME
TRAILER
PARK
ANEURIN
WRIGHT
...When You're 29 and Unemployed

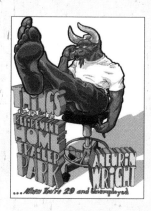

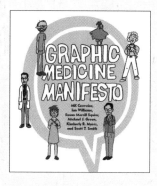

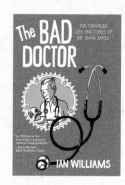

"Highly valuable for those facing illness in the family, caregivers, and anyone aspiring to live with empathy."
—Martha Cornog, *Library Journal*

GRAPHIC
MEDICINE
MANIFESTO
MK Czerwiec, Ian Williams, Susan Merrill Squier, Michael J. Green, Kimberly R. Myers, and Scott T. Smith

"It's becoming clear that graphic narratives can deepen understanding, not only of facts but of feelings, between patients, families, and professionals."
—Paul Gravett, author of *Comics Art*

The BAD DOCTOR
THE TROUBLED LIFE AND TIMES OF DR. IWAN JAMES
IAN WILLIAMS

"Ian Williams is the best thing to happen to medicine since penicillin."
—Alison Bechdel, 2014 MacArthur Fellow

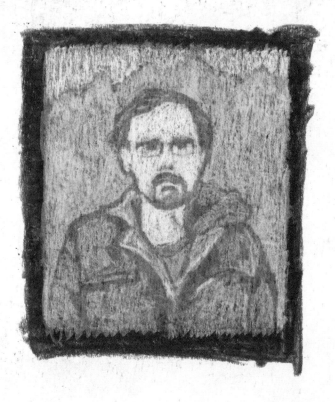

Gareth Brookes was born in Woking and studied Fine Art
at Newcastle University and the Royal College of Art.
An extract from his debut graphic novel, *The Black Project*,
won the Myriad First Graphic Novel Competition 2012, and
was published by Myriad in 2014. It also won Best Original
Graphic Novel at the Broken Frontier Awards. He has
self-published a number of handmade books including
The Land of My Heart Chokes on its Abundance.